Renal Nursing

This book is dedicated to my family

Commissioning Editor: Steven Black
Development Editor: Mairi McCubbin
Project Manager: Anne Dickie
Design Direction: George Ajayi
Illustration Manager: Bruce Hogarth
New illustrations for this edition: Antbits

Renal Nursing

THIRD EDITION

Edited by

Nicola Thomas

RGN BSc(Hons) MA

Senior Lecturer
City Community and Health Sciences
City University
London, UK

Foreword by

Jane Macdonald

Vice President of the British Renal Society

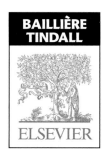

BAILLIÈRE TINDALL

ELSEVIER

EDINBURGH   LONDON   NEW YORK   OXFORD   PHILADELPHIA   ST LOUIS   SYDNEY   TORONTO   2008

BAILLIÈRE
TINDALL
ELSEVIER

BAILLIÈRE TINDALL
An imprint of Elsevier Limited

First edition 1997
Second edition 2002
Third edition 2008
  Reprinted 2008

ISBN: 978 0-7020-2839-7

British Library Cataloguing in Publication Data
A catalogue record for this book is available from the British Library

Library of Congress Cataloging in Publication Data
A catalog record for this book is available from the Library of Congress

Note
Knowledge and best practice in this field are constantly changing. As new research and experience broaden our knowledge, changes in practice, treatment and drug therapy may become necessary or appropriate. Readers are advised to check the most current information provided (i) on procedures featured or (ii) by the manufacturer of each product to be administered, to verify the recommended dose or formula, the method and duration of administration, and contraindications. It is the responsibility of the practitioner, relying on their own experience and knowledge of the patient, to make diagnoses, to determine dosages and the best treatment for each individual patient, and to take all appropriate safety precautions. To the fullest extent of the law, neither the Publisher nor the Editor assume any liability for any injury and/or damage to persons or property arising out of or related to any use of the material contained in this book.

The Publisher

Contents

List of contributors

Juliet Auer
Freelance writer, UK

Diane Blyton
Nurse Educator, Paediatric Nephrology, Children and Young Peoples Kidney Unit, Nottingham City Hospital NHS Trust, Nottingham, UK

Paul Challinor
Quality & Training Manager, B Braun Avitum UK, Caerphilly, UK

Charlotte Chalmers
Lecturer, School of Life Sciences, Napier University, Edinburgh, UK

Frances Coldstream
Consultant Nurse – Predialysis Management, London, UK

Jean–Yves De Vos
Dialysis Research Nurse/Dialysis Head Nurse, Ronse, Belgium

Barbara Engel
Tutor in Nutrition and Dietetics, School of Biomedical and Molecular Sciences, University of Surrey, Guildford, Surrey, UK

Judith Hurst
Senior Lecturer, City Community and Health Sciences, City University, London, UK

Shelley Jepson
Senior Nurse, Paediatric Nephrology, Children and Young Peoples Kidney Unit, Nottingham City Hospital NHS Trust, Nottingham, UK

Natasha McIntyre
Renal Consultant Nurse, Renal and Transplant Directorate, Nottingham City Hospital, Nottingham, UK

Althea Mahon
Renal Consultant Nurse, Renal Department, Barts and The London NHS Trust, London, UK

Fliss Murtagh
Research Training Fellow, Department of Palliative Care and Policy, Kings College London, London, UK

Nicola Thomas
Senior Lecturer, City Community and Health Sciences, City University, London, UK

Raymond Trevitt
Renal Transplant Nurse Specialist, Royal London Hospital, London, UK

Janet Wild
Clinical Education Manager, Baxter Healthcare Ltd, Berkshire, UK

Foreword

A third edition of *Renal Nursing* is much welcomed in light of recent advances in clinical knowledge and key national drivers such as the Renal National Service Frameworks (NSFs). Also the breadth of nursing care for people identified with kidney disease continues to evolve dramatically.

Part One of the Renal NSF (2004) challenged us to deliver timely and high-quality dialysis and transplant services to all children, young people and adults with identified and established renal failure. Part Two of the Renal NSF (2005) ensures that those at risk of developing or who are diagnosed with chronic kidney disease are identified, assessed, treated and followed-up. It is recognised that some of those people identified may be suffering from acute renal failure. Not all of those identified will either progress or choose to access dialysis therapy, but instead may prefer, in the latter case, to an agreed palliative care plan.

Indeed, the number of people on renal replacement therapy is expected to grow by at least 50% within less than 10 years. Delivery of care for those with renal disease has, therefore, expanded and includes a range of support staff such as Health Care Assistants and Assistant Practitioners, and qualified nurses through Specialist, Advanced and Consultant Nurse positions. The settings in which care is provided have also undergone a sea change, with early identification and management of chronic kidney disease being appropriately undertaken in primary care settings by the range of health care professionals who work in this field. Gaining new skills or underpinning existing proficiency in the UK and Europe has been supported by a range of publications and tools including competence frameworks, such as those developed by *Skills for Health*.

This edition of *Renal Nursing* rises to the challenge of articulating and capturing these changes and the knowledge required for those working in this domain. It celebrates and values the key role taken by nursing, whilst identifying its position in a clinical team that always strives to provide high-quality patient care. This significant and highly valued publication for all in renal care will be a much appreciated addition to your resources.

Jane Macdonald
Lead Nurse, Renal Services
Hope Hospital
Salford
Vice President, British Renal Society
Vice President, Kidney Alliance

Preface

I am delighted to have been asked to edit the third edition of this successful book for nurses working in nephrology, dialysis and transplantation. The past five years have seen tremendous changes in renal care in the UK: the publication of the National Service Framework for Renal Services in 2004/5; the introduction of international guidance on staging of chronic kidney disease (CKD); a new laboratory measurement of kidney function, the estimated glomerular filtration rate (eGFR); and in 2006 the introduction of CKD standards in the Quality and Outcomes Framework (QOF) for General Practice. The effect of these changes is that previously undiagnosed CKD has now been identified resulting in an increased workload for renal and primary care professionals. These recent developments are discussed in much more depth in this third edition, in particular, the chapter on predialysis care has been extended to include CKD. There is also a new chapter on end-of-life care, another very important aspect of renal care and management.

This book is mostly for those who are new to the renal specialty. Nurses who are studying on preregistration courses and practitioners who are commencing a postregistration course in renal nursing will find it particularly helpful. It also serves as a good foundation for nurses who wish to refresh their knowledge in a part of the renal field in which they are currently not practising, or for other members of the multi-professional team who are commencing a career in nephrology. This new edition is again written in a style that promotes renal nursing for what it is: a dynamic, varied and rewarding specialty.

Each chapter has been written by an expert in his or her field. Recognition must go to those authors who wrote chapters for the first or second edition, but were unable to contribute to this edition. They are Tim Armstrong, Gemma Bircher, Patricia Franklin, Jane Hattersley, Marianne Vennegoor, and Geraldine Ward. Thank you also to Toni Smith, editor of the first edition.

Renal nurses in the 21st century face a constant challenge to keep abreast of developments in care and management. They have to keep up-to-date with new technologies, respond to the rapid evolution in standards of care and use resources effectively. They have to manage an ever-increasing workload as a consequence of more accurate screening of those with chronic kidney disease. What does not change is the constant physical and psychosocial challenges that patients and their families have to face. This must always be in our minds. In my twenty-five years of practice as a renal nurse the repeated request from patients is that we should emphasise what *can* be done rather than what cannot. The word 'restriction' should not be part of a renal nurse's vocabulary: why not fluid or dietary *allowance*? As in the second edition, I have endeavoured to use a language in this book that puts patients at the centre of care. I hope that this latest edition will continue to encourage renal nurses to care for their patients with compassion, sensitivity and understanding.

Nicola Thomas
London March 2007

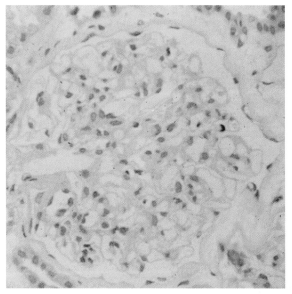

(a)

Plate 1
Renal histology from biopsy specimen (light micrographs). (a) A normal glomerulus. (b) A glomerulus from a patient with a diffuse proliferative (poststreptococcal) glomerulonephritis. Note how 'full' the glomerulus appears with a great increase in the number of cells due to inflammation. (See Ch. 2)

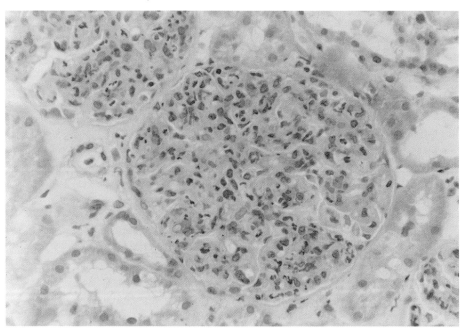

(b)

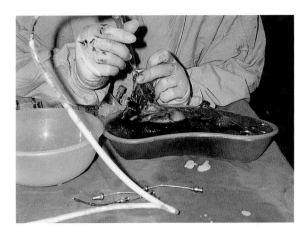

Plate 2
Kidney undergoing perfusion
(in ice) immediately after
harvesting (See Ch. 12.)

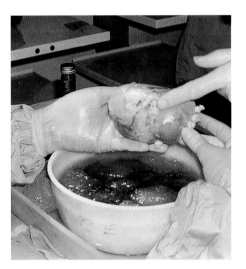

Plate 3
Cooled kidney in surgical glove,
ready for transplantation
(See Ch. 12.)

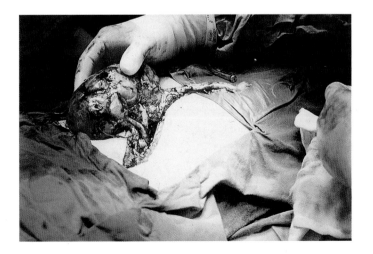

Plate 4
Transplanted kidney after
removal of clamps showing
'pinking up' and urine
formation (See Ch. 12.)

Chapter **1**

The history of dialysis and transplantation

Nicola Thomas

**LEARNING OUTCOMES
FOR THIS CHAPTER**

- To understand the evolution of haemodialysis, peritoneal dialysis and transplantation
- To appreciate the difficulties that healthcare professionals have had to overcome in the development of the nephrology specialty
- To evaluate the changing focus of renal care in the 21st century
- To identify the challenges for nephrology nursing in the future

INTRODUCTION

The introduction of dialysis as a life-saving treatment for kidney failure was not the result of any large-scale research programme, rather it emerged from the activities of a few pioneering individuals who were able to utilise ideas, materials and methods from a range of developing technologies.

Haemodialysis (HD) as a routine treatment for renal failure was initiated in the 1960s, followed by continuous ambulatory peritoneal dialysis in the late 1970s. The recognition of the need for immunosuppression in transplantation in the 1960s enabled it to become the preferred treatment for many patients.

HAEMODIALYSIS

THE BEGINNING

It was the Romans who first used a form of dialysis therapy by giving hot baths to patients to remove urea. The action of the hot water made the patient sweat profusely and this, together with the toxins diffusing through the skin into the bath water, would temporarily relieve symptoms. However, the Romans did not understand why the treatment worked. The effect was to leave the patient fatigued but, as the only hope, this treatment was still used on occasions into the 1950s.

The first time that the term 'dialysis' was used was in 1854 by Thomas Graham (Fig. 1.1), a Scottish chemist (Graham 1854). He used dialysis to describe the transport of solutes through an ox bladder and this was the catalyst for other researchers working in a similar field to focus on the membrane.

Membranes were made from a variety of substances, including parchment and collodion (Eggerth 1921). Collodion is a syrupy liquid that dries to form a porous film and allows the passage of small-molecular-weight substances, while being impermeable to substances with a molecular weight greater than 5 kDa. In 1889, BW Richardson referred to the use of collodion membranes in the dialysis of blood. So, by this method, living animals were dialysed in experimental conditions (Richardson 1889) but the limiting factor that prevented the treatment being used in humans at this time was the lack of suitable materials.

PRE-1920

It was not until 1913 that the first article on the technique of HD, named the 'artificial kidney', was reported. Experimental dialysis was performed on animals, by using variances in the composition of dialysis fluid (Abel et al 1914). Substances could be added to the solution to avoid their net removal. The main aim of the experiments was the removal of salicylates.

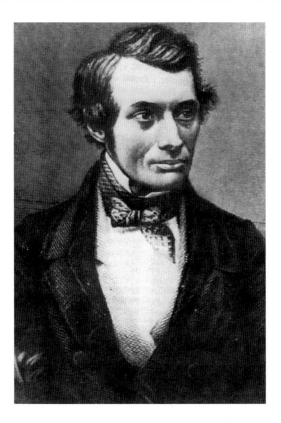

Figure 1.1
Thomas Graham 1805–1869.
(Engraving by C Cook after
photograph by Claudet.)

The removal of fluid and toxins accumulated owing to kidney disease
was not, at this time, considered.

In 1914, Hess & McGuigan were experimenting with dialysis in a pharmacology laboratory in Chicago. As a result, they were able to transfer
sugar from tissue to blood and from the blood across a collodion membrane. The design of the dialyser minimised the length of tubing from the
patient and a high blood flow was achieved by connection to the carotid
artery in an effort to minimise the necessity to use an anticoagulant.
A single U-shaped collodion tube was inserted into a glass cylinder with
a rubber stopper at one end. The blood flow both to and from the dialyser
was at one end with a port for adjusting the pressure inside the tube.
These experiments were still only performed on animals. The only anticoagulant available was in the form of an extract obtained from crushed
leech heads, called hirudin. This was far from satisfactory, even though
leeches were plentiful and readily available from the corner shop for
around $25 per 1000.

THE 1920s

The first dialysis performed on a human was carried out by the German
physician, Georg Haas, in Giessen in the latter half of the 1920s. He performed six treatments in six patients. Handmade collodion membranes
were used, and clotting was prevented by using hirudin and, later, a crude

form of heparin. Haas used multiple dialysers to increase the surface area of blood exposed to the dialysis fluid. This necessitated as many as six dialysers arranged in parallel and he found that the arterial pressure of the blood was insufficient to propel the blood through the entire extra-corporeal circuit; therefore, he introduced a pump into the circuit (Fig. 1.2). Haas was aware of the lack of support given to him by the hospital and his colleagues and, by the late 1920s, he gave up and the work was stopped. Georg Haas died in 1971 aged 85 years and was honoured as the pioneer of dialysis.

In spite of these treatments carried out from the 1920s to the 1940s, those with uraemia suffering from poor appetite and vomiting could be offered nothing more than bed-rest, and a bland salt-free diet composed mainly of vegetables, carbohydrate and fat to reduce protein metabolism. Dialysis was not considered a realistic option and the conservative therapy was only offered as a palliative measure.

Heinrich Necheles was the founder of the contemporary dialyser. In 1923, he experimented with the sandwiching of membranes, thus giving an increased surface area without the necessity for multiple dialysers. The membrane used was the peritoneum of a sheep and, because the membrane was prone to expansion, support sheets were placed between the layers of membrane, thus allowing a large surface area of membrane to come into contact with the dialysis fluid. Other features introduced by Necheles were a heater, the priming of the pathway for the blood and a filter to prevent clots returning to the patient.

THE 1930s

The 1920s and 1930s saw great advances in synthetic polymer chemistry, resulting in the availability of cellulose acetate, which could be used as a membrane for HD. It was in 1937 that the first synthetic membrane was used by the American scientist, William Thalhimer. The material,

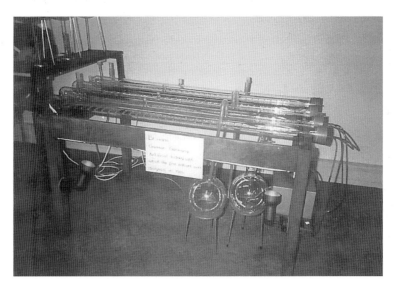

Figure 1.2
The equipment used by Georg Haas.

cellophane – a form of cellulose acetate, which was used extensively in the sausage industry – had potential that was not recognised for some years. In the mid-1930s came the purification of heparin, which could be used as an anticoagulant (Thalhimer et al 1938). Together these two advances gave rise to the next stage of development, which took place in 1943 in occupied Holland.

THE 1940s AND 1950s

Willem Kolff, a physician working in Groningen in Nazi-occupied Holland, had his attention drawn to the work of a colleague who was concentrating plasma by using cellulose acetate as a membrane and immersing it in a weak solution of sugar. Kolff noticed that toxins in the blood were altered by this method (Kolff 1950). He built a rotating drum dialyser (Figs. 1.3 and 1.4), which provided sufficient surface area for his first attempt at human dialysis (Kolff & Berk 1944). His machine consisted of 30 m of cellophane tube that was wound round a large cylinder. The cylinder was placed in a tank containing a weak solution of salts – the dialysate. The patient's blood was passed through the cellophane tube, the walls acting as a semipermeable membrane. Blood flow was achieved by the addition of a circuit containing a burette, which, when filled with blood, could be raised high enough to allow the blood to flow into the dialyser. The burette was then lowered, allowing the blood to drain back, and raised again to allow the blood to return to the patient. The slats in the construction of the cylinder were of wood owing to the shortage at this time of materials such as aluminium. (In retrospect, this was fortunate since the toxicity of aluminium is now appreciated.)

Six hours were required for the treatment and it is interesting to note that, with this method, similar efficiency of dialysis could be achieved as is possible with the dialysers in use today: a clearance of 170 ml min^{-1} urea could be achieved. Fluid could only be removed by increasing the osmotic pressure of the dialysate fluid by the addition of sugar, as an increase in pressure on the membrane would result in rupture (Kolff 1965). The whole procedure was very time-consuming and labour-intensive, as the process required attention at all times, to raise and lower the burette and observe the membrane for rupture, which happened frequently. Repairs to the membrane were carried out by inserting a glass tube at the point of rupture.

Kolff's first clinical experience was gained on a 29-year-old woman with chronic nephritis. The blood urea was kept stable for 26 days but, after 12 sessions of dialysis, her blood urea began to increase, and she subsequently died.

After the war, in 1945, Kolff's technique was widely used, particularly in Sweden and the USA. The treatment was initially for acute renal failure when kidney function could be expected to return to normal following a short period of dialysis treatment. It was also used widely in the Korean War in 1952 to treat trauma-induced renal failure. The group, led by Paul Teschan, trained to use the rotating drum dialyser and saved many lives by lowering the high potassium levels of the victims (Teschan 1955).

Figure 1.3
The Kolff rotating drum.

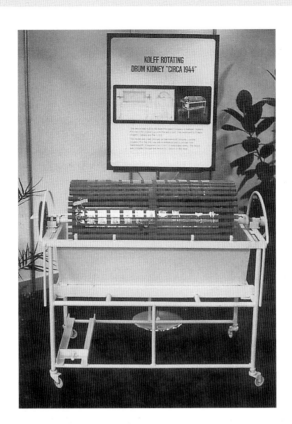

Figure 1.4
Diagram of the Kolff rotating
drum system.

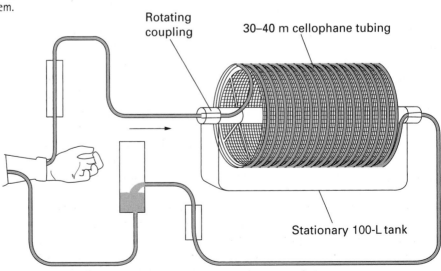

Some of the earliest research carried out on fluid removal from the blood using negative pressure was conducted by MR Malinow and W Korzon at Michael Reese Hospital in Chicago in 1946 (Malinow & Korzon 1947). The device used was the earliest version of a dialyser with multiple blood paths and negative pressure capacity. It had parallel sections of cellulose acetate tubing and, by adding layers of tubing, the surface area of the device could be increased. The diffusion properties of this device were not considered, as it was intended for the removal of water only from the blood. The device required a low priming volume and the circuit included a blood pump.

In the 1940s, interest in dialysis as a treatment for renal failure had spread throughout Europe and across to Canada, as the need was becoming widely recognised by the medical profession. After obtaining drawings of the Kolff dialyser, Russell Palmer and a colleague, from Vancouver in Canada, built a replica and dialysed their first patients in September 1947 (Palmer & Rutherford 1949).

Kolff was invited to take his artificial kidney to New York where he trained physicians in the operation of the life-saving device. There was resistance from hospital staff at the Mount Sinai Hospital, who only permitted the treatment to be administered in the surgical suite after normal surgical schedules were completed for the day. The first patient scheduled for treatment was a victim of mercuric chloride poisoning, but treatment was cancelled when a spontaneous diuresis occurred.

The first successful dialysis in Mount Sinai Hospital was in January 1948, in a female admitted to hospital having inserted mercury tablets into her vagina to induce an abortion (Fishman et al 1948). Eight hours after the first dialysis using the Kolff machine, the patient passed urine. The treatment had been a success. Victims of drug overdose were then regularly treated by use of the rotating drum dialyser until 1950.

To expand the use, the rotating drum would have to be modified to become easier to use. Kolff enlisted the help of Dr Carl Walter, who worked at the Peter Brent Brigham Hospital. Together with Edward Olson, an associate engineer from Fenwal, they set about designing and building a new version of the Kolff device. Stainless steel was used for the drum, and refinements included a hose for filling the pan with the 100 L of dialysate fluid, which was heated, and a hood to cover the drum. A tensioning device was used on the cellophane membrane as it had a tendency to stretch during use. The split connection for the patient's tubing was introduced, and this allowed the patient's tubing to remain stationary while the drum rotated. This was made leakproof and a Lucite hood was added to overcome heat loss from the extracorporeal blood. These improvements paved the way for wider acceptance of the use of dialysis treatment (Merrill et al 1950).

When the Kolff–Brigham kidney was used, the heparin dose ranged from 6000 to 9000 units, and was infused prior to the start of the treatment. The dialyser was primed with blood, and the blood flow to the dialyser was limited to 200 ml at a time to prevent hypotension. To assist blood flow, a pump was inserted in the venous circuit rather than in the arterial side to minimise the probability of pressure build-up in the membrane, which would cause a rupture.

This version of the Kolff–Brigham dialysis machine was used in 1948 and, in all, over 40 machines were built and exported all over the world. Orders for spare parts were still being received as late as 1974, from South America and behind the Iron Curtain.

THE 1950s

The Allis-Chalmers Corporation was one of the first companies to produce dialysis machines commercially. They were prompted into the manufacture when an employee developed renal failure. There was no machine available and so the firm turned its attention to producing a version of the Kolff rotating drum. The resulting machine was commercially available for $5600 and included all the sophistication available at the time. Allis-Chalmers produced 14 of these machines and sold them all over the USA into the early 1950s.

In October 1956, the Kolff system became commercially available, so the unavailability of equipment could no longer be used as an excuse for non-treatment of patients. Centres purchased the complete delivery system for around $1200 and the disposables necessary for the treatment were around $60. The system was still mainly used for reversible acute renal failure drug overdose, and poisoning (Fig. 1.5).

Figure 1.5
A typical dialysis machine from the 1950s: Fresenius.

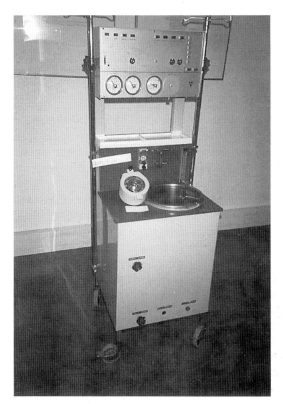

THE DEVELOPMENT OF THE DIALYSER

Jack Leonards and Leonard Skeggs produced a plate dialyser that would permit a reduction in the priming volume and allow negative pressure to be used to remove fluid from the patient's system (Skeggs et al 1949). A modification to this design included a manifold system, which allowed variation of the surface area without altering the blood distribution. Larger dialysers followed, which necessitated the introduction of a blood pump.

In the late 1950s, Fredrik Kiil of Norway developed a parallel plate dialyser, with a large surface area ($1\,m^2$) requiring a low priming volume (Fig. 1.6). A new cellulose membrane, Cuprophan, was used and this allowed the passage of larger molecules than other materials that were available at the time. The Kiil dialyser could be used without a pump. Kiil dialysed the patients using their own arterial pressure. This dialyser was widely used because the disposables were relatively inexpensive when compared with other dialysers at that time.

A crude version of the capillary-flow dialyser, the parallel dialyser using a new blood pump, and a more advanced version of the Alwall kidney was developed (MacNeill 1949). However, it was John Guarino who incorporated the important feature of a closed system, a visible blood pathway.

To reduce the size of the dialyser without reducing the surface area, William Y Inouye and Joseph Engelberg produced a plastic mesh sleeve to protect the membrane. This reduced the risk of the dialysis fluid coming into contact with the blood. Because this was a closed system, the

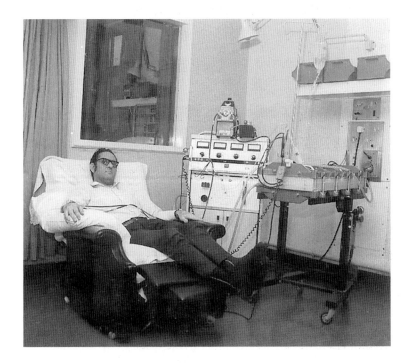

Figure 1.6
The Kiil dialyser. (Equipment on the far right of image).

effluent could be measured to determine the fluid loss of the patient. It is the true predecessor of the positive- and negative-pressure dialysers used today.

The first commercially available dialyser was manufactured by Baxter and based on the Kolff kidney. It provided a urea clearance of approximately 140 ml min^{-1}, equivalent to today's models, and was based on the coil design. The priming volume was 1200–1800 ml and this was drained into a container at the end of treatment, refrigerated and used for priming for the next treatment. It was commercially available in 1956 at $59.00.

The forerunner of today's capillary-flow dialyser was produced by Richard Stewart in 1960. The criteria for design of this hollow-fibre dialyser were a low priming volume and minimal resistance to flow. The improved design contained 11 000 fibres, which provided a surface area of 1 m^2.

Future designs for the dialyser will focus on refining the solute and water-removal capabilities, as well as reducing the size and priming requirements of the device, thus allowing an even higher level of precise individual care.

THE EMERGENCE OF HOME HAEMODIALYSIS

It was Scribner's shunt that provided vascular access, thus leading to the first dialysis unit to be established for chronic patients at the University of Washington Hospital. Belding Scribner also developed a central dialysate delivery system for multiple use and set this up in the chronic care centre, which had 12 beds. These beds were quickly taken and his plan for expansion was rejected. The only alternative was to send the patients home, and so patients and their families were trained to perform the dialysis and care for the shunts. Home dialysis was strongly promoted by Scribner (Fig. 1.7).

Stanley Shaldon reported in 1961 that a patient dialysing at the Royal Free Hospital in London was able to self-care by setting up his own machine, initiating and terminating dialysis; so home haemodialysis in the UK was made possible. The shunt was formed in the leg for vascular access, to allow the patient to have both hands free for the procedures. Hence Shaldon was able to report the results of his first patient to be placed on overnight home HD in November 1964. With careful patient selection, the venture was a success. Scribner started to train patients for home at this time, and his first patient was a teenager assisted by her mother. Home dialysis was selected for this patient, so that she would not miss her high-school education. The average time on dialysis was 14 h twice weekly. To allow freedom for the patient, overnight dialysis was widely practised. At first, emphasis was on selection of the suitable patient and family, even to the extent of a stable family relationship, before the patient could be considered for home training (Baillod et al 1965).

From these beginnings, large home HD programmes developed in the USA and in the UK, thus allowing expansion of the dialysis population without increasing hospital facilities. Many patients could now be considered for home treatment, often with surprisingly good results, as the

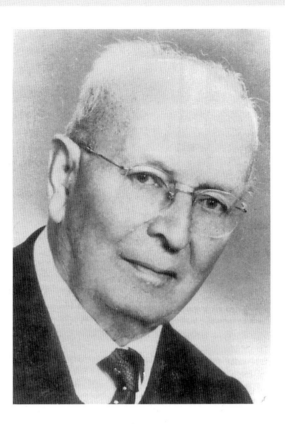

Figure 1.7
Belding H Scribner.

dialysis could be moulded to the requirements of the individual, rather than the patients conforming to a set pattern. However, with the development in the late 1970s and early 1980s of continuous ambulatory peritoneal dialysis (CAPD) as the first choice for home treatment, the use of home HD steadily dwindled; however, it is now receiving renewed interest. The National Institute for Health and Clinical Excellence (NICE) has published guidance on home versus hospital haemodialysis (NICE 2002), and recommends all suitable patients should be offered the choice between home haemodialysis or haemodialysis in a hospital/satellite unit.

VASCULAR ACCESS FOR HAEMODIALYSIS

It was Sir Christopher Wren, of architectural fame, who in 1657 successfully introduced drugs into the vascular system of a dog. In 1663, Sir Robert Boyle injected successfully into humans. Prison inmates were the subjects and the cannula used was fashioned from a quill. For HD to become a widely accepted form of treatment for renal failure, a way to provide long-term access to the patient's vascular system had to be found and, until this problem was solved, long-term treatment could not be considered. In order for good access to be established, a tube or cannula had to be inserted into an artery or vein, thus giving rise to good blood flow from the patient. The repeated access for each treatment quickly led to exhaustion of blood vessels for cannulation. The need for a system whereby a sufficiently large blood flow could be established for dialysis, without destroying a length of blood vessel every time dialysis was required, was imperative.

Teschan, in the 11th Evacuation Hospital in Korea, was responsible in the 1950s for developing a method of heparin lock for continuous access to blood vessels. The cannulae were made from Tygon tubing and stopcocks, and the blood was prevented from clotting by irrigation with heparinised saline. It was not a loop design, as the arterial and venous segments were not joined together.

In 1960 in the USA, George Quinton (an engineer) and Belding Scribner (a physician) used two new synthetic polymers (Teflon and Silastic) to make tubing capable of forming a connection between a vein and an artery. Thus they were able to re-route the blood outside the body (usually in the leg). This was known as the arteriovenous (AV) shunt. The tubing was disconnected at a union joint in the centre and each tube then connected to the lines of the dialysis machine. At the end of treatment, the two ends were then reconnected, establishing a blood flow from the artery to the vein outside the body. In this way, repeat dialysis was made possible without further trauma to the vascular system.

This external shunt, while successful, had drawbacks. It was a potential source of infection, often thrombosed and had a restrictive effect on the activity of the patient. This form of access is still occasionally used for acute treatment, although the patient's potential requirements for chronic treatment must be considered when the choice of vessels is made, so that vessels to be used in the formation of an AV fistula are not scarred. In 1966, Michael Brescia and James Cimino developed the subcutaneous radial artery-to-cephalic vein AV fistula (Cimino & Brescia 1962), with Cimino's colleague Kenneth Appel performing the surgery.

The AV fistula required less anticoagulation, had reduced infection risk and gave access to the bloodstream without danger of shunt disconnection. Subsequently, a number of synthetic materials have been introduced to create internal AV fistulae (grafts). These are useful when the patient's veins are not suitable to form a conventional AV fistula, such as in severe obesity, with loss of superficial veins owing to repeated cannulation, or in the elderly or those with diabetes.

Venous access by cannulation of the jugular or femoral veins has now largely replaced the shunt for emergency dialysis.

THE PRESENT

Monitoring and total control of the patient's therapy became more important as dialysis became widespread, and so equipment development continued. Sophisticated machines incorporated temperature monitoring, positive-pressure gauges and flow meters. Negative-pressure monitoring followed, as did a wide range of dialysers with varying surface areas, ultrafiltration capabilities and clearance values. Automatic mixing and delivery of the dialysate and water supply to the machine greatly increased the margin of safety for the procedure, and made the dialysis therapy much easier to manage. The patient system that has evolved provides a machine that monitors all parameters of dialysis through the use of microprocessors, allowing the practitioner to programme a patient's requirements (factors such as blood flow, duration of dialysis and fluid removal) so that the resulting treatment is a prescription for the individual's needs. Average dialysis time is reduced to 4 h three times weekly, or less if a high-flux (high-performance) dialyser is used.

The early 1970s saw the number of patients increase owing to the increased awareness brought about by the availability of treatment. Free-standing units for the sole use of kidney dialysis came into being, leading to dialysis becoming a full-time business. Committees for patient selection were disbanded and the problems concerned with inadequate financial resources came to the fore. Standards for treatment quality have now been set. Attempts continue to reduce treatment duration to enhance the patient's quality of life. Good nutrition has also emerged as playing a vital role in reducing dialysis morbidity and mortality. Dialysis facilities are demanded within easy reach of patients' homes, and this expectation has led to the emergence of small satellite units, managed and monitored by larger units, as a popular alternative to home HD treatment. In 2002, there were 101 satellite dialysis units in the UK.

PERITONEAL DIALYSIS

Peritoneal dialysis (PD) as a form of therapy for renal failure has been brought about by a climax of the innovative efforts and the tenacity of many pioneers over the past 2 centuries. It was probably the early Egyptian morticians who first recognised the peritoneum and peritoneal cavity as they embalmed the remains of their influential compatriots for eternity. The peritoneal cavity was described in 3000 BC in the Ebers papyrus as a cavity in which the viscera were somehow suspended. In Greek times, Galen, a physician, made detailed observations of the abdomen while treating the injuries of gladiators.

The earliest reference to what may be interpreted as PD was in the 1740s when Christopher Warrick reported to the Royal Society in London that a 50-year-old woman suffering from ascites was treated by infusing Bristol water and claret wine into the abdomen through a leather pipe (Warrick 1744). The patient reacted violently to the procedure and it was stopped after three treatments. The patient is reported to have recovered and was able to walk 7 miles (approximately 13 km) a day without difficulty. A modification of this was subsequently tried by Stephen Hale of Teddington in England: two trocars were used – one on each side of the abdomen – allowing the fluid to flow in and out of the peritoneal cavity during an operation to remove ascites (Hale 1744).

Subsequent experiments on the peritoneum (Wegner 1877) determined the rate of absorption of various solutions, the capacity for fluid removal (Starling & Tubby 1894) and evidence that protein could pass through the peritoneum. It was also noted that the fluid in the peritoneal cavity contained the same amount of urea that is found in the blood, indicating that urea could be removed by PD (Rosenberg 1916). This was followed by Tracy Putnam suggesting that the peritoneum might be used to correct physiological problems, when he observed that under certain circumstances fluids in the peritoneal cavity can equilibrate with the plasma and that the rate of diffusion was dependent on the size of the molecules. Research also suggested at this time that the clearance of solutes was proportional to their molecular size and solution pH, and that a high flow rate maximised the transfer of solutes, which also depended on peritoneal surface area and blood flow (Putman 1923).

George Ganter was looking for a method of dialysis that did not require the use of an anticoagulant (Ganter 1923). He prepared a dialysate solution containing normal values of electrolytes and added dextrose for fluid removal. Bottles were boiled for sterilisation and filled with the solution, which was then infused into the patient's abdomen through a hollow needle.

The first treatment was carried out on a woman who was suffering acute renal failure following childbirth. Between 1 and 3 L of fluid was infused at a time, and the dwell time was 30 min to 3 h. The blood chemistry was reduced to within acceptable limits. The patient was sent home, but unfortunately she died, as it was not realised that it was necessary to continue the treatment in order to keep the patient alive.

Ganter recognised the importance of good access to the peritoneum, as it was noted that instilling the fluid was easier than attaining a good return volume. He was also aware of the complication of infection, and indeed this was the most frequent complication he encountered. Ganter identified four principles, which are still regarded as important today:

- there must be adequate access to the peritoneum
- sterile solutions are needed to reduce infection
- glucose content of the dialysate must be altered to remove greater volumes of fluid
- dwell times and fluid volume infused must be varied to determine the efficiency of the dialysis.

There are reports of 101 patients treated with PD in the 1920s (Abbott & Shea 1946, Odel et al 1950). Of these, 63 had reversible causes, 32 irreversible and in two the diagnosis was unknown. There was recovery in 32 of 63 cases of reversible renal failure. Deaths were due to uraemia, pulmonary oedema and peritonitis.

Stephen Rosenak, working in Europe, developed a metal catheter for peritoneal access, but was discouraged by the results because of the high incidence of peritonitis. In Holland, PSM Kop, who was an associate of Kolff during the mid-1940s, created a system of PD by using materials for the components that could easily be sterilised: porcelain containers for the fluid, latex rubber for the tubing and a glass catheter to infuse the fluid into the patient's abdomen. Kop treated 21 patients and met with success in ten.

Morton Maxwell, in Los Angeles, in the latter part of the 1950s, had been involved with HD, and it was his opinion that HD was too complicated for regular use. Aware of the problems with infection, he designed a system for PD with as few connections as possible. Together with a local manufacturer, he formulated a peritoneal solution, and customised a container and plastic tubing set and a single polyethylene catheter. The procedure used was to instil 2 L of fluid into the peritoneum, leave it to dwell for 30 min and return the fluid into the original bottles. This would be repeated until the blood chemistry was normal. This technique was carried out successfully on many patients and the highly regarded results were published in 1959. This became known as the Maxwell technique (Maxwell et al 1959). This simple form of dialysis recognised that it was no longer necessary to have expensive equipment with highly specialised staff in a large hospital to initiate dialysis. All that was required was an understanding of the procedure and available supplies.

THE CATHETER

Up to the 1970s, PD was used primarily for patients who were not good candidates for HD, or who were seeking a gentler form of treatment. Continuous flow using two catheters (Legrain & Merrill 1953) was still sometimes used but the single-catheter technique was favoured because of lower infection rates.

The polyethylene catheter was chosen by Paul Doolan (Doolan et al 1959) at the Naval Hospital in San Francisco when he developed a procedure for the treatment to use under battlefield conditions in the Korean War. Because of the flexibility of the catheter, it was considered for long-term treatment. A young physician called Richard Ruben decided to try this procedure, known as the Doolan technique (Ruben et al, unpublished work), on a female patient who improved dramatically but deteriorated after a few days without treatment. The patient was, therefore, dialysed repeatedly at weekends and allowed home during the week, with the catheter remaining in place. This was the first reported chronic treatment using a permanent indwelling catheter.

Catheters were made from tubing available on the hospital ward and included gallbladder trocars, rubber catheters, whistle-tip catheters and stainless-steel sump drains. However, as with the polyethylene plastic tubes, the main problem involved kinking and blockage. Maxwell described a nylon catheter with perforations at the curved distal end and this was the catheter that became commercially available. Advances in the manufacture of the silicone peritoneal catheter by Palmer (Palmer et al 1964) and Gutch (1964) included the introduction of perforations at the distal end. Later, Tenckhoff included the design of a shorter catheter, a straight catheter and a curled catheter. He also added the Dacron cuff, either single or double, to help to seal the openings through the peritoneum (Tenckhoff & Schechter 1968). He was also responsible for the introduction of the trocar that gave easy placement of the catheter. Dimitrios Oreopoulos, a Greek physician, was introduced to PD in Belfast, Northern Ireland, during his training and he noted the difficulties encountered with the catheters there. He had been shown a simple technique for inserting the catheter by Norman Dean from New York City, which allowed the access to be used over and over again.

PERITONEAL DIALYSIS AT HOME

In 1960, Scribner and Boen (Boen 1959) set up a PD programme that would allow patients to be treated at home. An automated unit was developed which could operate unattended overnight. The system used 40-L containers that were filled and sterilised at the University of Washington. The bottles were then delivered to the patient's home, and returned after use. The machine was able to measure the fluid in and out of the patient by a solenoid device. An indwelling tube was permanently implanted into the patient's abdomen, through which a tube was inserted for each dialysis treatment. The system was open and, therefore, was vulnerable to peritonitis. A new method was then used, whereby a new catheter was inserted into the abdomen for each treatment and removed after the treatment ended. This was still carried out in the home, when a physician would attend the patient at home for insertion of the catheter, leaving once the treatment had begun. The carer was trained to discontinue the treatment and remove the catheter. The wound was covered by a dressing and the patient would be free of dialysis until the next week. This treatment was carried out by Tenckhoff et al (1965) in a patient for 3 years, requiring 380 catheter punctures.

The large 40-L bottles of dialysate were difficult to handle, and delivery to the home and sterilisation were not easy. Tenckhoff, at the University of Washington, installed a water still into the patient's home, thus providing a sterile water supply. The water was mixed with sterile concentrate to provide the correct solution, but this method was not satisfactory as it remained cumbersome and dangerous due to the high pressure in the still. Various refinements were tried using this method, including a reverse osmosis unit and this was widely used later for HD treatment.

Lasker, in 1961, realised the potential of this type of treatment and concentrated on the idea of a simple version by instilling 2 L of fluid by a gravity-fed system. This proved to be cheaper to maintain but was labour intensive. Later that year, he was approached by Ira Gottscho, a businessman who had lost a daughter through kidney problems, and together they designed the first peritoneal cycler machine. The refinements included the ability to measure the fluid in and out, and the ability to warm the fluid before the fill cycle. Patients were sent home using the automated cycler treatment as early as 1970, even though there was a bias for HD at that time.

In 1969, Oreopoulos accepted a position at the Toronto Western Hospital and, together with Stanley Fenton, decided to use the Tenckhoff catheter for long-term treatment. Because of a lack of space and facilities at the hospital, it was necessary to send the patients home on intermittent

PD. He reviewed the Lasker cycler machine and ordered a supply, and by 1974 was managing over 70 patients on this treatment at home. Similar programmes were managed in Georgetown University and also in the Austin Diagnostic Clinic in the USA.

THE BEGINNING OF CONTINUOUS AMBULATORY PERITONEAL DIALYSIS

It was in 1975, following an unsuccessful attempt to haemodialyse a patient at the Austin Diagnostic Clinic, that an engineer, Robert Popovich, and Jack Moncrief became involved in working out the kinetics of 'long-dwell equilibrated dialysis' for this patient. It was determined that five exchanges each of 2 L per day would achieve the appropriate blood chemistry, and that the removal of 1–2 L of fluid from the patient was needed per day. Thus came the evolution of CAPD (Popovich et al 1976).

The treatment was so successful that the Austin group were given a grant to allow them to continue dialysing patients with CAPD. Strangely, their first description and account of this clinical experience was rejected by the American Society for Artificial Internal Organs. At this time, the treatment was called 'a portable/wearable equilibrium dialysis technique'. The stated advantages compared with HD included:

- good steady-state biochemical control
- more liberal diet and fluid intake
- improvement in anaemia.

The main problems were protein loss (Popovich et al 1978) and infection. It was recognised that the source of infection was almost certainly related to the use of the bottles. Oreopoulos found that collapsible polyvinylchloride (PVC) containers for the solution were available in Canada. Once the fluid was instilled, the bag could then be rolled up and concealed under the clothing. The fluid could be returned into the bag during draining by gravity, without a disconnection taking place (Oreopoulos et al 1978). New spike connections were produced for access to the bag of fluid, and a Luer connection for fitting to the catheter, together with tubing devised for HD, greatly reduced the chances of infection. The patients treated on an intermittent basis (by intermittent peritoneal dialysis; IPD) were rapidly converted to CAPD and evaluation of the new treatment was rapid, owing to the large numbers being treated. Following approval by the US Food and Drug Administration, many centres were then able to develop CAPD programmes.

The first complete CAPD system was released on to the market in 1979, giving a choice of three strengths of dextrose solution. Included in this system were an administration line and sterile items packed together to form a preparation kit, to be used at each bag change in an attempt to keep infection at bay. The regime proposed by Robert Popovich and Jack

Moncrief entailed four exchanges over a 24-h period, three dwell times of approximately 4 h in the daytime and one dwell overnight of 8 h. This regime is the one mainly used today.

The systems are continually being improved, with connectors moving from spike to Luer to eliminate as far as possible the accidental disconnection of the bag from the line. A titanium connector was found to be the superior form of adaptor for connection of the transfer set to the catheter and probably led to a reduced infection rate for peritonitis. A disadvantage of this technique is the flow of fresh fluid down the transfer set along the area of disconnection, thus encouraging any bacteria from the disconnection to be instilled into the abdomen. The development of the Y-system (flush before fill) in the mid-1980s in Italy resulted in a further decrease in peritonitis.

AUTOMATED PERITONEAL DIALYSIS

Automated PD in the form of continuous cyclic peritoneal dialysis (CCPD) was further developed by Diaz-Buxo in the early 1980s to enable patients who were unable to perform exchanges in the day to be treated with PD overnight (Fig. 1.8).

Figure 1.8
The American Medical Products continuous cyclic peritoneal dialysis machine 1980.

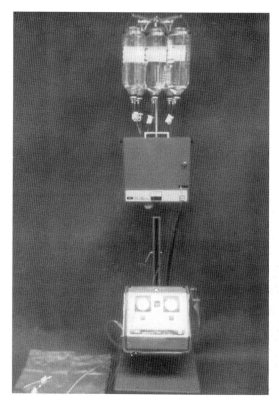

ADVANCES IN PERITONEAL DIALYSIS FOR SPECIAL NEEDS

Recent advances in CAPD treatment include a dialysate, which not only provides dialysis but contains 1.1% amino acid, to be administered to malnourished patients. This may be particularly useful for the elderly on CAPD, in whom poor nutrition is a well-recognised complication.

Those with diabetes were initially not considered for dialysis because of the complications of the disease. Carl Kjellstrand, at the University of Minnesota, suggested that insulin could be administered to those with diabetes by adding it to the PD fluid (Crossley & Kjellstrand 1971). However, when this suggestion was first put forward, it was not adopted because the 30-min dwell did not give time for the drug to be absorbed into the patient. It became viable later, when the long dwell dialysis was initiated and this gave the advantage of slow absorption, resulting in a steady state of blood sugar in the normal range, thus alleviating the need for painful injections (Flynn & Nanson 1979).

The realisation that patients are individuals, bringing their own problems associated with training, brought many exchange aid devices on to the market to assist the patient in the exchange procedure. These exchange devices were mainly used to assist such disabilities as blindness, arthritis (particularly of the hands) and patients prone to repeated episodes of peritonitis (Fig. 1.9).

THE FUTURE

In some centres, PD is usually the first choice of treatment for established renal disease and in many countries and, because of the lack of facilities for in-centre HD, will remain so. In 2004 in England and Wales, 26% of all patients on dialysis were on PD therapies (UK Renal Registry, 2005). However the relative prevalence of PD in the UK has been declining since

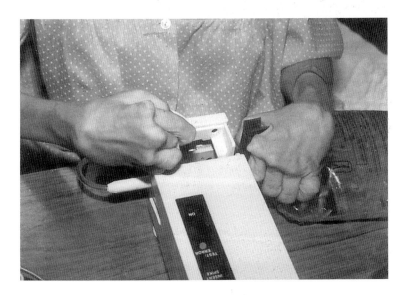

Figure 1.9
The Baxter ultraviolet exchange device.

its peak in the early 1990s, possibly because of the availability of satellite haemodialysis and a high level of PD technique failure.

TRANSPLANTATION

IN THE BEGINNING

Kidney transplantation as a therapeutic and practical option for renal replacement therapy (RRT) was first reported in published literature at the turn of the 20th century. The first steps were small and so insignificant that they were overlooked or condemned.

The first known attempts at renal transplantation on humans were made without immunosuppression between 1906 and 1923 using pig, sheep, goat and subhuman primate donors (Elkington 1964). These first efforts were conducted in France and Germany, but others followed. None of the kidneys functioned for long, if indeed at all, and the recipients all died within a period of a few hours to 9 days later.

Of all the workers at this time, the contribution made by Alixis Carrel (1873–1944) remains the most famous. His early work in Lyons, France and in Chicago involved the transplantation of an artery from one dog to another. This work later became invaluable in the transplantation of organs. In 1906, Carrel and Guthrie, working in the Hull Laboratory in Chicago, reported the successful transplantation of both kidneys in cats and later a double nephrectomy on dogs, reimplanting only one of the kidneys. He found that the secretion of urine remained normal and the animal remained in good health, despite having only one kidney (Carrel 1908). Carrel was awarded the Nobel Prize in 1912 for his work on vascular and related surgery.

While at this stage there was no clear understanding of the problem, some principles were clearly learned. Vascular suture techniques were reviewed and the possibility of using pelvic implantation sites was investigated and practised. No further renal heterotransplantations (animal to human) were tried until 1963 when experiments using kidneys from chimpanzee (Reemtsma et al 1964) and baboon were tried, with eventual death of the patients. This ended all trials using animal donation.

The first human-to-human kidney transplant was reported in 1936, by the Russian Voronoy, when he implanted a kidney from a cadaver donor of B-positive blood type into a recipient of O-positive blood type, a mismatch that would not be attempted today. The donor had died 6h before the operation and the recipient died 6h later without making any urine. The following 20 years saw further efforts in kidney transplantation, all without effective immunosuppression (Groth 1972). The extraperitoneal technique developed by French surgeons Dubost and Servelle became today's standard procedure.

THE FIRST SUCCESSES

The first examples of survival success of a renal transplant can probably be attributed to Hume. Hume placed the transplanted kidney into the thigh of the patient, with function for 5 months. Then at the Peter Bent Brigham Hospital in Boston, USA, in December 1954, the first successful identical-twin transplant was performed by the surgeon Joseph E Murray in collaboration with the nephrologist John P Merrill (Hume et al 1955). The recipient survived for more than two decades. The idea of using identical twins had been proposed when it was noted by David C Miller of the Public Health Service Hospital, Boston, that skin grafts between identical twins were not rejected (Brown 1937). The application of this information resulted in rigorous matching, including skin grafting, prior to effective immunosuppression.

Over the period between 1951 and 1976 there were 29 transplants performed between identical twins, and the survival rate for 20 years was 50%. Studies of two successfully transplanted patients, who were given kidneys from their non-identical twins, were also reported (Merrill et al 1960). The first survived 20 years (died of heart disease) and the second, 26 years (died of carcinoma of the bladder). Immunosuppression used in these cases was irradiation.

IMMUNOSUPPRESSION

It was Sir Peter Medawar who appreciated that rejection is an immunological phenomenon (Medawar 1944), and this led to research into weakening the immune system of the recipients to reduce the rejection. In animals, corticosteriods, total body irradiation and cytotoxic drug therapy were used. Experiments in animals were still far from successful, as were similar techniques when used in humans. It was concluded that the required degree of immunosuppression would lead to destruction of the immune system and finally result in terminal infections.

A few patients were transplanted between 1960 and 1961 in Paris and Boston, using drug regimes involving 6-mercaptopurine or azathioprine with or without irradiation. They all died within 18 months. Postmortem examination of failed kidney grafts showed marked changes in the renal histology, which at first were thought unlikely to be due to immunological rejection, but later it was convincingly shown that this was indeed the underlying process.

In the early days of kidney transplantation, the kidney was removed from either a living related donor or a cadaver donor and immediately transferred to the donor after first flushing the kidney with cold electrolyte solution, such as Hartman's solution. In 1967, Belzer and his colleagues developed a technique for continuous perfusion of the kidney using oxygenated cryoprecipitated plasma, which allowed the kidney to be kept up to 72 h before transplantation. This machine perfusion required constant supervision, and it was found that flushing the kidney with an electrolyte solution and storage at 0°C in ice saline allowed the kidney to be preserved for up to 24 h or more (Marshall et al 1988). This was a major development in transplantation techniques.

During the 1950s it was recognised that many of the survivors of the Hiroshima atomic bomb in 1945 suffered impairment to their immune system. It was concluded that radiation could, therefore, induce immunosuppression and clinical total body irradiation was used to prolong the survival of renal transplants in Boston in 1958. This did improve the survival of some transplants; however, the overall outcomes were poor. There was clearly a need for a more effective form of immunosuppression than irradiation.

A breakthrough in immunosuppressive therapy occurred in 1962 in the University of Colorado, when it was discovered that the combination of azathioprine and prednisone allowed the prevention and, in some cases, reversal, of rejection (Starzl et al 1963). Transplantation could at last expand. A conference sponsored by the National Research Council and National Academy of Sciences in 1963 in Washington resulted in the first registry report, which enabled the tracing of all the early non-twin kidney recipients. In 1970 work commenced on the development of ciclosporin by Sandoz in Basle, Switzerland, after the drug's potential was recognised (Borel et al 1976). Clinical trials carried out in Cambridge, UK (Calne et al 1979), showed that outcomes on renal transplantation were greatly improved, both with graft and with patient survival. Ciclosporin revolutionised immunosuppression treatment for transplant patients, even though it is itself nephrotoxic and its use needs close monitoring.

Tissue typing is a complex procedure and, as yet, is far from perfect. The use of the united networks for organ sharing has increased the efforts of matching donor and recipient, and data available from these sources show a significant gain in survival of well-matched versus mis-matched cadaver kidneys. Cross-matching remains as important today as it was 25 years ago at its conception. None of the immunosuppressive measures available today can prevent the immediate destruction of the transplanted organ by humoral antibodies in the hyperacute rejection phase. This was recognised as early as 1965 (Kissmeyer-Neilsen et al 1966) and it may be that this phenomenon holds the key to the future of successful heterotransplantation.

BLOOD TRANSFUSIONS

It was observed in the late 1960s that patients who had received multiple blood transfusions before organ transplantation did not have a poorer graft survival than those who had not been transfused. In 1974, Opelz & Terasaki observed that patients who had received no transfusions whatsoever were more likely to reject the transplant. It became evident, therefore, that a small number of blood transfusions resulted in an improved organ survival and so the transfusion policies for non-transfused recipients were changed throughout the world. This 'transfusion effect' is of much less importance with the ciclosporin era.

PRESENT

Renal transplantation has been a dramatic success over the past 30 years, with patient survival rates not less than 97% after 6 months' transplantation for both living related and cadaver transplants. Although short-term survival for the graft is good – around 90% expectation of survival of the graft at 1 year – cadaveric graft survival at 5 years of around 60%

is less impressive, with a substantial minority losing their renal graft after 10 years.

THE FUTURE

There is no doubt that renal transplantation is the treatment of choice for many patients requiring RRT as, in general, it gives a better quality of life than dialysis. However, organs are in short supply. From April 2005 to March 2006, 1799 patients received a kidney transplant, although the number of patients registered on the active transplant list at 31 March 2005 for a kidney or kidney and pancreas transplant has increased by 32% since 1996 (United Kingdom Transplant 2005). A change in the law may result in more kidneys becoming available for transplantation, by allowing easier access to donors or removing the need for relatives' consent. However, until a significant breakthrough is achieved, there will continue to be a waiting list for transplantation and it will be necessary to continue to improve the techniques of dialysis.

SUMMARY

The Kidney Alliance (an umbrella body representing all organisations involved in renal services) suggested in 2001 that acceptance rates for renal replacement therapy (RRT) are rising, but there remain geographical inequalities. Some areas in the UK do not have autonomous renal services or satellite dialysis units. In 2005, the total estimated acceptance rate for RRT in adults in the UK was 108 per million population (pmp) (UK Renal Registry, 2006). Acceptance rates in some areas have been lower than in other European countries (Fig. 1.10).

Figure 1.10
End-stage renal failure (ESRF) patients treated by renal replacement therapy. HD, haemodialysis; PD, peritoneal dialysis; pmp, per million population. (From Kidney Alliance 2001, with permission.)

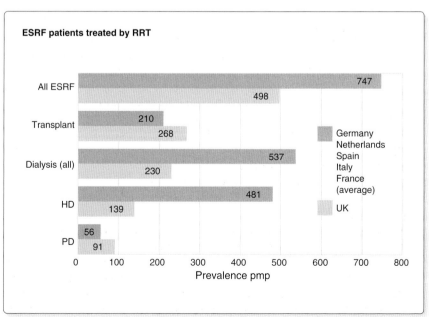

It has been predicted that there will be substantial growth in the RRT population to 2010 and that the numbers receiving RRT will not plateau for at least 20 years. Even with an optimistic increase in transplant supply (11% pa for 5 years), numbers on haemodialysis (HD) will continue to rise substantially, especially in older people (Roderick et al 2004). Another challenge is the difficulty in recruiting and retaining nursing staff skilled in dialysis care.

Dialysis has come a long way from the small beginnings of the hot baths in Rome. Refinements and improvements continue, most recently with the emergence of erythropoietin in the late 1980s to correct the major complication of anaemia in these patients. Improvements in access for both HD and peritoneal dialysis will emerge. The challenge of adequate dialysis for all who need treatment remains.

Transplantation is still not available for all those who are eligible and changes in the law may help with the availability of donor organs.

Multidisciplinary teams will continue to strive to give patients the best possible quality of treatments until there is a revolutionary breakthrough in the prevention of renal failure.

ACKNOWLEDGEMENT

With grateful thanks to Toni Smith who was the original author of this chapter.

References

Abbott WE, Shea P. Treatment of temporary renal insufficiency (uraemia) by peritoneal lavage. Am J Med Sci 1946; 211: 312.

Abel JJ, Rowntree LG, Turner BB. The removal of diffusable substances from the circulating blood of living animals by dialysis. J Pharmacol Exp Ther 1914; 5: 275–316.

Baillod RA, Comty C, Ilahi M et al. Proceedings of the European Dialysis and Transplant Association 2. Amsterdam: Excerpta Medica 1965: 99.

Boen ST. Peritoneal dialysis. Amsterdam: Van Gorcum 1959: 26.

Borel JF, Feurer C, Gubler HU et al. Biological effects of cyclosporin A. A new antilymphocytic agent. Agents Actions 1976; 6: 468–475.

Brown JB. Homografting of the skin. With report of success in identical twins. Surgery 1937; 1: 558–563.

Calne, RY, Rolles K, White DJG et al. Cyclosporin A initially as the only immunosuppressant in 34 recipients of cadaveric organs: 32 kidneys, 2 pancreases, and 2 livers. Lancet 1979; 1: 1033–1036.

Carrel, A. Results of the transplantation of blood vessels, organs and limbs. JAMA 1908, 51: 1662–1667 (Reprinted in JAMA 1983; 250: 994–953).

Cimino, JE, Brescia MJ. Simple venepuncture for haemodialysis. N Engl J Med 1962; 267: 608–609.

Crossley K. Kjellstrand CM. Intraperitoneal insulin for control of blood sugar in diabetic patients during peritoneal dialysis. Br Med J 1971; 1: 269–290.

Doolan PD, Murphy WP Jr, Wiggins RA et al. An evaluation of intermittent peritoneal lavage. Am J Med 1959; 26: 831–844.

Eggerth AH. The preparation and standardization of collodion membranes. J Biol Chem 1921; 48(1): 203–221.

Elkington JR. Moral problems in the use of borrowed organs artificial and transplanted. Ann Intern Med 1964; 60: 309–313.

Fishman AP, Kroop IG, Leiter HE et al. Management of anuria in acute mercurial intoxication. NY State J Med 1948; 48: 2393–2396.

Flynn CT, Nanson, JA. Intraperitoneal insulin with CAPD – an artificial pancreas. Trans Am Soc Artif Intern Organs 1979; 25: 114–117.

Ganter G. About the elimination of poisonous substances from the blood by dialysis. Munch Med Wochenschr 1923; 70: 1478–1480.

Graham T. The Bakerian lecture – on osmotic force. Phil Trans R Soc Lond 1854; 144: 177–228.

Groth CG. Landmarks in clinical renal transplantation. Surg Gynecol Obstet 1972 134: 323–328.

Gutch CF. Peritoneal dialysis. Trans Am Soc Artif Intern Organs 1964; 10: 406–407.

Hale S. A method of conveying liquors into the abdomen during the operation of tapping. Phil Trans R Soc 1744; 43: 20–21.

Hess CLV McGuigan H. The condition of the sugar in the blood. J Pharmacol Exp Ther 1914; 6: 45–55.

Hume DM, Merrill JP, Miller BF et al. Experience with renal homotransplantation in the human. Report of nine cases. J Clin Invest 1955; 34: 327–382.

Kidney Alliance. End-stage renal failure – a framework for Planning and Service Delivery. Kidney Alliance 2001.

Kissmeyer-Neilsen F, Olsen S, Peterson VP et al. Hyperacute rejection of kidney allografts, associated with pre-existing humoral antibodies against donor cells. Lancet 1966; 2: 662–665.

Kolff WJ, Berk HT. The artificial kidney: a dialyser with a great area. Acta Med Scand 1944; 117: 121–134.

Kolff WJ. Artificial kidney – treatment of acute and chronic uraemia. Cleveland Clin Q 1950; 17: 216–228.

Kolff WJ. First clinical experience with the artificial kidney. Ann Intern Med 1965; 62: 608–619.

Legrain M Merrill JP. Short term continuous transperitoneal dialysis. N Engl J Med 1953; 248: 125–129.

MacNeill AE. Some possible uses of blood dialysers. Surgeons practice meeting. New England Surgical Society Sept 23 1949. Bretton Woods, NH: Proceedings of the New England Surgical Society 1949: 3.

Malinow MR, Korzon W. Experimental method for obtaining an ultrafiltrate of the blood. J Lab Clin Med 1947; 31: 461–471.

Marshall VC, Jablonski P, Scott DF. Renal preservation. In: Morris PJ, ed. Kidney transplantation: principles and practice, 3rd edn. Philadelphia: WB Saunders 1988: 151–182.

Maxwell MH, Rockery RE, Kleeman CR. Peritoneal dialysis, techniques and application. JAMA 1959; 170: 917–924.

Medawar PB. The behaviour and fate of skin autografts and skin homografts in rabbits. J Anat 1944; 78: 176–199.

Merrill JP, Murray JE, Harrison JH et al. Succesful homotransplantation of the kidney between non-identical twins. N Engl J Med 1960; 262: 1251–1260.

Merrill JP, Thorn GW, Walter CW et al. The use of an artificial kidney. 1. Technique. J Clin Invest 1950; 29: 412–424.

NICE Technology Appraisal No. 48: Guidance on home compared with hospital haemodialysis for patients with end-stage renal failure 2002. www.nice.org.uk/page.aspx?o=TA048guidance

Odel HM, Ferris DO, Power H. Peritoneal lavage as an effective means of extrarenal excretion. Am J Med 1950; 9: 63–77.

Opelz G, Terasaki PI. Poor kidney transplant survival in recipients with frozen-blood transfusions or no transfusions. Lancet 1974; 2: 696–698.

Oreopoulos DG, Robson M, Izatt S et al. A simple and safe technique for continuous ambulatory peritoneal dialysis. Trans Am Soc Artif Organs 1978; 24: 484–489.

Palmer RA, Quinton WE, Gray JF. Prolonged peritoneal dialysis for chronic renal failure. Lancet 1964; 1: 700–702.

Palmer RA, Rutherford PS. Kidney substitutes in uraemia: the use of Kolff's dialyser in two cases. Can Med Assoc J 1949; 60: 261–266.

Popovich RP, Moncrief JF, Decherd JF et al. The definition of a novel portable/wearable equilibrium peritoneal dialysis technique. Abstract Trans Am Soc Artif Organs 1976; 5: 64.

Popovich RP, Moncrief JW, Nolph KD et al. Continuous ambulatory peritoneal dialysis. Ann Intern Med 1978; 88: 449–456.

Putman T. The living peritoneum as a dialysing membrane. Am J Physiol 1923; 63: 548–555.

Reemtsma K, McCracken BH, Schlegel JU et al. Renal heterotransplantation in man. Ann Surg 1964; 160: 384–410.

Richardson BW. Practical studies in animal dialysis. Asclepiad (Lond) 1923; 6: 331–332.

Roderick, P, Davies R, Jones C et al. Simulation model of renal replacement therapy: predicting future demand in England. Nephrol Dial Transplant 2004 19: 692–701.

Rosenberg M. Nitrogenous retention of substances in the blood and in other body fluids in the core of the kidneys. J Berl Klin Wochenshr 1916; 53: 1314–1316.

Skeggs LT Jr, Leonards JR, Heisler CR. Artificial kidney: 11. Construction and operation of an improved continuous dialyser. Proc Soc Exp Biol Med 1949; 72(3): 539–543.

Starling EH, Tubby AH. On the paths of absorption from the peritoneal cavity. J Physiol 1894; 16: 140.

Starzl TE, Marchioro TL, Waddell WR. The reversal of rejection in human renal homografts with subsequent development of homograft tolerance. Surg Gynecol Obstet 1963; 117: 385–395.

Tenckhoff H, Schechter H. A bacteriologically safe peritoneal access device. Trans Am Soc Artif Intern Organs 1968; 14: 181–186.

Tenckhoff H, Shilipetar G, Boen ST. One year experience with home peritoneal dialysis. Trans Am Soc Artif Intern Organs 1965; 11: 11–14.

Teschan PE. Haemodialysis in military casualties. Trans Am Soc Artif Intern Organs 1955; 2: 52–54.

Thalhimer W, Solandt DY, Best CH. Experimental exchange transfusion using purified heparin. Lancet 1938; 11: 554–555.

UK Renal Registry: Ninth annual report of the UK Renal Registry. Bristol: UK Renal Registry 2006.

United Kingdom Transplant (UKT). Transplant Activity in the UK 2004–2005. 2005. www.uktransplant.org.uk/ukt/statistics/transplant_activity_report/current_activity_reports.jsp/ukt/tx_activity_report_2005_uk_complete-v2.pdf

Warrick C. An improvement in the practice of tapping, whereby that operation instead for the relief of symptoms, became an absolute cure for ascites, exemplified in the case of Jane Roman. Phil Trans R Soc 1744; 43: 12–19.

Wegner G. Surgical comments on peritoneal cavity with special emphasis on ovariotomy. Arch Klin Chir 1877; 20: 53–145.

Chapter 2

Applied anatomy and physiology and the renal disease process

Charlotte A Chalmers

CHAPTER CONTENTS

LEARNING OUTCOMES FOR THIS CHAPTER	■ To understand the structure and main functions of the kidney ■ To explain the basic renal processes of filtration, reabsorption and secretion ■ To identify the main conditions causing chronic and established renal failure ■ To analyse the clinical features of these conditions and explain the principles of care management

INTRODUCTION

This chapter provides the reader with a detailed discussion on all aspects of renal physiology, together with the relationship to important patho-physiological processes in renal disease and some brief discussion on related nursing observations. The first part of the chapter explores the normal renal anatomy and physiology and the second part deals with disease processes causing established renal failure. This is not intended as a complete reference to all kidney diseases, rather to illustrate how altered renal physiology can affect the whole body, and indeed how other diseases can impact on kidney function.

STRUCTURE AND FUNCTIONS OF THE KIDNEY

The kidneys are paired organs lying behind the peritoneum, on either side of the vertebral column. The upper pole of the kidney is at the spinal level of T12 and the lower pole at approximately L3. The right kidney is a little lower owing to the presence of the liver on that side. Usually, the kidneys are oriented with the concave surface facing the spine. However, owing to developmental aberrations, other orientations of the kidney may occasionally exist (e.g. lying in the pelvis) but these do not usually affect function. Each kidney is approximately 11 cm long and weighs about 150 g (Fig. 2.1).

On the concave surface of the kidney lies the hilus, from which the ureter and the main blood vessels and nerves access the kidney. The cut surface of the kidney reveals two distinct regions: a dark outer region, the cortex, and a pale inner region called the medulla. The outer cortex

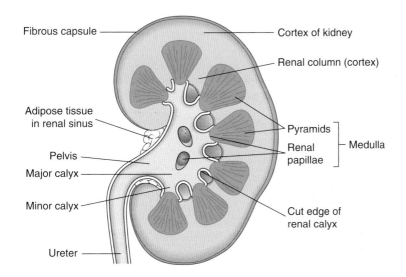

Figure 2.1
Coronal section of a kidney.
(After Hinchliff SM, Montague
SE. Physiology for nursing
practice. London: Baillière
Tindall, 1988, with permission
of Baillière Tindall.)

is covered by a fibrous capsule and the whole kidney is surrounded by
a pad of fat that offers some protection against injury. Broadly speaking, the cortex contains the filtering and reabsorptive components of
the nephrons, while the medulla contains the concentrating and diluting components of the nephrons and a system of collection ducts. These
ducts funnel the urine into the pelvis at the heart of the medulla, from
where it moves down the ureter into the bladder (Fig. 2.2).

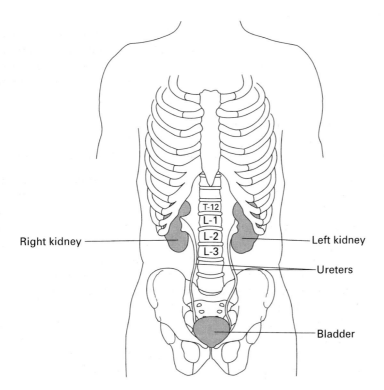

Figure 2.2
Relative position of the kidneys
in the body.

THE NEPHRON

The nephron is the functional unit of the kidney and each kidney contains approximately 1 million nephrons (Fig. 2.3). The unique structure of the nephron is critically related to its complex functions and contains five components, each performing a distinct process:

- the Bowman's capsule – forming a blind-ending capsule around a knot of capillaries called the glomerulus (the site of filtration)
- the proximal convoluted tubule (the site of bulk-phase reabsorption and some secretion)
- the loop of Henle (where the concentration and dilution of urine mainly occur)
- the distal convoluted tubule (the site of 'fine-tuning' reabsorption and more secretion)
- the collecting duct (also important for the concentration of urine and for carrying urine into the renal pelvis).

Figure 2.3
Microanatomy of nephron.
(From Hinchliff SM, Montague SE, Watson R. Physiology for nursing practice. London: Baillière Tindall, 1999, with permission of Baillière Tindall.)

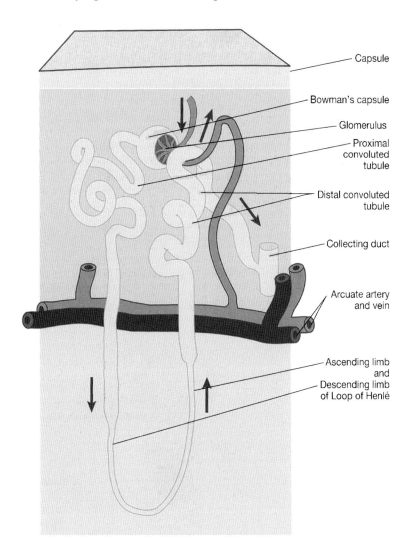

Capsule

Bowman's capsule

Glomerulus

Proximal convoluted tubule

Distal convoluted tubule

Collecting duct

Arcuate artery and vein

Ascending limb and Descending limb of Loop of Henlé

These processes do not occur in isolation, but are interdependent and intimately related to each other by the shape of the nephron. The importance of this fact will become clear when the renal processes are discussed in more detail.

There are broadly two types of nephron found in the kidney (Fig. 2.4). Approximately 85% of nephrons are cortical nephrons, which have short loops of Henle that are contained in the cortex of the kidney. The other 15% of nephrons are called juxtamedullary nephrons and they have long loops of Henle, which extend deep into the medulla of the kidney. It is the long loops of Henle that enable concentration of urine; animals adapted to arid environments have long loops of Henle compared with those that have a lesser requirement to conserve water. These loops, together with the collecting ducts that also pass through the medulla, give the pyramids of the medulla a striated appearance.

The main functions of the kidney are to rid the body of the end-product of metabolism and to regulate the electrolytes found in the body fluids. A more detailed list of the functions of the kidney can be found in Box 2.1. Before looking at how the kidney achieves its functions, there follows a discussion on the impressive versatility of urine.

THE VERSATILITY OF URINE

When the immense variability in the qualities of urine that can be produced in order to control our internal environment is considered, one cannot fail to be impressed by the complexities of the workings of the kidney. Broadly speaking, there are three parameters that can be varied in order to maintain the constancy of our bodily fluids: urinary volume, urinary concentration and urinary content.

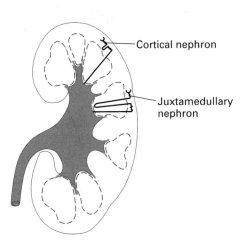

Cortical nephron

Juxtamedullary nephron

Figure 2.4
The position of the nephrons in the kidney.

Box 2.1   The functions of the kidney

Excretory
Excretion of metabolic waste products, e.g. urea and creatinine

Regulatory
Regulation of:

- Body water volume
- Body fluid osmolality
- Electrolyte balance
- Acid–base balance
- Blood pressure

Metabolic
Activation of vitamin D
Production of renin
Production of erythropoietin

Urinary volume

In a healthy person, the volume of urine produced per day can vary from as little as 300 mL, if no water is ingested or there is excessive water loss from the body (as in diarrhoea), up to a maximum of 23 L in cases of excessive fluid ingestion. In health, urine output cannot drop below 300 mL day^{-1} because this is the absolute minimum water volume required to excrete the daily load of toxic waste products. If the amount of waste products to be removed by the kidney rises, then the minimum urine volume must also rise. However, the average urine output per day is approximately 1500 mL. The kidneys' ability to vary the volume of daily urine output over such a wide range is essential if we are to maintain a constant body fluid volume in the face of adverse factors such as excessive heat, which causes sweating; colonic infections causing diarrhoea; or excessive thirst and water ingestion, as seen in the condition psychogenic polydipsia (Table 2.1).

Urinary concentration

Though the volume of urine can vary over a wide range, the amount of solutes to be excreted by the kidney each day is much less variable. Thus, in order to excrete a fairly fixed volume of solutes each day in a very variable volume of water, the kidney must have the ability to concentrate or dilute the urine. On a hot summer's day when very little fluid has been drunk, urine is dark in colour and of low volume, whereas if liberal amounts of beer have been consumed at a party, large volumes of watery urine are passed all evening. In fact this diuretic effect of beer is not wholly due to the volume imbibed, but also to the fact that the alcohol present in the beer suppresses the secretion (from the posterior pituitary gland) of antidiuretic hormone (ADH; also known as vasopressin), a hormone which would normally prevent diuresis. The hangover suffered the next day is, therefore, caused by dehydration.

Inputs (mL)		Outputs (mL)	
Water	1500	Urine[a]	1500
Food	500	Insensible loss	
		lungs	400
		skin[b]	400
Water of	400	Faeces[c]	100
metabolism			
Total	2400		2400

[a] Urinary volume is the only factor that can be regulated by the body to balance fluid inputs.
[b] This insensible loss of fluid through the skin is by simple evaporation (not sweat). Sweat is called 'sensible loss' and may reach up to 5 L h⁻¹, for example, when a person is exercising excessively.
[c] Loss of fluid with the faeces can be as high as several litres per day in the presence of severe colonic infections such as cholera.

Table 2.1
Normal fluid inputs and outputs

The ability of the kidneys to excrete all the body's excess solutes in varying amounts of water by concentrating or diluting the urine is essential for maintaining a constant body osmolality (Box 2.2). The mechanism in the kidney that controls the concentration or dilution of urine is often affected early on in renal disease, making it difficult for the individual to control both body fluid volume and osmolality in response to changes in fluid inputs and outputs. This can result in the individual tipping back and forth from states of dehydration to fluid overload.

Box 2.2 Concepts of osmosis and body osmolality

- Water can move between the different body fluid compartments across semipermeable membranes by the process of osmosis
- The more concentrated a solution, the more water will be drawn into this solution
- Any solute that can cause the movement of water across a semipermeable membrane is said to be 'osmotically active'
- The osmotic activity of substances in solution is dependent on the number of dissolved particles in the solution and not on their size or charge
- Sodium chloride (NaCl) dissociates in solution into Na^+ and Cl^- ions, so the number of osmotically active particles is almost double the number of NaCl molecules (but not exactly double, since the dissociation is not complete;

the solution consists of NaCl, Na^+ and Cl^- particles)
- Osmotically active particles in solution are measured by the unit called the osmole or milliosmole (mosmol)
- Osmolality is measured in milliosmoles per kilogram of water (mosmol kg water⁻¹) and is a measure of the potential osmotic activity of dissolved solutes in solution
- Normal body fluid osmolality is 285 mosmol kg water⁻¹
- The concentration (rather than the osmotic activity) of individual electrolytes is measured in mmol (millimoles) or μmol (micromoles) rather than mosmol (e.g. normal fasting blood glucose range = 3.6–5.8 mmol L⁻¹)

Urinary content

The range of substances that can be constituents of urine is varied and includes the following.

- Ions: sodium, potassium, calcium, magnesium, chloride, bicarbonate, phosphate and ammonium.
- Metabolic waste: urea, creatinine and uric acid.
- Drug metabolites: most metabolites of pharmacological agents are eventually excreted from the body through the kidneys; many are detoxified in the liver first.
- Other products of normal metabolism: metabolites of hormones can be detected in the urine by appropriate assays and may be a diagnostic aid, for example, the appearance of human chorionic gonadotrophin in the urine in the early stages of pregnancy forms the basis of the pregnancy test.

Normal urine is clear in appearance, though it may vary in colour from pale to dark amber, depending on its concentration. It has no unpleasant odour, though urine that has been standing a long time may develop a strong ammonia smell. Finally, normal urine has a pH that is slightly acidic (around pH 6), although urine can have a pH in the range 4.0–8.0 in cases of severe acidosis or alkalosis, respectively.

BASIC RENAL PROCESSES

GLOMERULAR FILTRATION

This is a process of filtration of plasma across the glomerular basement membrane from the glomerulus into the Bowman's capsule (Fig. 2.5).

Figure 2.5
The glomerulus and Bowman's capsule.

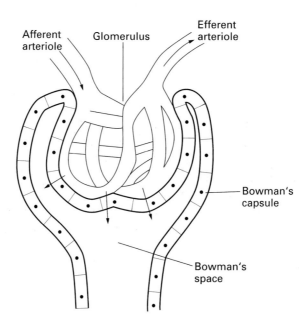

The glomerular filtration surface is a unique structure composed of three layers:

- the endothelial lining of the glomerular capillaries
- the basement membrane
- the epithelial cells of the Bowman's capsule, or podocytes. Filtration occurs between the slits formed by the finger-like processes of these cells (called pedicels) that surround the glomerular capillaries (Fig. 2.6).

These three layers are fused together and act as a barrier to the filtration of large-molecular-weight molecules such as proteins.

Blood enters the glomerulus from a series of branches of the renal artery, ending in the afferent arteriole. Blood then leaves the glomerulus through the efferent arteriole rather than a vein. In the majority of nephrons (those situated in the cortex), the efferent arteriole from the glomerulus divides up into capillaries, which cover the surfaces of the convoluted tubules. The capillaries finally empty into the venous system. In the deeper juxtamedullary nephrons the efferent arteriole from the glomerulus divides to form loops that lie parallel to the loops of Henle and so run down into the medulla. These vessels are called the vasa recta and are concerned with the process of concentration of the urine (Fig. 2.7). Blood then leaves the kidney through a series of larger converging veins, ending in the renal vein, which returns the blood to the vena cava.

In effect, the nephrons contain two capillary beds, one within the glomerulus and a second, which surrounds the convoluted tubules of the nephrons. This unusual arrangement of two capillary beds in tandem enables a pressure gradient to exist within the nephron, with high pressure in the glomerulus, favouring filtration, and a relatively low pressure in the peritubular capillaries, favouring reabsorption.

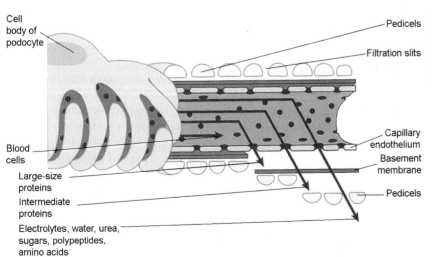

Cell body of podocyte

Blood cells

Large-size proteins

Intermediate proteins

Electrolytes, water, urea, sugars, polypeptides, amino acids

Pedicels

Filtration slits

Capillary endothelium

Basement membrane

Pedicels

Figure 2.6
Schematic representation of the filtration barrier. (Redrawn from Creager JG. Human anatomy and physiology. CA: Wodsworth, 1983, with permission.)

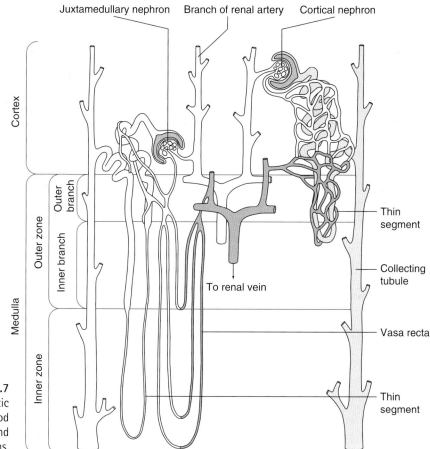

Juxtamedullary nephron   Branch of renal artery   Cortical nephron

Cortex

Medulla

Outer zone — Outer branch / Inner branch

Inner zone

To renal vein

Thin segment

Collecting tubule

Vasa recta

Thin segment

Figure 2.7
Diagrammatic representation of the blood supply to cortical and juxtamedullary nephrons. (From Lamb JF, Pitman RM. Essentials of physiology, 3rd edn. London: Blackwell Scientific, 1991, with permission.)

The formation of a filtrate from plasma flowing through the glomerulus occurs due to Starling's forces (Fig. 2.8). These are the same forces that cause the filtration and reabsorption of tissue fluid in other capillary beds in the body, but with some important adaptations. In the glomerulus, fluid is forced across the glomerular basement membrane because of the high hydrostatic pressure of blood flowing through the afferent arteriole. This pressure is greater than the oncotic pressure opposing it. Oncotic pressure is essentially osmotic pressure, exerted by proteins in the blood. In an ordinary capillary bed, this filtrate would be almost entirely reabsorbed back into the capillary at the venule end because the hydrostatic pressure would have fallen to below the oncotic pressure of the capillary, which would then pull the fluid back in by osmosis. However, in the glomerulus, because blood leaving enters another arteriole (the efferent arteriole) rather than a venule, a high hydrostatic pressure is maintained and oncotic pressure is insufficient to draw fluid back into the capillary. This situation is obviously desirable so that large amounts of filtrate can be made. All of the filtrate formed in the glomerulus passes into the Bowman's capsule and is often referred to as tubular urine (Fig. 2.8).

a) Muscle capillaries

Arteriole end

Outward pressure:
Capillary hydrostatic
pressure = 35mm Hg

Inward pressure:
Protein oncotic
pressure = 25mm Hg

**Net outward
pressure** = 10mm Hg

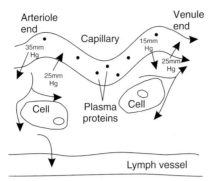

Venule end

Outward pressure:
Capillary hydrostatic
pressure = 15mm Hg

Inward pressure:
Protein oncotic
pressure = 25mm Hg

**Net inward
pressure** = 10mm Hg

b) Glomerular capillaries

**Afferent arteriole
end**

Outward pressure:

Capillary hydrostatic
pressure = 45mm Hg

Inward pressure:

Protein oncotic
pressure = 25mm Hg

Bowman's capsule
hydrostatic
pressure = 10mm Hg

**Net outward
pressure** = 10mm Hg

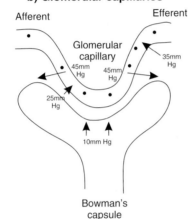

**Efferent arteriole
end**

Outward pressure:

Capillary hydrostatic
pressure = 45mm Hg

Inward pressure:

Protein oncotic
pressure = 35mm Hg

Bowman's capsule
hydrostatic
pressure = 10mm Hg

**Net inward
pressure** = 0mm Hg

Figure 2.8
Comparison of Starling's
forces between muscle
capillaries and glomerular
capillaries.
(a) Starling's forces
operating in muscle
capillaries, resulting in the
formation and reabsorption
of tissue fluid.
(b) Starling's forces
operating in glomerular
capillaries, resulting in the
formation of glomerular
filtrate.

Amount and composition of glomerular filtrate

The amount of glomerular filtrate formed per minute is referred to as the glomerular filtration rate (GFR), and in the average healthy person is approximately 125 mL min^{-1}. This volume is the sum amount from all 2 million nephrons in the kidneys and thus the amount from each nephron is relatively small. A quick calculation shows that at a GFR of 125 mL min^{-1}, the total amount of filtrate formed per day is 180 L – approximately 60 times the circulating plasma volume. Obviously, the majority of this must be reabsorbed to prevent severe dehydration.

The 'average' GFR quoted is generally only average for a young adult. Children have a lower GFR than this because their nephrons are still increasing in size (all nephrons are present at birth). After the age of about 30 years, the number of functioning nephrons starts to decrease because of the ageing process, thus the GFR decreases proportionately. However, this only becomes significant to health when the GFR falls to around 5 mL min^{-1} – a situation that only occurs in a diseased kidney. The GFR can be calculated clinically by measuring the creatinine clearance rate. This requires a 24-h urine sample and blood sample from the patient. The principles of this test are described in Chapter 6.

The composition of the initial glomerular filtrate is that of a plasma ultrafiltration; that is, without proteins. The main determinant of what can pass through the glomerular basement membrane is molecular size, although the molecular shape and charge are also important. The passage of strongly negatively charged molecules, such as albumin, tends to be retarded because of the presence of fixed negative charges in the basement membrane, which repel their movement. Albumin, a small protein, has a molecular weight of 69 kDa, a weight just below the cut-off point for filtration. It can therefore cross the filter, but does so only in minute quantities, since it is also hindered by its negative charge. It is because of this free permeability of small molecules that the composition of the initial glomerular filtrate is the same as that of the plasma for small molecules, and will include the major ions sodium, potassium, chloride, bicarbonate, calcium and phosphate; glucose, amino acids and the toxic waste products of urea and creatinine. Any albumin filtered is reabsorbed through the proximal tubule into the renal lymph system and returned to the blood stream.

SELECTIVE REABSORPTION

Reabsorption is a process that involves the movement of water and dissolved substances from the tubular fluid back into the bloodstream. The term 'selective' infers a regulatory function to this process, as indeed not all of the filtered substances are returned to the blood. Any substances not reabsorbed will pass with the urine into the bladder to be excreted from the body. The main sites for reabsorption in the nephron are the proximal and distal convoluted tubules.

Mechanisms of reabsorption

Broadly speaking, there are three mechanisms in the nephron for the reabsorption of water and solutes: osmosis, diffusion and active transport. Osmosis is the movement of water from an area of low concentration to a more concentrated solution across a membrane, which allows water molecules through but is selectively permeable to solute molecules (a semipermeable membrane).

Diffusion occurs where a concentrated solution meets one that is less concentrated. The solute will equilibrate throughout the solvent. This may occur across a membrane so long as the membrane is permeable to the solute. Diffusion may also occur through specialised 'protein carriers' in the membrane. This is sometimes known as 'facilitated diffusion'. In these cases, the number of protein carriers in the membrane is limited, meaning that movement of the solute will be limited. This is true for tubular reabsorption of glucose (which is also linked to sodium transport). Once all the carriers are active, reabsorption of glucose has reached its maximum. If the filtered load of glucose is excessive, not all can be reabsorbed and glucose will appear in the urine, as happens in untreated diabetes mellitus.

Active transport is so named because it is an energy-requiring process. The energy source is adenosine triphosphate (ATP). Active transport can move solutes against a concentration gradient. Cells that carry out a lot of active transport will have many mitochondria present (the 'power-generating' organelles of cells).

In the proximal tubule cells, where most reabsorption is by active transport, the cells are packed with mitochondria. Proximal tubule cells also have a large brush border on their luminal surface (the surface facing into the tubule) to increase their surface area for reabsorption. In contrast, cells lining the descending loop of Henle are comparatively thin, have no brush border and have relatively few mitochondria. This suggests that these cells are not very metabolically active and are adapted for reabsorption by passive diffusion. The epithelial cells of the distal tubule are similar to those of the proximal tubule but with a less well-defined brush border and fewer mitochondria. This suggests that these cells are capable of active transport of substances but in much lesser quantities than in the proximal tubule. This again illustrates how each segment of the nephron is anatomically adapted to carry out its unique functions. The different cell types lining the tubules are illustrated in Figure 2.9.

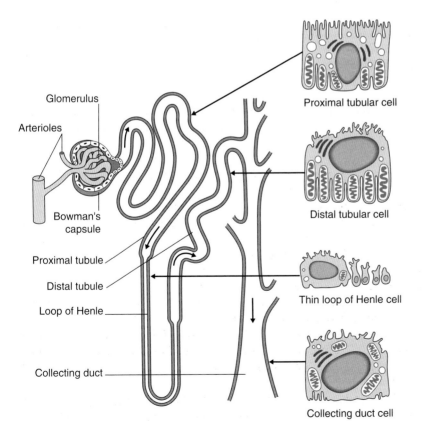

Glomerulus

Arterioles

Proximal tubular cell

Bowman's capsule

Distal tubular cell

Proximal tubule

Distal tubule

Thin loop of Henle cell

Loop of Henle

Collecting duct

Collecting duct cell

Figure 2.9
Essential features of the structure of a nephron. (After Hinchliff SM, Montague SE. Physiology for nursing practice. London: Baillière Tindall, 1988, with permission of Baillière Tindall.)

Reabsorption in the proximal convoluted tubule – the site of bulk–phase reabsorption

Approximately 65% of all reabsorption occurs in the proximal tubule (hence the term 'bulk phase') and is obligatory rather than regulatory. Most substances here are reabsorbed by active transport mechanisms, including sodium, chloride, potassium, glucose, amino acids, phosphate and bicarbonate. Urea is absorbed by passive diffusion and water is reabsorbed by osmosis. Some substances are reabsorbed almost entirely in the proximal tubule, such as glucose and amino acids, which do not appear in the urine, whereas others have only between 60 and 70% reabsorption, such as sodium, water and potassium. Approximately 50% of urea is reabsorbed here but creatinine is not reabsorbed at all. However, for all substances that are reabsorbed, the proximal tubule is the site where the bulk of this reabsorption occurs.

Reabsorption in the distal convoluted tubule – the site of fine-tuning reabsorption

This is the site where more specific regulation of substances occurs according to the needs of the body. In order for the distal tubule to be aware of precisely what the body's reabsorptive needs are, a method of communication between the cells of the distal tubule and the rest of the body is required. This communication system is via a range of hormones that form part of a negative-feedback system for the homeostatic control of ions and water. For example, sodium and water reabsorption are under the control of aldosterone (secreted by the adrenal cortex) and ADH secreted by the posterior pituitary gland. Potassium reabsorption is also controlled by aldosterone, whereas calcium and phosphate are controlled by parathyroid hormone (PTH). The precise mechanisms for controlling the electrolytes outlined above will be dealt with in later sections in this chapter.

SECRETION

The process of secretion occurs in both the proximal and distal tubules, and involves the movement of substances from blood flowing through the peritubular capillaries, through the tubule wall cells, into the tubular fluid. In this respect, secretion is the opposite process to reabsorption. Substances that are secreted into the tubules are excreted in the urine. Though creatinine is freely filtered at the glomerulus, total creatinine excretion is increased by 20% by the process of secretion. Ions that are transported into the tubules by secretion are hydrogen, which is secreted in both the proximal and distal tubules, and is important in acid–base control, and potassium, which is secreted in the distal tubule in exchange for sodium reabsorption. The hormone involved is aldosterone.

EXCRETION OF DRUGS AND DRUG METABOLITES

Many drugs and their metabolites are finally excreted from the body through the kidneys by the processes of glomerular filtration and secretion. Like other filtered substances, the rate of filtration of drugs will depend on their molecular size and charge: smaller molecules are filtered more rapidly than larger ones. Drugs that bind to plasma proteins are filtered very slowly because of the size of the complex. Some drugs are cleared from the blood purely by glomerular filtration and thus the rate of clearance cannot exceed the GFR of 125 mL min⁻¹, whereas other drugs are excreted by a combination of filtration and secretion, such as benzylpenicillin, which achieves a total clearance rate of 480 mL min⁻¹ (Laurence & Bennett 1987).

CONCENTRATION AND DILUTION OF URINE

The components of the nephron that are involved in the concentration and dilution of the urine are the loop of Henle and the collecting ducts. The concentration of urine is measured in units of osmolality (mosmol kg water⁻¹). The most dilute urine that humans can produce is approximately 60 mosmol kg water⁻¹, but this situation occurs in the pathological condition of diabetes insipidus in which the pituitary gland fails to produce ADH. The most concentrated urine that can be produced is approximately 1400 mosmol kg water⁻¹, which is greater than four times more concentrated than plasma (plasma osmolality = 285 mosmol kg water⁻¹) and requires maximum ADH secretion. The average range of urine osmolality in people with normal kidneys is between 300 and 500 mosmol kg water⁻¹.

COUNTERCURRENT MECHANISM OF URINARY CONCENTRATION

The countercurrent mechanism is a complex physiological process that will not be discussed in great detail.

In order to concentrate the urine the following factors are required:

- the creation and maintenance of a local environment in the kidney that allows large quantities of water to be reabsorbed by osmosis from the collecting duct back into the blood
- a mechanism that can influence the opening and closing of water channels in the collecting ducts in order to control the exact amount of water reabsorbed.

CREATION OF THE LOCAL ENVIRONMENT (FIG. 2.10)

This local environment consists of an increasing hyperosmotic medullary interstitium as one moves towards the tip of the loops of Henle. In other words, the tissue spaces between the loops of Henle in the medulla of the kidney must be made hyperosmotic compared to the fluid in the collecting duct. As the collecting ducts pass through the medulla on their way to the renal pelvis, water can be pulled out by osmosis, resulting in less water entering the urine.

This hyperosmotic environment is created by the active and passive transport of ions (mainly sodium and chloride) out of the tubular fluid as it passes through the loop of Henle into the medullary interstitium. The build-up of ions here gradually increases and becomes more concentrated

Figure 2.10 Countercurrent mechanism. Thick horizontal arrows, active transport; PCT, proximal convoluted tubule; DCT, distal convoluted tubule; thin horizontal arrows, passive transport. (From Hubbard JL, Mechan DJ. Physiology for health care students. Edinburgh: Churchill Livingstone, 1987, with permission.)

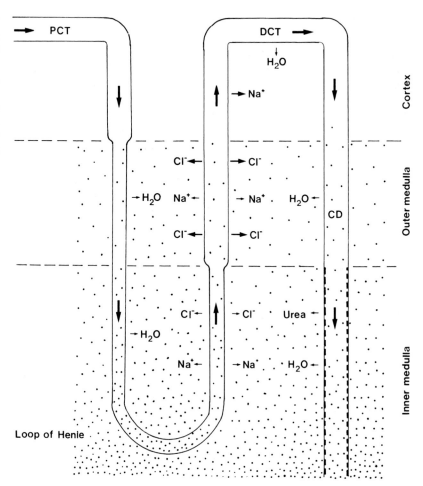

as the loop of Henle descends into the medulla. The tip of the medulla can reach osmolalities of up to 1400 mosmol kg water^{-1}. Water does not follow the transport of ions into the medullary interstitium by osmosis because the thick ascending limb of the loop of Henle is impermeable to water. Urea also makes an important contribution to the creation of the hyperosmotic environment. Urea can diffuse passively through the walls of the tubules at most points along the nephron, but urea diffusion is greatly enhanced across the collecting tubule wall in the presence of even small amounts of ADH. Thus large amounts of urea become concentrated in the medullary interstitium.

MAINTENANCE OF THE LOCAL ENVIRONMENT: THE COUNTERCURRENT MECHANISM

It could be thought that as fast as the hyperosmotic environment is created it will be washed out by processes of diffusion and reabsorbed back into blood. However, the environment is maintained because of the unique arrangement of the looped vasa recta capillaries around the loops of Henle (Figs. 2.7 and 2.11). The vasa recta are only supplied with 1–2% of the blood entering the kidneys, so there is very little blood flow for ions to be reabsorbed back into. In addition, the vasa recta lie with their ascending and descending limbs in very close proximity. This close proximity allows for rapid exchange of water and solutes between the two limbs. So, as blood flows down the descending limb of the vasa recta, the high concentration of ions in the medullary interstitium enables ions to diffuse into the vasa recta (markedly increasing their concentration), and water to move out by osmosis, but as the blood moves into the ascending limb of the vasa recta, the high concentration of ions in the blood then enables ions to diffuse back out into the medullary interstitium (and water back into the blood), maintaining the hyperosmotic environment.

THE REGULATION OF BODY FLUID VOLUME AND OSMOLALITY

Sodium is the main extracellular cation (positively charged ion) and is intimately related to extracellular volume. An increase in body sodium content could lead to an increase in extracellular fluid volume, leading to hypertension and oedema; and a decrease in body sodium content could lead to a decrease in extracellular fluid volume leading to hypotension and dehydration. Thus, it is vitally important that body sodium content is kept at a constant level, if body fluid volume is to remain constant. Fortunately, the healthy kidney conserves sodium very efficiently in shortage, and can excrete $10-150 \, \text{mmol day}^{-1}$ when sodium is in excess.

Sodium levels, and hence fluid volume, are regulated by three hormones: ADH, aldosterone and atrial natriuretic peptide.

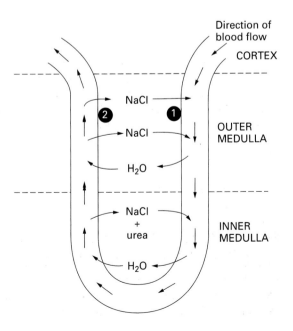

Figure 2.11
Maintenance of the hyperosmotic environment. (1) As blood flows down the descending limb of the vasa recta, the high concentration of sodium chloride and urea in the medullary interstitium causes passive diffusion of these ions into the blood, while water diffuses out of the blood by osmosis. (2) As blood enters the ascending limb, the high concentration of sodium chloride and urea that has accumulated in the tip of the vasa recta then diffuses back out into the interstitium, while water is osmotically attracted back into the blood, thus maintaining the hyperosmotic environment in the medullary interstitium. The net result of this process is that solutes circulate around in the vasa recta but are not washed out into the main circulation.

Antidiuretic hormone

Antidiuretic hormone is secreted from the posterior pituitary gland in response to a rise in plasma osmolality. Osmoreceptors in the hypothalamus detect small changes in the plasma osmolality and send signals to the posterior pituitary to secrete more or less ADH. Since sodium, along with its associated anion (negatively charged ion) chloride (Cl^-), contributes approximately 95% of the extracellular fluid osmolality, sodium concentration of extracellular fluid is obviously important in determining ADH secretion.

Antidiuretic hormone receptors are found in the collecting ducts of kidney tubules and ADH acts to open water channels found here. Remember that the collecting ducts pass through the inner medulla of the kidney – a region of high osmolality. If water channels in the walls of the collecting ducts open, water will move out of the collecting duct into the medullary interstitium and finally into the circulation. The fall in plasma osmolality then leads to a slowing down of ADH secretion by negative feedback (Fig. 2.12).

Aldosterone

Aldosterone is a steroid hormone secreted from the adrenal cortex. It has its effect on the distal tubule of the nephron: the more aldosterone is secreted, the more sodium is reabsorbed. Aldosterone, however, is not the sole determinant of body sodium balance, although in extreme cases of oversecretion of aldosterone, such as in Cushing's disease, hypertension may result from over-retention of sodium and water.

The secretion of aldosterone, unlike ADH, is not directly triggered by extracellular osmolality but is regulated by a peptide, angiotensin II. The function of this peptide is described in the section on the renin–angiotensin system, below.

Figure 2.12
Negative-feedback loop for antidiuretic hormone (ADH) release and control of plasma osmolality.

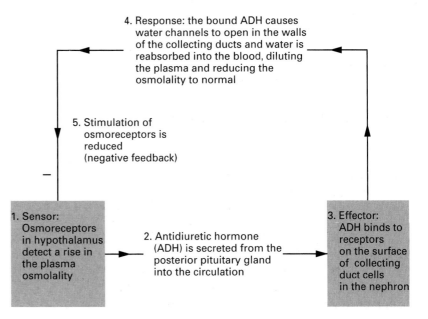

4. Response: the bound ADH causes water channels to open in the walls of the collecting ducts and water is reabsorbed into the blood, diluting the plasma and reducing the osmolality to normal

5. Stimulation of osmoreceptors is reduced (negative feedback)

1. Sensor: Osmoreceptors in hypothalamus detect a rise in the plasma osmolality

2. Antidiuretic hormone (ADH) is secreted from the posterior pituitary gland into the circulation

3. Effector: ADH binds to receptors on the surface of collecting duct cells in the nephron

This peptide is released from cardiac atrial cells in response to an increased atrial stretch. It has five known major effects:

Atrial natriuretic peptide

- inhibition of aldosterone secretion by the adrenal cortex
- reduction of renin release by the kidney
- reduction of ADH release from the posterior pituitary
- vasodilation
- natriuresis and diuresis.

All of these effects result in the excretion of sodium and water through the kidney, reducing the extracellular fluid volume back to normal. Other factors that may be important in sodium regulation are renal prostaglandins, kinins and the renal nerves. Failure to regulate the extracellular fluid volume occurs commonly in people with renal disease and leads to hypertension.

THE RENIN–ANGIOTENSIN SYSTEM

The distal convoluted tubule forms a unique contact with the glomerulus, passing in the angle between the afferent and efferent arterioles. At this point, specialised cells called the macula densa in the wall of the distal tubule make contact with cells in the endothelium of the arterioles, which release a hormone called renin (Fig. 2.13). The macula densa and the renin-releasing cells are collectively called the juxtaglomerular apparatus or complex.

The juxtaglomerular apparatus is responsible for maintaining a constant blood flow through the glomerulus and thus a constant GFR despite fluctuations in arterial pressure. This is achieved through a tubule feedback mechanism in which a fall in GFR results in a fall in the chloride ion concentration in the distal tubule. This stimulates the macula densa cells, which send 'signals' to the renin-secreting cells to release renin. Renin acts via the renin–angiotensin system (Fig. 2.14) to produce both local vasoconstriction of the efferent arteriole (increasing GFR) and peripheral vasoconstriction to increase arterial blood pressure. In addition, salt and water retention increase due to the effects of aldosterone.

ALDOSTERONE AND THE CONTROL OF BODY POTASSIUM CONTENT

Potassium is the main intracellular cation. Only about 2% of the total body potassium content is extracellular. Potassium ions are freely filtered at the glomerulus: 65% of reabsorption takes place in the proximal tubule. However, the renal handling of potassium ions is not as efficient as that of sodium, nor is potassium conserved so well when there is a shortage. The secretion of potassium is also linked to that of sodium and hydrogen ions. Unlike sodium regulation, where aldosterone is just one factor in the regulation of sodium content, aldosterone is the only hormone involved in the control of potassium content and thus has a very important regulatory role. Small increases in extracellular potassium

Figure 2.13
The juxtaglomerular apparatus showing the macula densa. (From Hinchliff SM, Montague SE, Watson R. Physiology for nursing practice. London: Baillière Tindall, 1988, with permission of Baillière Tindall.)

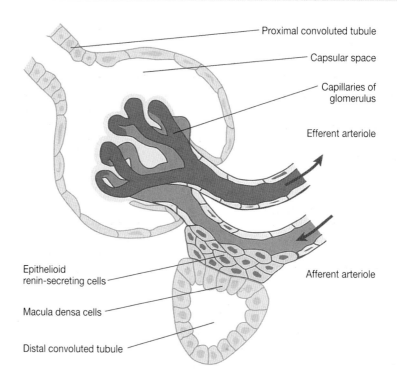

Figure 2.14
The renin–angiotensin system. GFR, glomerular filtration rate. (From Hinchliff SM, Montague SE, Watson R. Physiology for nursing practice. London: Baillière Tindall, 1988, with permission of Baillière Tindall.)

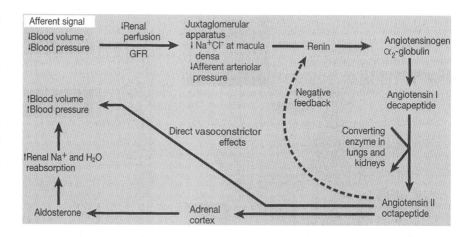

concentration directly stimulate aldosterone secretion from the adrenal cortex. The effect of aldosterone in the distal tubule of the nephron is to increase the secretion of potassium into the urine. When aldosterone levels fall, the reverse occurs and less potassium is secreted. The release of aldosterone stimulated by rises in extracellular potassium concentration is strongly controlled by a negative-feedback system. Once the potassium concentration returns to normal the stimulus to secrete aldosterone is quickly switched off.

The hormone aldosterone increases sodium reabsorption in exchange for potassium or hydrogen ions. If excess potassium ions need to be secreted, then fewer hydrogen ions can be secreted and vice versa. Clinically, this phenomenon results in an association between metabolic acidosis and hyperkalaemia (or conversely, metabolic alkalosis and hypokalaemia), since in patients with acidosis the distal tubules will increase the rate of hydrogen ion secretion (to prevent a fall in plasma pH) by reducing the rate of potassium ion secretion, which results in the retention of potassium ions in the blood, leading to hyperkalaemia.

HYPOKALAEMIA AND HYPERKALAEMIA

Potassium is important in maintaining the membrane potential of nerve and muscle cells and hence affects their excitability. Disturbances in potassium balance show their effects in abnormal nerve and muscle function, and may be life threatening.

Changes in muscle tone and in the electrocardiogram (ECG) may indicate an altered potassium balance. The diet almost invariably contains adequate potassium, so hypokalaemia generally occurs owing to excessive losses. Persistent vomiting, diarrhoea or the use of certain prescribed diuretics are the most likely causes of low blood potassium. Dialysis using an inappropriate concentration of potassium may also result in hypokalaemia. Treatment of hypokalaemia by the administration of a potassium salt must be undertaken with care since this may result in hyperkalaemia. The uptake of potassium into cells is also dependent on the acid–base balance in the patient. Acidosis (low blood pH) causes the release of potassium from cells so acid–base disturbances must first be corrected.

Hyperkalaemia can occur as a result of decreased potassium excretion in the renal patient. Insulin promotes uptake of potassium into cells, so insulin deficiency may lead to hyperkalaemia, as can excessive tissue breakdown following trauma.

REGULATION OF CALCIUM, PHOSPHATE AND MAGNESIUM

Calcium and phosphate are the main mineral constituents of bone, and thus the majority of calcium and phosphate in the body is found in the skeleton. However, small amounts of both these ions are found in extracellular fluid. Calcium exists in the plasma in two forms: approximately 50% exists in the free ionised form ($1.25\,mmol\,L^{-1}$), and the other 50% in a bound form, mainly bound to protein, particularly albumin ($1.25\,mmol\,L^{-1}$). Usually when serum calcium levels are measured, the total calcium concentration is measured ($2.5\,mmol\,L^{-1}$). This total calcium is then 'corrected' depending on the blood albumin level, since it is the ionised form of the calcium that is important in the extracellular fluid in controlling nerve and muscle conduction. Any condition which leads to a fall in the ionised calcium concentration (even if total calcium remains normal) will lead to the classic symptoms of hypocalcaemia – tetany, muscle cramps and even convulsions. In situations of hypercalcaemia, the main effects seen are pruritus, extraskeletal calcification, renal calculi, peptic ulceration and changes in mental function, such as memory loss and depression.

Inorganic phosphate (i.e. those ions carrying a charge) exists in several forms –'acid' phosphate ($H_2PO_4^-$) and 'alkaline' phosphate HPO_4^-. The normal plasma range of total inorganic phosphate is $0.87–1.45\,mmol\,L^{-1}$. Phosphate is important in buffer systems to maintain the plasma pH and exists in equilibrium with calcium.

Both calcium and phosphate are freely filtered at the glomerulus. When the plasma phosphate level is below $1\,mmol\,L^{-1}$, all the filtered phosphate is reabsorbed in the early proximal tubule. However, once the plasma phosphate level rises above $1\,mmol\,L^{-1}$, the amount of phosphate excreted in the urine rises in proportion to the plasma concentration. Further excretion of phosphate in the distal tubule (by secretion) can occur in response to the rise in the circulating level of PTH. Calcium reabsorption is very similar to that of sodium, in that approximately 65% occurs in the proximal tubule, and a further 20–25% in the ascending limb of the loop of Henle, leaving around 10–12% of filtered calcium being delivered to the distal tubule. How much more calcium is reabsorbed in the distal tubule depends on the levels of circulating PTH.

Magnesium is an important intracellular cation involved in energy storage and production. In all, 55% of total body magnesium is found within bones, so it is not surprising that magnesium balance is linked to that of calcium.

Parathyroid hormone increases tubular reabsorption of magnesium. Under normal circumstances, gastrointestinal absorption and urinary excretion of magnesium are equal. Gastrointestinal disorders may, therefore, decrease magnesium uptake but this is matched by a decrease in renal excretion. Most diuretics, and alcohol, increase renal magnesium excretion.

THE RENAL HANDLING OF CALCIUM AND PHOSPHATE – THE ROLES OF PARATHYROID HORMONE, VITAMIN D AND CALCITONIN

The mechanisms by which plasma calcium and phosphate are regulated are closely interrelated. The two major regulators are PTH and vitamin D. Calcium and phosphate can enter the plasma from the gut and from the bone. Indeed, almost all of the approximately 1 kg of calcium in a 70-kg person is found in the bone. Of this, a few grams exchange daily with the plasma calcium pool. Calcium and phosphate can leave the plasma by being redeposited in bone, or by renal excretion.

Parathyroid hormone is secreted by the parathyroid glands situated next to the thyroid. Secretion is stimulated by a decrease in plasma calcium concentration and reduced when plasma calcium levels rise. Its effect is to raise plasma calcium concentration, mainly by increasing bone breakdown (resorption), releasing calcium ions. PTH also acts in the kidney, stimulating one step in the conversion of vitamin D to its active metabolite, calcitriol or 1,25-dihydroxycholecalciferol.

Vitamin D is a steroid that enters the body either through dietary intake or by the effect of sunlight on the skin. However, this is an inactive form of the vitamin called cholecalciferol. To become activated, it needs to undergo two metabolic conversions, one in the liver and one in the kidney. These conversions result in the formation of calcitriol. This active form has its effect in the gut, kidney and (in the presence of PTH) on bone, raising plasma calcium levels. The actions of vitamin D are summarised in Figure 2.15.

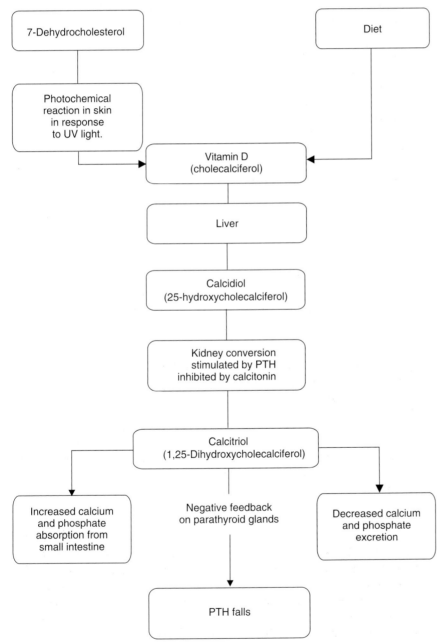

Figure 2.15
The actions of vitamin D. UV, ultraviolet; PTH, parathyroid hormone. (From Lote CJ. Principles of renal physiology, 3rd edn. London: Croom and Helm, 1994, with kind permission from Kluwer Academic Publishers.)

The effects of both vitamin D and PTH are to increase the plasma calcium concentration. However, these effects are carefully controlled by a negative-feedback system, which prevents the calcium level rising too high. The negative-feedback system is outlined in Figure 2.16. Only if calcium levels suddenly rise (as after a high-calcium meal) is calcitonin stimulated to be released from the C cells of the thyroid gland, causing calcium to be redeposited in the bone. This is a rapid and relatively short-acting effect. The control of calcium and phosphate levels is essential for the maintenance of normal bone. In renal disease, the production of calcitriol is reduced, thus removing the negative-feedback effect on PTH. The result is a rise in PTH leading to loss of calcium from bone and the complications of renal bone disease. Renal bone disease is discussed in Chapter 5.

Calcium ions play an important role in the regulation of nerve and muscle function, and in blood clotting. Hypocalcaemia is characterised by increased excitability of muscles leading to tetany, when skeletal muscles go into spasm. Hypercalcaemia is a common finding in an individual with renal failure.

ACID–BASE CONTROL

Acid–base balance is about maintaining the constancy of the pH of the body's fluids. The pH scale is a logarithmic scale (range 1–14) that measures the concentration of free hydrogen ions in a fluid. In fact, the scale is reciprocal, which means that, as the pH becomes lower, the hydrogen ion concentration gets increasingly greater. Thus at acidic pH levels (below 7),

Figure 2.16
Negative-feedback loop for parathyroid hormone release and calcium and phosphate control.

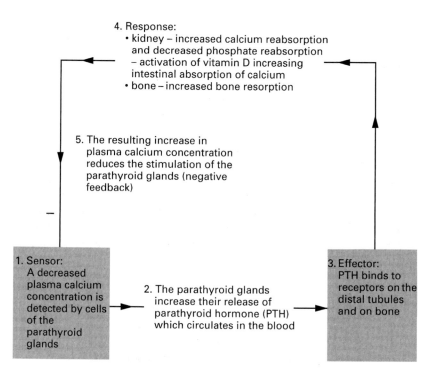

4. Response:
   • kidney – increased calcium reabsorption and decreased phosphate reabsorption – activation of vitamin D increasing intestinal absorption of calcium
   • bone – increased bone resorption

5. The resulting increase in plasma calcium concentration reduces the stimulation of the parathyroid glands (negative feedback)

1. Sensor:
   A decreased plasma calcium concentration is detected by cells of the parathyroid glands

2. The parathyroid glands increase their release of parathyroid hormone (PTH) which circulates in the blood

3. Effector:
   PTH binds to receptors on the distal tubules and on bone

the hydrogen ion concentration of the fluid is very high relative to that at basic pH levels (above 7). In fact, for each point on the scale there is a tenfold difference in the hydrogen ion concentration. When we consider that the normal pH range of our bodily fluids is between 7.35 and 7.45, this appears very narrow but actually represents over a 20% difference in the hydrogen ion concentration! It is doubtful we would tolerate a 20% change in our sodium ion concentration with such ease.

So what are acids and bases? Simply put, acids are molecules that in the right environmental conditions will give up or donate a hydrogen ion to the solution it is in, and a base is a molecule that mops up or accepts free hydrogen ions from the solution. Thus, in order to maintain a constant hydrogen ion concentration (and hence constant pH), both acids and bases need to be present in the solution to donate or accept free hydrogen ions as required. Acids and bases working together in this way to minimise changes in pH are called buffers.

Though there are several buffering systems in the body, including haemoglobin, plasma proteins, organic and inorganic phosphates, the most important one physiologically is the bicarbonate buffering system and it is this one that will be described.

BICARBONATE BUFFERING SYSTEM

To understand the bicarbonate buffering system, the following reaction sequence needs to be understood:

$$CO_2 + H_2O \leftrightarrow H_2CO_3 \leftrightarrow H^+ + HCO_3^-$$

This equation explains how the components of the buffering system are generated in the plasma. Carbon dioxide is generated by cells as an end-product of metabolism and diffuses into the plasma. The CO_2 dissolves in water to form carbonic acid (H_2CO_3), which is the acid component of the buffering system. The carbonic acid, in turn, is in equilibrium with the hydrogen (H^+) and bicarbonate ions (HCO_3^-). This forms the basic component of the buffering system. This reaction sequence can run in either direction, thus if there is a build-up of CO_2 in the plasma, then more carbonic acid will be formed and the reaction will be driven to the right in order that more bicarbonate ions can be formed to minimise changes in the pH. However, if an excess of hydrogen ions builds up (from metabolic processes), then the reaction will be driven to the left, resulting in CO_2 and water forming. The excess CO_2 can then be blown off in the lungs. Since this reaction sequence constantly runs backwards and forwards to maintain a constant pH, then it follows that pH must be dependent on the relative proportions of CO_2 to bicarbonate ions. This can be shown in the following equation:

$$pH \propto HCO_3^-/PCO_2$$

Both components of this equation can be controlled by the body. The bicarbonate ion concentration is carefully controlled by the kidneys, whereas the PCO_2 is controlled by the lungs. Thus the lungs and the kidneys are the two main organs that together control the acid–base balance of the body.

CONTROL OF BICARBONATE ION CONCENTRATION BY THE KIDNEY

Bicarbonate ions are freely filtered in the glomerulus. When the plasma bicarbonate concentration is normal ($25\,mmol\,L^{-1}$), then all of the filtered bicarbonate is reabsorbed: 90% reabsorption occurs in the proximal tubule and 10% in the distal tubule. However, if plasma bicarbonate concentration is higher than normal, then this excess bicarbonate is lost in the urine.

The reabsorption of bicarbonate ions in the nephron is not a straightforward transport of ions from the tubular fluid into the plasma, as with other ions, but involves various chemical reactions inside the tubular wall cells. The filtered bicarbonate in the tubule undergoes the whole reaction sequence identified above for the bicarbonate buffering system so that CO_2 and water are formed. This is catalysed by the enzyme carbonic anhydrase, which is found in the brush border of the proximal tubular cells. The resulting CO_2 then diffuses into the tubular cell, where it undergoes the same reaction sequence, reforming the bicarbonate ion plus a hydrogen ion. The hydrogen ion is secreted into the tubule to be excreted and the bicarbonate ion diffuses into the plasma. This process is sometimes referred to as bicarbonate 'trapping' (Fig. 2.17).

This process preserves bicarbonate ions in the blood, but to excrete excess hydrogen ions, substances must take up these ions in the kidney tubule to prevent their reabsorption into the blood. This is the role of the phosphate ions (HPO_4^{2-}) and the ammonia ions (NH_3), both of which take up one hydrogen ion to form $H_2PO_4^-$ and NH_4^+, respectively. The process also generates HCO_3^- ions, which can be reabsorbed. NH_4^+ ions cannot

Figure 2.17
Bicarbonate reabsorption in the kidney tubules.

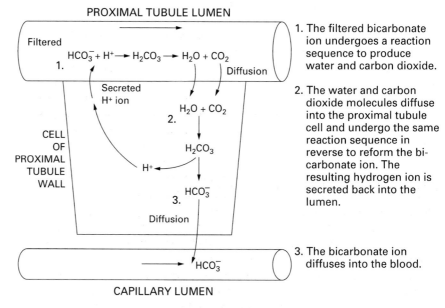

PROXIMAL TUBULE LUMEN

Filtered
$$HCO_3^- + H^+ \longrightarrow H_2CO_3 \longrightarrow H_2O + CO_2$$
1.   Diffusion

Secreted H$^+$ ion
$$H_2O + CO_2$$
2.
$$H_2CO_3$$
$$H^+$$
CELL OF PROXIMAL TUBULE WALL
$$HCO_3^-$$
3.
Diffusion

$$HCO_3^-$$

CAPILLARY LUMEN

1. The filtered bicarbonate ion undergoes a reaction sequence to produce water and carbon dioxide.

2. The water and carbon dioxide molecules diffuse into the proximal tubule cell and undergo the same reaction sequence in reverse to reform the bicarbonate ion. The resulting hydrogen ion is secreted back into the lumen.

3. The bicarbonate ion diffuses into the blood.

readily diffuse back across cell membranes, so the H^+ ions are effectively trapped in the tubule lumen.

CORRECTING ACID–BASE FLUCTUATIONS IN THE HEALTHY INDIVIDUAL

Fall in plasma pH

This is a condition called acidaemia or, more commonly, acidosis. This problem arises when there are excess hydrogen ions in the body fluids. In the absence of respiratory or renal disease, the initial response to control pH is for the excess hydrogen ions to drive the bicarbonate reaction sequence to the left to produce CO_2 and water. The lungs can then deal with this excess CO_2 by increasing the respiratory rate to 'blow off' the CO_2. This process gives a quick short-term compensation to the problem but not long-term correction. The rise in hydrogen ion concentration is then corrected by the kidneys secreting the excess hydrogen into the urine and in the process generating further bicarbonate for reabsorption into the plasma.

Rise in plasma pH

This condition is called alkalaemia or alkalosis, and arises when there is a reduction in the hydrogen ion concentration of the body fluids. The kidney plays the main role in correcting this problem by reducing the amount of hydrogen ion secretion. However, because hydrogen ion secretion and bicarbonate reabsorption are coupled together, this also results in a reduction in the plasma bicarbonate level. The plasma bicarbonate concentration is then corrected by a reduction in ventilation rate by the lungs, which leads to a build-up of CO_2, which drives the reaction sequence to the right to generate more bicarbonate ions.

Although the above compensatory and correction processes buffer the small fluctuations that occur in the acid–base balance in the healthy individual, larger fluctuations in acid–base balance tend to occur when there is either respiratory or metabolic disease. This is because the normal correction mechanisms are blocked. For example, in disorders of ventilation, a respiratory acidosis or, rarely, alkalosis may develop, whereas in disorders of metabolism (including renal disease) a metabolic acidosis or alkalosis may develop. Descriptions of these disorders are beyond this chapter, but the reader is referred to Box 2.3 for a brief outline of the causes and symptoms of the metabolic acidosis of renal failure.

ERYTHROPOIETIN PRODUCTION BY THE KIDNEY

The final important role that the kidney has is the production of the hormone erythropoietin. Erythropoietin is a glycoprotein that promotes the proliferation and differentiation of erythrocyte precursors in the bone marrow. Thus, erythropoietin is necessary for the maintenance of a normal red cell count and prevention of anaemia. The erythropoietin-producing cells of the kidney have been identified as being peritubular cells, most likely endothelial cells of the cortex and outer

> **Box 2.3**   Metabolic acidosis
>
> **Causes of acidosis in renal failure**
> - Reduced renal excretion of acids
> - Reduced renal reabsorption of bicarbonate
>
> **Markers and symptoms**
> - Fall in plasma pH (as hydrogen ion concentration rises)
> - Fall in plasma bicarbonate concentration
> - Increased anion gap (difference between the plasma concentration of cations Na^+ and K^+, and anions Cl^- and HCO_3^-)
> - Possible hyperkalaemia, which may lead to fatal cardiac arrhythmias
> - Depressed central nervous system causing coma
> - Respiratory compensation, hyperventilation (Kussmaul's breathing)
> - Possible development of renal bone disease

medulla (Lacombe et al 1991). Erythropoietin production is stimulated by hypoxia and inhibited when the hypoxia is corrected, thus its production is controlled by the negative-feedback principle. The kidney is not the only site of erythropoietin production. Approximately 20% of erythropoietin is produced at extrarenal sites, thought mainly to be the liver. However, in the presence of severe renal disease, this extrarenal production of erythropoietin is insufficient to maintain the red cell count at normal levels, achieving only one-third to one-half the normal level. Anaemia is therefore a problem in most patients with chronic and established renal failure, although this has now been overcome with the use of recombinant erythropoietin. See Ch. 5 for nursing management of anaemia in renal disease.

CONDITIONS CAUSING CHRONIC AND ESTABLISHED RENAL FAILURE

In this part of the chapter the reader is introduced to some of the common causes of chronic and established renal failure and the altered physiology that results from, or may lead to, renal dysfunction. It is not intended as a complete guide to chronic kidney disease, but as a starting point for understanding how important the kidneys are and how their function interacts with other body systems.

Chronic kidney disease is a result of a number of pathological processes causing irreversible damage to kidney tissue. There is a mass destruction of nephrons, so that the kidneys are unable to maintain fluid and electrolyte balance and excrete waste products from the body.

Chronic kidney disease is caused by a slow progressive kidney disease over a course of many years (perhaps 10–20). There may be an insidious onset of renal failure with the minimum of symptoms developing in the patient on the approach to established renal failure. Unlike acute renal failure, where a full recovery of renal function can occur, in chronic kidney disease the kidneys are permanently damaged and the disease is usually progressive. Chronic kidney disease is defined by the Kidney Disease Quality Outcome Initiative (K/DOQI) as kidney damage or glomerular filtration rate of $< 60\,\mathrm{mL\,min^{-1}\,1.73\,m^{-2}}$ for 3 months or more, irrespective of cause (Levey et al 2005).

THE RELATIONSHIP BETWEEN BLOOD PRESSURE AND RENAL FUNCTION

Despite normal fluctuations in the systemic blood pressure, the kidneys are to some extent able to autoregulate the pressure of blood entering the glomerular capillaries. This ensures that the glomerular hydrostatic pressure remains constant and GFR is maintained. In addition, the kidneys are the source of the hormone renin, which has a direct effect on blood pressure via the renin–angiotensin pathway (see Fig. 2.14). If the blood pressure entering the glomerulus drops, then more renin is released, resulting in a rise in systemic blood pressure.

If the filtering mechanism of the kidney is impaired by a drop in hydrostatic pressure within the glomeruli or by damage to glomerular tissue, the ability of the kidney to excrete nitrogenous waste products and to regulate water and electrolytes may be impaired. This will ultimately result in symptoms associated with renal failure, including fluid retention, which leads to hypertension.

Conversely, if blood pressure is persistently raised (hypertension), there is a risk of damage to blood vessels throughout the body, but particularly those in the brain (leading to stroke), coronary vessels and renal vessels. The renal artery, or smaller renal arteries, may become narrowed by arteriosclerosis (e.g. renal artery stenosis or renovascular disease). This will lead to impaired renal blood flow, which will stimulate the release of renin, and the cycle of hypertension is worsened.

Hypertension may, therefore, be the cause and the result of renal failure.

RENAL ARTERY STENOSIS

In renal artery stenosis there is a major reduction in renal perfusion. This alteration results in increased renin secretion and activation of the renin–angiotensin system. If left untreated, accelerated hypertension will develop, resulting in further pathological changes and damage to the kidneys. The changes that take place in arterial stenosis include the following.

- Atherosclerosis: lipids and fibrous tissue lining the main renal artery and its larger branches.
- Hyaline arteriolar sclerosis: thickening vessel walls owing to the deposition of hyaline material, narrowing the lumen. This occurs naturally after 50 years of age, but is also seen earlier in diabetics.

- Thickening of small arteries: increase of fibrous tissue in the media of arteries, narrowing the lumen.

Obstruction to the renal blood flow can also be caused by the following.

- Vasculitis: necrosis and inflammation of the vessel walls because of immunological changes.
- Embolism: the kidney is a common site of embolism from circulating cardiac thrombi.
- Thrombosis: intravascular coagulation in the arterioles and glomerular capillaries of the kidney, which will result in renal tissue infarction (Figs. 2.18–2.21).

Figure 2.18
Renal arteriograms. (a) Digital subtraction arteriogram following injection of contrast material into the aorta, showing renal artery stenosis. The right renal artery is absent. The left renal artery is stenosed (arrow), but contrast medium has passed the stenosis and the developing nephrogram can be seen. The abdominal aorta is severely irregular and atheromatous. (b) In another patient, a catheter has been passed beyond a stenosis at the ostium of the right renal artery in preparation for balloon dilatation/stenting. (From Davison AM, Cumming AD, Swainson CP et al. Diseases of the kidney and urinary system. In: Haslett CC, Chilvers ER, Hunter JAA et al (eds) Davidson's principles and practice of medicine, 18th edn. Edinburgh: Churchill Livingstone, 1999: 417–470, with permission.)

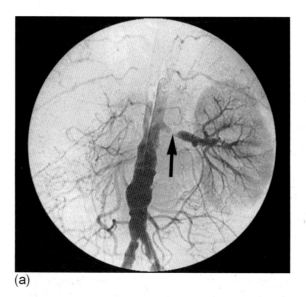

(a)

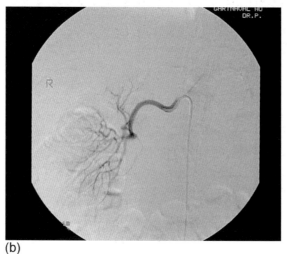

(b)

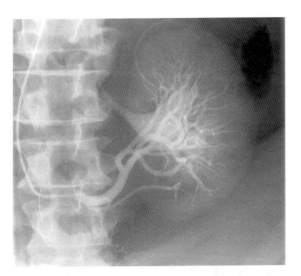

Figure 2.19
Conventional angiogram
showing a normal right renal
artery. Contrast material has
been injected into the renal
artery by means of a catheter,
seen just to the left of the
vertebral column.

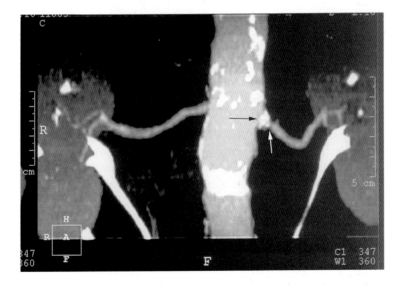

Figure 2.20
Computed tomography scan
showing left renal artery
stenosis. The black arrow
points to a calcified plaque at
the origin of the artery with
narrowing of the artery distal
to the plaque (white arrow).
Heavy calcification is seen in
the aorta (bright patches).

DISEASE PROGRESSION AND PROGNOSIS

It is estimated that renal artery stenosis accounts for 25% of established
renal failure in dialysis patients aged over 60 years (Scoble 1999).

Hypertension resulting from renal artery stenosis may be treated by
drugs to reduce blood pressure or by lipid-lowering treatment. The stenosis
itself can be treated by angioplasty of the renal artery with intra-arterial balloon catheters, by insertion of a stent or by surgical bypass of the narrowed
vessel (McLaughlin et al 2000).

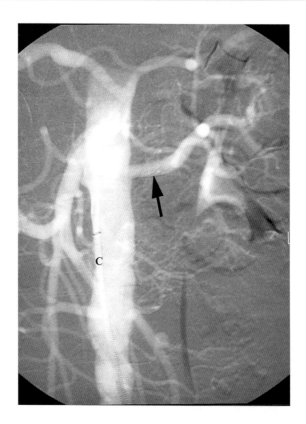

Figure 2.21
Digital subtraction angiogram of the same patient shown in Figure 2.20 following treatment by insertion of a metallic stent (black arrow) to improve the blood flow to the left kidney. C, catheter.

NEPHROSCLEROSIS

Hypertension can cause nephrosclerosis and is a major precipitating factor of renal disease. Hypertension that is not treated leads to sclerosis of the renal arterioles and the blood supply to glomeruli, tubules and interstitium gradually decreases. Scar tissue develops in the kidney, resulting in loss of renal function and eventually chronic kidney disease.

BLOOD PRESSURE CONTROL

The control of hypertension is the treatment of priority in patients with chronic kidney disease in preventing the progression of renal failure and cardiovascular complications. Health education pertaining to cessation of smoking and alcohol, healthy eating and regular exercise for weight control is just as important in patients with chronic kidney disease as in other patients with hypertension.

NEPHROTIC SYNDROME

The nephrotic syndrome is not a disease but a collection of symptoms. It is characterised by:

- heavy proteinuria (> 3.5 g in 24 h)
- a reduction in plasma proteins
- severe and generalised oedema.

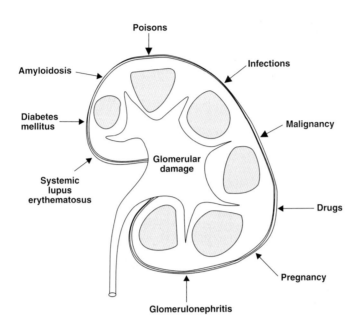

Figure 2.22
Causes of the nephrotic
syndrome.

The nephrotic syndrome may develop in a patient with a primary renal disease of unknown cause (idiopathic nephrotic syndrome) or it may be associated with other conditions in which kidney involvement is secondary, such as amyloidosis or diabetes mellitus (Fig. 2.22).

PATHOLOGY

The nephrotic syndrome is the result of glomerular damage increasing the glomerular basement membrane permeability, allowing large amounts of small albumin molecules to pass through into the urine. It should be remembered that the size of the albumin molecule is just at the cut-off point in size of particle that may pass through the glomerular filter (see Fig. 2.6). As the disease progresses, proteins of larger molecular weight leak through the glomerular basement membrane and GFRs may also reduce as the glomerular damage increases.

As the protein continues to be excreted, the serum albumin decreases (hypoalbuminaemia). This in turn leads to a low plasma oncotic pressure and diffusion of fluid into the tissue spaces causing generalised oedema (see Fig. 2.8a).

A reduction in the circulating blood volume stimulates the release of renin from the kidney, resulting in more aldosterone being released from the adrenal cortex, which is responsible for the retention of sodium and water. Retained fluid also passes out of the capillaries into the tissue, causing more oedema (Fig. 2.23).

In the early stages of the nephrotic syndrome, the protein leak may be the only disorder of renal function, but with some glomerular lesions the disease progresses and nephrons are destroyed. This will lead to established renal failure and the patient will require dialysis.

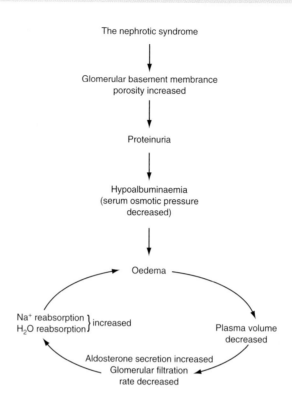

Figure 2.23
Oedema formation in the
nephrotic syndrome.

COMMON CAUSES OF ESTABLISHED RENAL FAILURE

The most common causes of established renal failure in the UK are diabetes mellitus (approximately 20% of all new patients), glomerulonephritis, pyelonephritis, polycystic kidney, renal vascular disease and hypertension (Ansell & Feest 2000).

DIABETIC NEPHROPATHY

Diabetic nephropathy is the term used to describe damage to the kidney structure and function that occurs as a result of the long-term complications of diabetes mellitus. Type 1 and Type 2 diabetes mellitus are characterised by raised blood glucose levels and sustained hyperglycaemia. This is associated with glycosylation of proteins, glycosylated haemoglobin (HbA_{1C}) being an example. These biologically active molecules are known as advanced glycosylation end-products (AGEs) and it is these compounds that cause vascular tissue damage. Patients with diabetes are therefore at increased risk of suffering renal and cardiovascular insufficiency (Makita et al 1994). Diabetic nephropathy develops in 30–40% of patients with Type 2 diabetes and has become the single most common cause of established renal disease in the Western world (Rossing et al 2005).

Pathology

Patients initially develop microalbuminuria (i.e. $30–300\,mg\,24\,h^{-1}$). This may not occur for up to 10 years after the diagnosis of type 1 diabetes mellitus, but diabetes mellitus may go undetected for so long that micro-albuminuria is present at diagnosis. After 1–5 years, proteinuria becomes clinical, even to nephrotic levels (> 3.5 g day^{-1}). With good blood pressure and glycaemic control, and with prescription of angiotensin-converting enzyme (ACE) inhibitors or angiotensin receptor blockers (ARBs), it is possible to delay the progression from microalbuminurea to macroalbu-minurea and to slow the decline in glomerular filtration rate. In practice, there is little evidence that the incidence of diabetic nephropathy is declin-ing (Steffes 1997). Ritz et al (1999) have highlighted that the incidence of those with established renal failure and diabetes mellitus has increased progressively in the past decade, and have argued that the challenge for the future will be better patient management in the earlier phases of neph-ropathy.

The kidneys may be of normal size or slightly larger than normal. In Type 1 diabetes, the most important structural changes involve the glomerulus, whereas in patients with Type 2 diabetes, tubulointersti-tial and vascular lesions are more common (Vestra and Fioretto 2003). The pathologies associated with diabetes mellitus are listed below.

- Pyelonephritis: the most common lesion found in those with diabe-tes mellitus, causing chronic kidney disease and a result of autonomic neuropathy in the bladder.
- Diffuse intercapillary glomerulosclerosis: causing thickening and sclerosis of the basement membrane of the glomerular capillary and proliferation of the mesangial cells.
- Nodular glomerulosclerosis (or Kimmelstiel–Wilson nodules): the glomerulus becoming increasingly replaced and destroyed by the deposition of nodules of a glycoprotein material.
- Arteriosclerosis, which develops in the arteries supplying the glomer-ulus due to hyaline deposits in the afferent and efferent arterioles, causing ischaemia and accelerating the disease process.
- Papillary necrosis.

RENAL FAILURE AND GLUCOSE CONTROL

The kidneys have an important role in the metabolism of insulin and, as the GFR decreases in renal failure, so does the delivery of insu-lin to the proximal tubule cells where it is metabolised; consequently, the circulating half-life of insulin increases with higher levels in the body after any given dose. Insulin requirements or oral hypoglycae-mic agents should therefore be decreased so that hypoglycaemia does not occur.

Intensive diabetes management with the goal of achieving near-nor-mal blood glucose levels has been shown to delay the onset of micro-albuminuria in Type 1 and Type 2 diabetes. The American Diabetes Association (2006) has published a position statement on diabetic neph-ropathy, which has useful care recommendations. Early diagnosis of diabetes is also important. Finne et al (2005) found that children diag-nosed with diabetes before the age of 5 years have the most favourable prognosis in terms of progression to established renal failure.

GLOMERULONEPHRITIS

The term glomerulonephritis covers a group of conditions in which inflammation in the glomerulus occurs, either as a primary disease or as part of a systemic illness. It is therefore important to consider the possibility of an underlying systemic condition if glomerulonephritis is diagnosed. See Couser (1999) for further reading.

Glomerular disease occurs when the structure or function of the glomerular capillary network have been damaged as a result of antigen–antibody reactions in the glomeruli. There are contributions from lymphocytes, macrophages, antibodies, immune complexes and inflammatory mediators. The glomerular cells may proliferate, basement membrane may thicken or exudates of leukocytes and platelets may build up in the glomerulus. These tissue reactions result in changes in the filtration properties of the glomerulus, leading to proteinuria, haematuria, impaired excretory renal function and hypertension.

Any age group may be affected, though some types are particularly common in children. The estimated incidence of glomerulonephritis in the UK is 17–60/million population. See Plate 1 for histopathology, Box 2.4 for histopathology and clinical manifestations, and Box 2.5 for specific nursing observations.

In some cases, an underlying cause of the autoimmune response can be identified and eradicated. For example, drugs, tumours or infectious agents (e.g. streptococci) may result in glomerulonephritis, which may resolve on removal of the tumour or drug. Treatment for glomerulonephritis tends to involve anti-inflammatory and/or immunosuppressive drugs. In rare conditions with rapid deterioration of renal function, plasma exchange may be used.

The prognosis depends to a large extent on the particular subtype of glomerulonephritis, identified by the pattern of glomerular injury involved:

- minimal-change glomerulonephritis (renal biopsy normal by light microscopy)
- membranous nephropathy
- immunoglobulin A (IgA) nephropathy
- focal segmental glomerulosclerosis
- focal necrotizing glomerulonephritis (associated with syndrome of rapidly progressive glomerulonephritis)
- mesangiocapillary glomerulonephritis
- postinfection glomerulonephritis.

Minimal change glomerulonephritis

These patients (usually children between 2 and 6 years) typically present with rapid-onset nephrotic syndrome. The condition is very rarely associated with impairment of excretory renal function and is occasionally secondary to drug use (particularly non-steroidal anti-inflammatory drugs; NSAIDs) or malignancy (e.g. lymphoma). Severe oedema may be present but without associated hypertension.

Box 2.4   Glomerular disease

Glomerulonephritis is the term used to describe a variety of disorders that principally affect the glomeruli in the kidney. Such glomerulopathies may arise as primary disorders of the glomerulus, or as part of a systemic disorder, such as systemic lupus erythematosus (SLE) or diabetes mellitus.

Histopathology

Glomerular damage may be manifest as one or more of the following tissue reactions:

- Cellular proliferation – leading to an increase in the number of cells in the glomerular tufts.
- Leukocyte infiltration of inflammatory cell – mainly neutrophils and monocytes.
- Basement membrane thickening – as occurs in diabetes mellitus, or this may be a response caused by precipitated immune complexes.
- Hyalinisation and sclerosis – hyalinisation is the accumulation of homogeneous, amorphous substance in the glomerular tuft composed of mesangial matrix, basement membrane and plasma protein. Sclerosis is the total obliteration of structural detail in the glomerular tuft and is the end-result of glomerular damage.

Clinical manifestations

Clinical presentation of glomerular disease may range from an acute onset of disease with a reversible outcome, to a chronic insidious onset that eventually leads to renal failure after several decades. A number of syndromes of glomerular disease are defined:

- Proteinuria – occurs if the glomerular basement membranes are damaged so that they leak protein.
- Nephrotic syndrome – occurs if the basement membranes are damaged more severely and increase the protein leak to > 3.5 g protein 24 h^{-1}. This in turn induces a low serum albumin and generalised oedema. Hyperlipidaemia usually also occurs.
- Haematuria – occurs if capillary walls are disrupted, allowing red cells to pass into the urine. This may be microscopic or macroscopic. However, most forms of haematuria are non-glomerular in origin.
- Nephritic syndrome – occurs when basement membrane damage and red blood cell leakage are present together, leading to proteinuria and haematuria, accompanied by generalised oedema and mild hypertension.
- Renal failure (acute or chronic) – occurs when damage to the glomeruli is severe enough to impair the normal filtering function of the glomerulus, resulting in an accumulation in the blood of substances such as urea, creatinine and potassium.

Box 2.5   Glomerular disease: specific nursing observations

Parameter	Rationale
Temperature	Patients with nephrotic syndrome are prone to infection, which exacerbates the disease if not detected and treated promptly
Blood pressure	Hypertension or hypotension may be present, depending on the patient's fluid and cardiac status. One should also monitor for a postural drop
Respiration	Rapid, shallow breaths may indicate pulmonary oedema. Severely acidotic patients may develop Kussmaul's respirations (deep, sighing hyperventilation)
Daily weight	Serial measurements of the patient's weight (at the same time each day) give the clearest indication of changes in fluid status
Urinalysis	The urine should be tested for protein and blood as indicators of glomerular disease. Urinary volume should also be monitored, and the urine sent for culture if infection is suspected
Skin	The skin should be observed for: oedema, dehydration, pruritus, flaking and dryness, pressure sores and rashes. A skin rash may indicate a systemic disease, such as systemic lupus erythematosus, vasculitis or Henoch–Schönlein purpura

Management of care Diuretic therapy may clear the oedema. Most patients respond to high-dose corticosteroids, but relapse is common as the dose is reduced and up to 50% of patients remain corticosteroid-dependent. In these patients, alkylating agents, such as cyclophosphamide, are sometimes successful. Ciclosporin is also effective (Macanovic & Mathieson 1999).

Prognosis Subsequent relapses in the condition can be treated with simiar protocols. Patients do not usually develop chronic kidney disease.

Membranous glomerulonephritis These patients typically present with proteinuria, which may be asymptomatic or severe enough to cause nephrotic syndrome. Microscopic haematuria, hypertension and/or impaired excretory renal function may also be associated. It is seen in adults rather than in children. Onset is insidious and the disease develops slowly, over the course of 20 years in some cases.

There is widespread thickening of the capillary wall in the glomerulus (but without proliferation of the cells), which seems to result from the deposition of immune complexes in the kidney. This can occur as a result of drug use (particularly NSAIDs, gold and penicillamine), secondary to tumours (e.g. carcinoma of bronchus or breast), infection (particularly hepatitis B) or hypothyroidism.

Management of care The prognosis of the secondary forms of the disease depends on the prognosis of the underlying condition. Complete resolution may be expected on withdrawal of the offending drug, whereas membranous glomerulonephritis that is secondary to a tumour has a poorer prognosis unless the tumour is eradicated.

At least 25% of patients undergo spontaneous remission of proteinuria without treatment. For those with a poorer prognosis, a combination of treatment with a steroid and an immunosuppressant (chlorambucil) given in alternating cycles may prove beneficial. There is a particular risk of thrombosis in membranous glomerulonephritis, so anticoagulants may also be prescribed (Macanovic & Mathieson 1999).

Prognosis Glomerular filtration rate may be normal for the first few years, but then may slowly deteriorate as the sclerosis of the glomerulus increases. If no primary cause of the disease is found and eradicated, dialysis or organ transplant may be inevitable in the long term.

IgA nephropathy This is the most common type of glomerulonephritis worldwide. Patients present with haematuria, sometimes with associated proteinuria, hypertension and impaired renal excretory function. The immunoglobulin IgA is deposited in the glomerulus, and there is sometimes proliferation of the glomerular cells. The cause of the deposits is not known, but it seems the problem is in the IgA system rather than in the kidney. An associated glomerular change is seen in Henoch-Schönlein purpura, a condition more common in children which is associated with a purpuric rash, joint and gastrointestinal involvement.

There is no proven treatment for this form of glomerulonephritis, although in patients with heavy proteinuria, steroids may be used successfully to reduce the protein loss. Antihypertensives (e.g. ACE inhibitors) may also be used.

Management of care and prognosis for the patient

Focal segmental glomerulosclerosis

This condition is named after the areas of scarring that occur in the glomeruli. The sclerotic changes affect some glomeruli but not others (focal), and may affect only parts of each glomerulus (segmental). The patient will typically present with nephrotic syndrome (hypertension, haematuria and impaired excretory renal function).

Treatment with prolonged courses of corticosteroids may induce remission of nephrotic syndrome, but the disease often progresses and established renal failure develops in about 50% of patients within 10 years.

Management of care and prognosis for the patient

Focal necrotising glomerulonephritis

Also known as rapidly progressive glomerulonephritis, this condition is associated with rapid but progressive deterioration in renal function, and the presence of oliguria or anuria. Haematuria and proteinuria also occur. If pulmonary haemorrhage is present, this is known as Goodpasture's syndrome. Without effective treatment, established renal failure will develop in weeks and months, rather than years.

Acute inflammation in the glomerulus is the underlying cause, sometimes with the formation of crescents when the glomerulus is squashed by cells, which fill the Bowman's space. In some cases, antibodies to the glomerular basement membrane are present but, in most cases, no immunoglobulin is identified in the glomerulus.

If specific antibodies are identified (by a serological test), plasma exchange followed by corticosteroid and immunosuppressant therapy will remove the offending antibodies and prevent further proliferation. The prognosis in these cases is directly related to the amount of damage already done to the glomeruli.

Management of care and prognosis

Mesangiocapillary or membrane–proliferative glomerulonephritis

Three subtypes of this condition are recognised, identifiable only by electron microscopy. In all cases, the presentation of the patient is similar, with proteinuria, haematuria, hypertension and impaired renal function. There are no known causes. All types tend to have a progressive course and up to 50% of patients develop chronic kidney disease within 10 years. Treatment focuses on blood pressure control and use of corticosteroids.

Postinfection glomerulonephritis

Poststreptococcal glomerulonephritis (e.g. following a throat infection) was a common cause of renal failure in the pre-antibiotic era and is still common in some parts of the world. Immune complexes that arise following infection with group A haemolytic streptococci deposit in the glomerular capillary wall, resulting in proteinuria, haematuria and hypertension.

Glomerulonephritis may complicate infection with a range of organisms. Infection with *Staphylococcus*, influenza B, hepatitis B and C, and human immunodeficiency virus (HIV) may all result in renal damage.

PYELONEPHRITIS

This is a bacterial infection of kidney tissue, with the infection beginning in the lower urinary tract and ascending to the kidney(s). Acute pyelonephritis is commonly associated with pregnancy, obstruction, instrumentation or trauma to the urinary tract, and patients with a chronic illness.

Chronic pyelonephritis is the result of repeated infections of the urinary tract. There is widespread destruction of nephrons and replacement with scar tissue, which eventually causes established renal failure. For the majority of patients, the disease starts in early childhood and is due to ureteric reflux and infection, but symptoms of the disease may not present clinically until adulthood. In adults, chronic pyelonephritis is a complication of obstruction in the renal tract, because stone formation and structural abnormalities both cause stasis of urine.

Clinical features and management of care

The patient will present with pyrexia and rigors, and loin pain over the affected kidney(s). Symptoms of a lower urinary tract infection may also be present.

Antibiotics can be given to treat the acute phase of the infection, but there is little evidence to prove that prophylactic antibiotics slow down the onset of chronic kidney disease. A high fluid intake (up to 3L day^{-1}) is important.

Disease progression and prognosis

If the chronic infections are only affecting one kidney, the disease is usually prolonged but benign. Bilateral chronic infection will ensure that chronic kidney disease is of rapid onset.

Reflux nephropathy is a congenital anatomical abnormality where there is incompetence of the sphincter at the junction of the ureter with the bladder, allowing the reflux of urine back up the ureter and into the renal pelvis. Infection may develop and the formation of scar tissue will eventually cause chronic kidney disease. If identified early, surgical correction will be needed. Recurrent urinary tract infection during childhood should always be fully investigated and treated.

POLYCYSTIC KIDNEY DISEASE

Polycystic kidney disease is one of a number of cystic diseases of the kidney. Polycystic disease refers to two hereditary cystic diseases – autosomal recessive polycystic kidney disease and autosomal dominant polycystic kidney disease. Both conditions may occur in children, although the recessive disease is more commonly seen in this age group. The following descriptions will refer to autosomal dominant polycystic kidney disease, one of the most common genetic disorders, which is responsible for approximately 10% of patients with established renal failure.

Genetics

The autosomal dominant form of the disease is one of the most common genetic disorders, affecting an estimated 80/100 000 of the population (Davison et al 1999). The condition occurs equally in men and women and is transmitted by both sexes. If one parent is affected, 50% of the offspring will develop the disease, although symptoms may not develop until patients reach their 20s. The mean age of starting dialysis treatment is 57 years. However, by the age of 80, virtually all individuals who carry the gene will manifest some form of the disease.

Three genes appear to be responsible for the condition: currently, location of two of the genes is known (Murcia et al 1998). Work is also in progress to identify genes responsible for the recessive form of the disease (in which two copies of the affected genes must be inherited, one from each parent).

Pathology

Both kidneys are considerably enlarged and consist of a compact mass of cysts, which are scattered equally throughout the cortex and medulla (Fig. 2.24). The cysts increase in size and eventually rupture, allowing infection and scar tissue formation, and reducing the number of functioning nephrons. The enlarged cysts compress the normal renal tissue and hypertensive changes and glomerulosclerosis occur. Cysts are filled with watery fluid, which may be clear, bloodstained from a recent haemorrhage, brown from an old haemorrhage or filled with pus (Figs. 2.25–2.27).

Liver cysts may be found in patients with polycystic kidneys and there is also a significant association with aneurysms of the cerebral arteries.

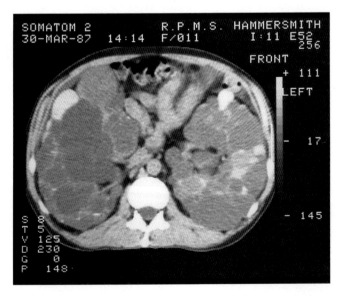

Figure 2.24
Polycystic kidney disease. Two very large polycystic kidneys, shown by computed tomography. (From Davison AM, Cumming AD, Swainson CP et al. Diseases of the kidney and urinary system. In: Haslett CC, Chilvers ER, Hunter JAA et al (eds) Davidson's principles and practice of medicine, 18th edn. Edinburgh: Churchill Livingstone, 1999: 417–470, with permission.)

Figure 2.25
Ultrasound of a normal left kidney.

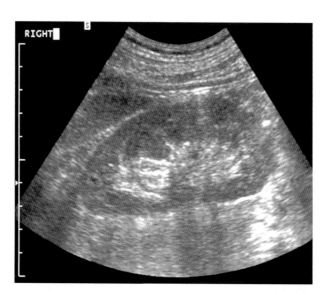

Figure 2.26
Ultrasound of a polycystic kidney showing how the normal tissue is replaced by multiple fluid-filled cysts (C).

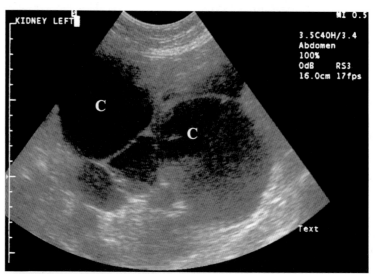

Figure 2.27
Computed tomography scan showing a polycystic left kidney; the cysts are marked by C. The white arrows point to normal renal tissue. The right kidney has been removed.

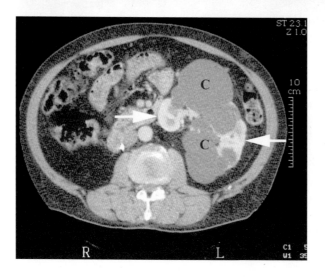

1. Pain: the patient may complain of abdominal distension or discomfort following minor physical trauma and this may cause frank or microscopic haematuria. Pain in the flank is associated with the large cysts rupturing and any blood clots that are passed will cause the patient to experience colic. Mild analgesia may be sufficient to relieve discomfort, but pain caused by cysts rupturing or from clot retention may require opiates.
2. Haematuria and proteinuria: microscopic or frank haematuria is seen in more than 50% of patients. Chronic blood loss does not usually result in anaemia, since the erythropoietin production by the kidneys is increased. Patients may be advised to alter their lifestyle if they are prone to physical abdominal trauma, which may cause cysts to rupture. Mild proteinuria is always present in the mid to late stages of the disease and may be the first abnormality that draws attention to the condition during a routine medical examination.
3. Urinary tract infections: repeated urinary tract infections are common complications and may affect the cysts. Unnecessary urological investigation should be avoided and female patients should receive health education regarding perineal hygiene. All patients should be advised on the importance of a high fluid intake to prevent urinary stasis and how to recognise the signs of a urinary tract infection.
4. Hypertension: secondary hypertension is common in patients with polycystic disease and may deteriorate as established renal failure approaches. It is treated aggressively, not only because it may accelerate deterioration of renal function but because it may increase the risk of intracerebral haemorrhage in these patients (Ecder et al 2000).

Clinical features and management of care

MULTISYSTEM DISEASES AFFECTING THE KIDNEY

The kidney may be affected in many ways by disease processes that are not directly associated with renal function. This vulnerability is, in part, due to the high blood supply of the kidneys; together the kidneys receive 25% of the cardiac output. The glomerular capillaries, because of their filtering properties, come into close contact with all blood constituents.

The effects of diabetes mellitus and of systemic infections in the kidney have already been mentioned. The following are some more examples of multisystem diseases that may affect the kidney.

This is an autoimmune inflammatory disease which affects joints, blood vessels, skin and the nervous system, as well as the kidneys. Glomerular inflammation may result in proteinuria, haematuria and hypertension; renal involvement often occurs within 3 years of diagnosis of the disease. Non-renal manifestations of the disease are usually present, such as arthralgia, rash and haematological disorders.

Systemic lupus erythematosus

Amyloidosis is the term given to a group of chronic infiltrative disorders characterised by the presence of deposits of an abnormal protein called amyloid. Two groups of protein deposit exist, AL amyloid or AA amy-

Renal amyloidosis

loid, but renal involvement occurs with both. AA amyloid deposits are a complication of many chronic inflammatory diseases, occurring in up to 10% of patients with rheumatoid arthritis; AL amyloid deposits may occur secondary to myeloma or as the primary condition, AL amyloidosis. This is a systemic disease that affects the heart, peripheral nervous system, liver and kidney.

A common site of deposition of the insoluble amyloid fibrils is in the walls of the renal arterioles and glomerular capillaries. The result is usually nephrotic syndrome followed by progressive renal failure.

Scleroderma or systemic sclerosis

This is a multisystem condition that causes gradual hardening and tightening of the skin and increased binding to subcutaneous tissue. Renal involvement is one of the less common but most serious complications of the disease and, in the past, was a major cause of mortality. Patients often present with the features of malignant hypertension and rapidly deteriorating renal function. Diastolic pressure may exceed 130 mmHg. Antihypertensives, particularly ACE inhibitors, improve the renal outlook of these patients, but there is no treatment for the underlying condition.

Polyarteritis nodosa

More common in men than women, this condition usually presents in later life. It is characterised by widespread inflammation of small and medium arteries and aneurysm formation. Thrombosis in these arteries can lead to complications that particularly affect the gut, peripheral nervous system and kidneys. The renal presentation is that of progressive renal impairment caused by renal infarction and hypertension. Treatment is with corticosteroids, and renal prognosis depends on early diagnosis and treatment, since organ damage is irreversible.

CLINICAL FEATURES AND MANAGEMENT OF CARE

OEDEMA

In the early stages of the nephrotic syndrome, swollen eyes at the start of the day and swollen feet and ankles at the end of the day may be observed. As the disease progresses, or as a result of poor symptom control, the oedema becomes more generalised, causing pleural and peritoneal effusions, resulting in breathlessness and congestion of the gastrointestinal tract.

Fluid removal will be the treatment of priority for patients, but diuretic therapy needs to be administered carefully as profound hypoalbuminaemia may cause a reduced circulating blood volume, triggering a hypotensive response in some patients following the administration of large doses of intravenous diuretics. Infusions of small volumes of intravenous salt-poor albumin prior to the administration of diuretics will increase plasma volume and restore a diuretic response in the patient. In the majority of patients the albumin is excreted after 24–48 h.

All patients with severe oedema and receiving aggressive diuretics should be weighed daily and have 4-hourly lying and standing blood pressure recordings to observe for deficits caused by a reduced plasma volume.

PROTEINURIA

Urine has a frothy appearance owing to the high protein content (losses greater than 3.5 g in 24 h) and as a consequence hypoalbuminaemia develops. The loss of immunoglobulins increases the risk of infection. Hyperlipidaemia is also a clinical sign of the nephrotic syndrome, as a result of the liver synthesising more cholesterol and lipids. This makes the plasma milky in appearance.

Care for those with nephrotic syndrome can be very challenging for the renal care team. Fogo (2000) explored the significance and consequences of proteinuria in nephrotic syndrome and this paper is useful for further reading on the management of this disease.

MUSCLE WASTING

The loss of skeletal muscles becomes apparent when the generalised oedema has subsided. Muscle wasting is a result of protein mobilisation into the blood to counteract protein lost in the urine.

WEIGHT LOSS AND MALNUTRITION

Chronic nausea, vomiting and poor appetite may result from congestion in the gastrointestinal tract owing to oedema. Weight loss also results from proteinuria and muscle wasting. A dietetic referral should be made, and the patient encouraged to take a high-calorie diet with a protein allowance compensating for the protein loss.

TIREDNESS AND LETHARGY

These symptoms may be attributed to a combination of reduced calorie intake, to muscle wasting and to the generalised oedema, which may increase body weight by up to 10 kg. Patients should be encouraged to take plenty of rest.

INTRAVASCULAR CLOTTING

There is a risk of spontaneous intravascular clotting in a patient with nephrotic syndrome owing to the increase in circulating clotting proteins along with venous stasis in the legs and a reduction in plasma volume. During episodes of hospitalisation and immobility, prophylactic anticoagulants may be used (e.g. subcutaneous heparin). The use of antiembolic stockings increases venous return and reduces venous stasis.

References

American Diabetes Association. Standards of medical care in diabetes – 2006: nephropathy screening and treatment. Diabetes Care 2006, 29(Suppl 1): 521. care.diabetesjournals.org/content/vol29/suppl_1/

Ansell D, Feest T (eds). UK Renal Registry report. Bristol: UK Renal Registry, 2000.

Couser WG. Seminar. Glomerulonephritis. Lancet 1999; 353: 1509–1515.

Davison AM, Cumming AD, Swainson CP et al. Diseases of the kidney and urinary system. In: Haslett CC, Chilvers ER, Hunter JAA et al (eds) Davidson's principles and practice of medicine, 18th edn. Edinburgh: Churchill Livingstone, 1999: 417–470.

Eadington D, Plant, W, Winney R. Chronic renal failure. The Practitioner 1993; 237: 64–69.

Ecder T, Edelstein CL, Fick Brosnahan GM et al. Progress in blood pressure control in autosomal dominant polycystic kidney disease. Am J Kidney Dis 2000; 36: 266–271.

Finne P, Reunanen A, Stenman S, Groop PH, Gronhagen-Riska C. Incidence of end-stage renal disease in patients with type 1 diabetes. JAMA 2005; 294(14): 1782–1787.

Fogo A. Nephrotic syndrome: molecular and genetic basis. Nephron 2000; 85: 8–13.

Lawrence DR, Bennett PN. Clinical pharmacology, 6th edn. Edinburgh: Churchill Livingstone, 1987.

Levey AS, Eckardt KU, Tsukamoto Y et al. Definition and classification of chronic kidney disease: A position statement from Kidney Disease: Improving Global Outcomes (KDIGO). Kidney International 2005; 67: 2089–2100.

Macanovic M, Mathieson PW. Glomerulonephritis. Medicine 1999; 27: 59–62.

Makita Z, Bucala R, Rayfield EJ et al. Reactive glycosylation endproducts in diabetic uraemia and treatment of renal failure. The Lancet 1994; 343: 1519–1522.

McLaughlin K, Jardine AG, Moss JG. ABC of arterial and venous disease. Renal artery stenosis. Br Med J 2000; 320: 1124–1127.

Murcia NS, Woychik RP, Avner ED. The molecular biology of polycystic kidney disease. Pediatr Nephrol 1998; 12: 721–726.

Ritz E, Rychlik I, Locatelli F et al. End-stage renal failure in type 2 diabetes: a medical catastrophe of worldwide dimensions. Am J Kidney Dis 1999; 34: 795–808.

Rossing K, Mischak H, Parving H-H et al. Impact of diabetic nephropathy and angiotensin II receptor blockade on urinary polypeptide patterns. Kidney International 2005; 68: 193–205.

Scoble JE. Renovascular disease. Medicine 1999; 27: 100–102.

Steffes MW. Diabetic nephropathy: incidence, prevalence, and treatment. Editorial. Diabetes Care 1997; 20: 1059–1061.

Vestra MD, Fioretto P. Diabetic nephropathy: renal structural studies in type 1 and type 2 diabetic patients. International Congress Series 2003; 1253: 163–169.

Chapter 3

Psychological perspectives

Juliet Auer

■ To appreciate the far-reaching effects of renal failure on every aspect of life
■ To explore the psychological pressures experienced by patients and carers
■ To demonstrate differences between stresses of treatment in different age groups
■ To emphasise the importance of information-giving to promote active
  involvement of patient and carer
■ To evaluate the multidisciplinary approach to patient care
■ To promote understanding of the reasons for non-adherence to dialysis therapy
■ To explore issues surrounding withdrawal from treatment and the
  sympathetic management of the dying patient

**LEARNING OUTCOMES
FOR THIS CHAPTER**

INTRODUCTION

Ever since dialysis and renal transplantation were introduced in the USA in the late 1950s and early 1960s, and in the UK in the mid-1960s, psychologists and psychiatrists have been involved in studying the impact of living on a life-supporting machine or with a donor kidney, and with the problems encountered by patients, their families and also the staff who support them over years of survival against the odds (Abram 1969, 1970, Abram et al 1971, Kaplan de Nour & Czackes 1968, Shambaugh & Kanter 1969).

Much research has been done into the psychological aspects of dialysis and the quality of life of these patients, and numerous studies have been published by those most active in this field over the past 20 years, particularly Atara Kaplan de Nour, Roberta Simmons, Norman Levy, Howard Burton, Nancy Kutner and Roger Evans. As dialysis came to be offered to a wider age range in the 1980s, the adjustment of elderly patients has been studied by Westlie et al (1984), Kline et al (1986) and Neu & Kjellstrand (1986) in North America, and by Auer (1986) and Quarello et al (1992) in Europe, concluding that there is no reason why there should be any age limit to treatment, and that many patients in their eighth and even ninth decade can achieve good quality of life. In the 1980s and 1990s, as concern grew over the seemingly limitless demands of the healthcare budget, a number of studies focused on cost-benefit aspects of quality of life on dialysis, and the need to ration resources (Gudex 1986, Loomes & McKenzie 1989, Stanton 1999, Williams 1985). In the view of the health economist, dialysis is an expensive way of prolonging a life that may lack quality by objective measures, such as vocational rehabilitation and functional capacity. These conclusions, however, raise questions about the validity of objective measures in an area that may be better approached from a subjective stance; that is, do patients see their life on dialysis as worthwhile?

In the present chapter, a brief overview of some of the important findings is given, but chiefly attention is drawn to some of the everyday experiences of patients, gathered largely from working in a busy dialysis and transplant unit over a 20-year period. This will allow the reader to recognise some of the patients' reactions and the reasons for them, and provide a practical insight useful to those working with patients and families.

Every aspect of life is affected by renal failure and its treatment, and the effects spread to all those closely involved with the patient. Greater understanding of the day-to-day stresses and concerns of patients allows staff in renal units to respond with appropriate support. This needs to begin as early as possible, to prevent problems, whether practical (as in employment or finances) or emotional (as in relationship problems and unnecessary fears about prognosis or treatment; Bradley & McGee 1994).

THE PREDIALYSIS STAGE

Unfortunately, only about half of the patients who enter renal replacement programmes are followed in a predialysis clinic during the decline of their renal function towards end-stage. The remaining patients present acutely in established renal failure (ERF), or in acute-on-chronic renal failure, previously undiagnosed, which progresses rapidly to end-stage. Older patients (> 70 years) with acute renal failure are less likely to regain function than those less than 70 years of age. Those patients who have time to adjust over a period of months, or even years, to the fact that dialysis and/or transplantation will become necessary, seem to adjust more smoothly to treatment.

Increasingly, renal units are using this time to good effect, by preparing patients for the transition from chronic kidney disease to ERF and the need for dialysis, not only medically but also psychologically and socially. Such predialysis education may even delay the need for dialysis (Binik et al 1993), perhaps as a result of promoting better understanding of antihypertensive medication.

The subjects that need to be addressed vary according to age and circumstances, but may include:

- the importance and purpose of medication and diet
- choosing the treatment best suited to the patient's social situation and lifestyle
- problems with employment and finances owing to the illness
- problems with housing, taking treatment needs into consideration
- role changes within relationships, and effects on family members or carers
- difficulties in sexual and affectionate relationships (Stout et al 1985)
- effect of ERF on leisure activities and holidays.

In the case of younger patients, the effects can be far-reaching and devastating to contemplate, involving disruption of the overall life plan, including gaining independence from parents, higher education and training, career prospects, marriage and having children. Older patients usually face less fundamental losses.

PREDIALYSIS AND PRETRANSPLANT GROUPS

With few exceptions, the more information and preparation that can be provided, the better patients are able to adjust, especially if the knowledge acquired enables them to choose the treatment modality best suited to their circumstances (Bradley & McGee 1994). This preparation also benefits the spouse or carer, who is often more worried than the patient, having not always had the opportunity of talking to the doctor on clinic visits. Spouses are affected by the effects of the illness on the patient. These effects may include:

- lethargy and tiredness
- inability to concentrate
- irritability
- apathy/depression or anxiety
- reduced ability to show affection or sexual interest
- withdrawal and lack of communication

- constant complaints about symptoms, such as itching, loss of appetite or breathlessness
- sleep disturbance.

Spouses have frequently expressed frustration that symptoms are minimised or not reported to the medical team on clinic visits. Patients who are trying to come to terms with their own feelings often find it hard to spare extra energy to cope with the feelings of those close to them. They also feel guilty that the illness is affecting others, making it hard to relate to those they are 'letting down'. As a result, many spouses, who are facing the same worries about the future as the patient, feel unsupported and unappreciated.

Many units run predialysis and pretransplantation groups to assist both patients and their families during this period. Most have also appointed a predialysis nurse to coordinate various aspects of predialysis care, including information and liaison with the access nurse, dietitian and social worker as needed. In the author's renal unit, predialysis counselling was undertaken on an individual basis by the dietitian, social worker and nurses until the mid-1980s. This always included a visit to the patient's home by the social worker to assess which type of treatment was most likely to suit the individual's requirements. A social report was then prepared for medical and nursing staff, assessing the housing, way of life, employment, social supports, financial position, and any particular strengths and weaknesses inherent in the patient's situation. Such factors are far better explored away from the hospital in the patient's own environment. Ideally, this would still be the practice in most cases, but the increase in workload in renal units, certainly in the UK, has made it impractical to visit all patients at home before the need for dialysis treatment.

The solution chosen in an increasing number of units is to invite patients and families to attend sessions where as much information and teaching as possible can be given, to the greatest number, in the most time- and cost-effective way. In some hospitals, these groups are run by nursing staff, in others by the social worker. The most effective groups seem to be run on a multidisciplinary basis, with input from medical, nursing, dietetic and social work staff, and include teaching from established dialysis and transplant patients themselves (Bradley & McGee 1994).

The objective of these groups is in line with the Department of Health (DOH) concept of The Expert Patient – an initiative proposed in 2000, to make those with chronic conditions experts in their care and management, promoting independence and greater well-being (Department of Health 2001). Between 2004 and 2007 the DOH is planning to establish 'user-led self-management courses to allow people with chronic diseases to develop the confidence, knowledge and skills to manage their conditions better, and thereby gain a greater measure of control and independence to enhance their quality of life'. They acknowledge that in many longstanding conditions, such as diabetes, arthritis, asthma, multiple sclerosis and heart disease, the patient comes to know more about their individual condition than most professionals, and represent an 'untapped resource'. A small number of renal units are setting up renal-specific self-management programmes. It could be said that patients with kidney disease have been way ahead of the DOH for many years. In many ways, the first 'expert patients' were the early home dialysis patients, who, in the 1960s, were performing a highly technological treatment that was mysterious to any but renal doctors. Their own general practitioners (GPs) would visit to learn about the treatment. The patient with kidney disease has always become his or her own expert, and is an active participant in treatment rather than a passive recipient. By including patients as teachers in the information groups, this status is actively recognised and encouraged.

There are a number of different agendas and types of communication that can be used in an information group, which are listed below.

- Straightforward teaching: information about the causes and effects of renal failure, and the methods of treatment-medication, diet and dialysis/transplantation.
- Group support.
- Reassurance: the dispelling of myths about renal failure and treatment, ensuring that the patient's concerns are realistic, focusing on the real problems rather than rumours or hearsay (e.g. a number of patients have asked whether it is true that one can only survive a short period on dialysis and can expect to die unless transplanted quickly).
- Encouraging active participation in treatment, by establishing a climate of cooperative interaction between patients and staff, rather than passive acceptance.
- Introducing topics and encouraging questions, especially on subjects that many patients feel inappropriate to raise with busy medical staff at clinic appointments. This gives validity to a number of concerns that patients and relatives may consider outside the scope of the unit, for example:
  – depression
  – anxiety
  – relationship difficulties
  – body image
  – sexuality.

Once these are placed on the agenda, patients feel able to approach staff for individual discussion, if necessary.

In order to fulfil a number of these criteria at once, patients are taught partly by staff and partly by other patients, thus giving the role of 'patient' both status and an active and positive connotation. It also means that the information given has greater credibility, since it comes from someone who has first-hand experience. The informal support provided by the experienced patient to those not yet receiving dialysis is reassuring and valuable (Klang et al 1999). Questions to 'patient teachers' are often more freely expressed and wider-ranging than those put to staff. The overall impression created is one of teamwork, with the patient as part of the team rather than the passive object of attention.

A continuous ambulatory peritoneal dialysis (CAPD) exchange may be demonstrated by a patient, using a minimum of special equipment (i.e. no special work surface, bag warmer or hospital drip stand), allowing a brief overview of what is involved from a technical point of view. This demonstration gives a clear message that the treatment is portable, flexible and does not require either a clinical setting or the 'safety' of home. It is also shown to be something that can be done without embarrassment in front of others. All these messages are relayed without even needing to be mentioned. Most of the demonstrators used are middle-aged (50s plus), and are in employment, at least part-time – again giving a positive image of the treatment. Demonstrators are often asked whether they 'skip a treatment from time to time' or break the rules – and they usually give a truthful answer in the affirmative, in spite of the presence of staff – again helping to set the atmosphere for honest and realistic interaction with members of the team.

The teaching session includes a visit to the haemodialysis unit, where predialysis patients and relatives are encouraged to talk to patients on dialysis. Many have not previously entered the unit, and most are relieved and pleasantly surprised to find that the treatment is neither painful nor terrifying. The message conveyed by seeing patients eating, reading, dozing, knitting or watching television during treatment is a powerful one, emphasising the normality that is possible under these circumstances rather than the clinical procedure itself. It is also reassuring for those in the predialysis stage to be told that only a small amount of blood is outside the body at any one time. They see a number of different types of dialysis access and haemodialysis machines, and can be introduced to patients preparing for home treatment. There is often animated discussion with those on treatment, and many practical questions are asked, diverting thoughts from the general dread of needing a life-support treatment towards the reality of coping effectively with the situation.

By presenting the options for treatment, patients feel involved in the choice of dialysis modality. In some cases there are strong medical arguments for the choice of one or other type of dialysis, but patients should, nevertheless, feel that they have been presented with as much choice and information as possible. It is also empowering to patients to be given some control over a situation that has, in many ways, removed their options and self-determination – there can be few more limiting experiences than dependence on a life-support system. The patients who appear most successful, in the sense of making the most of a life that is being sustained against the odds, are those who maintain a sense of control over their treatment rather than being at the mercy of their situation. There is increase in confidence in patients encouraged to perform self-monitoring of weight and blood pressure rather than relying on staff. The more empowered patients feel, the less dependent and helpless they will feel. The goal is to give the patient as much self-respect and self-determination as possible, in a life that seems ruled by the illness and by healthcare professionals (Kutner 1994). A sense of control over the situation should include the knowledge and ability to 'bend the rules' within safe limits from time to time (e.g. missing an occasional peritoneal dialysis exchange in order to attend a special event, or knowing how to overstep the dietary restrictions for a special occasion without risking hyperkalaemia or serious fluid overload). These well-considered events should not be considered as non-compliant behaviour; rather, as the exceptions that prove the rule. It can be hard for staff to encourage flexibility, fearing abuse of any latitude allowed; yet, as in parenting, it is important to encourage an attitude of sensible and responsible independence. Slavish adherence to limiting regimes is probably responsible for more problems and unhappiness than occasional well-judged 'lapses'.

HOW MUCH INFORMATION SHOULD BE PRESENTED?

The information presented at this type of meeting needs to cater for a mythical 'average' patient, neither giving unrealistically high expectations by presenting an exceptionally fit, active and well-adjusted patient as an example, nor offering the point of view of a very depressed and disabled patient.

It is useful for those in the predialysis phase to hear from somebody who has experienced problems with one type of dialysis and has subsequently done well on another. It is also beneficial to introduce a transplant patient who has experienced the failure of a first graft and has later had a successful one.

Honesty is an important part of the contract between the patient and the team and, for this reason, the possible complications of treatments, such as CAPD peritonitis, hernias, leaks, need for resiting catheters, failure of a fistula to develop, or the side-effects of immunosuppression post-transplant, need to be openly discussed where appropriate. Staff are not helping or respecting patients if they are overprotective or overoptimistic about what they have to offer. Staff may use denial when interacting with patients – indeed, patients are likely to feel a 'failure' if staff present an idealised picture and they do not 'achieve' in line with expectations (Kaplan de Nour 1983). It is, however, possible to be honest without being unduly negative, and to present a balanced picture of possible benefits and drawbacks.

The philosophy behind information groups is, therefore, to present a realistic but not overdetailed picture, which sets the scene for a cooperative and interactive relationship with the team. It is always stated that individual problems and questions can be discussed on a one-to-one basis with an appropriate member of staff following the session or in clinic. The timing of sessions is quite important, since an adjustment period of at least 6 months is desirable. This allows time for considerations such as:

- negotiating with employers to arrange changes in hours or duties that will fit the future demands of treatment
- making adaptations to housing or moving house – this is especially important for older patients, who may wish to apply for sheltered

accommodation or for a transfer to a bungalow or ground-floor flat (letters from the hospital can often expedite such arrangements in the UK)

- early application for relevant Social Security benefits (e.g. disability living allowance) to minimise financial problems.

Although there is no hard and fast rule, it is usually appropriate to invite those with a creatinine of more than 300 mmol L^{-1} or an estimated GFR (eGFR) of less than 20–30, and whose renal function is declining, to attend information groups.

CONSERVATIVE MANAGEMENT AND SUPPORTIVE CARE

This chapter has so far concentrated on those who choose to have renal replacement therapy when they reach ERF. As professionals in the field, it is natural that we should believe in what we are offering to patients and even in some cases to 'oversell' dialysis treatments. As the dialysis population has aged, and the range of co-morbidity has increased, renal unit staff are increasingly questioning whether enthusiasm for dialysis treatment is always in the best interests of some patients. Part of predialysis education is, therefore, to offer the option of no dialysis.

A whole chapter in this book (Chapter 9) is concerned with end-of-life care, but there are particular challenges and perspectives from counsellors and social workers in this field, so these are discussed here.

It is very important to discuss possible dialysis options at some length with the individual patient and family, preferably in home surroundings but, if this is not possible, in the hospital. A multidisciplinary approach is needed with social work/counselling, medical and nursing input. The aim of conservative management is to improve quality of life by treating uraemic symptoms through diet and medication, including erythropoietin to correct anaemia, while supporting the patient and family both physically and psychologically (Levy et al 2004). Some patients opt for a trial of dialysis. In some cases, this goes well and the patient chooses to continue. If, however, it does not go well, the patient has the worst of both worlds, in that there have been hospital admissions for access, frequent travelling for treatment and an upsetting experience for no gain. Making the decision to stop the treatment is usually more difficult than deciding not to start, even if the patient feels unwell on dialysis.

The greatest psychological need of the patient opting for conservative management is the continued support of renal unit staff. Some feel that in 'rejecting' dialysis they are going it alone, whereas in fact their need for advice, information, monitoring and reassurance is as great or greater than if they had chosen to dialyse. Ideally there should be home visits from time to time, but in practical terms a regular telephone call is the best means of maintaining contact. Spouses need to know that they can contact the unit with their concerns, without being labelled as tiresome.

With good dietary management, blood pressure and fluid control, tablets for itching and for nausea and correction of anaemia, patients may feel better than for many months, and able to enjoy their remaining time. They will be aware that this is limited, and may want to deal with 'unfinished business' or the resolution of family conflicts as well as making time to see friends and family.

It is important to establish with patient and family where terminal care should take place. Some feel safer in a hospital or hospice, while others prefer to be at home under the care of the GP. Much will depend on the degree of social support available, and the feelings of the spouse or carer.

THE PSYCHOLOGICAL IMPACT OF RENAL REPLACEMENT THERAPY

ACCESS SURGERY

The reality of approaching dependence on dialysis is brought home to the patient by the creation of venous and/or peritoneal access. The anxious response to this admission for surgery can, therefore, seem out of proportion to the procedures themselves, which are comparatively trivial. The creation of access is an unmistakable signal that dialysis treatment is imminent. It is also the appropriate time for final psychological preparation. During admission for access, the patient can be given literature and information, talk to the dietitian about current and future nutrition, and to the social worker or nurse counsellor about feelings, psychosocial, housing, employment, family or financial concerns. It is also a good time to discuss future leisure activities and holidays, because the patient is usually most aware of contracting horizons and limitations at this point, and needs to be reminded that the object of dialysis is to enable life to be lived and to provide a life that is worth living, not simply to keep the patient alive to be dialysed.

Providing good psychological support and preparation involves spending time with patients and, however good one's communication skills and intentions, there is seldom the chance to do everything one would like. In this situation there is sometimes the temptation to abandon even the attempt to talk to patients about their concerns on the grounds that, if it cannot be done 'properly', it is not worth doing at all. This is very far from the case. Excellent and sensitive counselling can often be given with two minutes of listening and responding to a particular worry, provided one remains aware of needs and fears, and able to pick up the cues provided.

The creation of haemodialysis access is often a disfiguring experience for patients. Staff become so used to seeing central venous catheters, fistulae and grafts that they can forget that these cause turned heads and curious glances outside the hospital. Women in particular are sensitive to the appearance of access sites, not because of greater vanity, but because their normal clothing is less likely to cover the arms, shoulders and neck than a man's shirt and jacket. Most patients will have seen the well-developed fistulae of long-standing haemodialysis patients at clinic visits and these can be off-putting. Staff, particularly nurses, need to recognise the patient's feelings, advise on clothing, and help to make the lines and dressings as unobtrusive as possible.

Some haemodialysis access surgery is performed under local anaesthetic and can take a long time. In spite of adequate premedication, it can be an anxious and uncomfortable time for the patient, who may benefit from the presence of a familiar nurse to talk to during the procedure.

The Tenckhoff catheter in preparation for peritoneal dialysis (PD) is less noticeable to the outside world but arouses many private concerns, mostly involving body image and the reaction of the spouse or partner. Many patients fear that they will no longer be attractive to their partner, partly because of the catheter itself and partly because of abdominal distension, which changes the figure. Some patients, aware of the problems of colostomies and ileostomies, fear that the catheter will have a detectable smell. Before patients leave hospital, it is useful for the nurse to make sure that the partner has seen the exit site, and understands about the dressing and taping of the catheter securely to the side, whether or not the partner will be involved in assisting with treatment. It should be possible to explain to the couple at this stage that CAPD need not interfere with sexual relations. Some nurses feel comfortable with addressing this subject, while others do not, particularly if the couple are old enough to be the nurse's parents. If possible, discussions touching on sexuality should be left to someone who is at ease with the topic, since reluctance or embarrassment is hard to disguise, and easily transmitted to the patient.

HAEMODIALYSIS IN HOSPITAL

Patients go through a recognisable series of stages following the diagnosis of renal failure, similar to the responses to bereavement described by Kubler Ross (1970). These responses represent a process of adjustment to loss, starting with shock and numbness, followed by denial, bargaining, grief and anger, before reaching a degree of acceptance. Abram (1970) identified a second process of adjustment to the start of dialysis treatment. The stages may overlap, or fluctuate, as with the stages of bereavement, but can usually be identified by both staff and the patients themselves. At its most simple, the process has three phases as discussed below.

First phase: euphoria

Initially there is usually a sense of relief, for several reasons. First, after months or years of waiting in a kind of limbo, the hurdle of dialysis has been reached and cleared. Second, the patient may feel the benefit of treatment immediately, especially if uraemia was symptomatic, causing nausea and itching, or if breathlessness from pulmonary oedema was a problem. Third, the experience of haemodialysis is usually less traumatic than the patient had expected.

Second phase: depressive reaction

The second stage follows fairly quickly. The novelty of treatment wears off; the limitations, frustrations and the time involved begin to take their toll and the realisation that this situation will continue indefinitely starts to sap patients' reserves of endurance. In addition, although no longer frankly uraemic, patients are aware that dialysis cannot make them feel fully well. Tiredness, lack of energy and enthusiasm for life, irritability, poor sleep and low-grade depression make life on dialysis hard to tolerate, especially for those who expected to feel miraculously better. The partner and family are also likely to feel the strain and relationships may suffer. The effort of trying to continue with work while under these pressures may seem to be too much, and the patient doubts whether employment will be possible, and fears the financial and family consequences if work has to be abandoned. Those who had been full of determination not to let dialysis affect or interfere with their lives have to concede defeat: it is not possible to remain unaffected. This stage may last weeks or months, and needs to be handled with tolerance and understanding by all staff.

Third phase: realistic adjustment

If adjustment goes to plan, the patient gradually accepts the inevitable limitations, while making the most of the remaining possibilities. Hobbies, habits and roles at home may have to change. Alternative sources of satisfaction and enjoyment need to be discovered and exploited, but all this takes time and may need to be actively encouraged by staff. In the interim, support and consistency from the team provide the framework within which the patient learns to come to terms with a changed lifestyle.

It is not surprising that, during this period of adjustment, the patient may be low in mood, irritable, quick to take offence and sometimes unwilling to follow medical advice. It is easy for staff to find this unattractive and 'ungrateful', especially when dialysis is a scarce and expensive resource, and staff are themselves highly pressurised and doing their best. Most patients do not find the dialysis itself a difficult ordeal, unless there are persistent problems with access or cramps, or frequent battles over excessive interdialytic weight gain. The factors most likely to produce irritation are delays, especially caused by the transport system or machines not being ready, changes of schedule due to pressures on dialysis places, and the unpredictability of minor setbacks such as access problems. The time involved in the whole process becomes a central focus for many patients, who resent the proportion of their life now dedicated to dialysis, in spite of the fact that it is dialysis that is making life possible at all. Some frustration is directed at staff, but patients are usually anxious not to alienate those who are caring for them, and to be 'good'. As a result, the spouse and family may take the brunt of the negative feelings and often lament that on hospital visits, the patient claims that all is well yet complains of numerous physical problems at home (Auer 1990b).

This pattern of reaction in the early months of haemodialysis applies to all age groups, but the negative effects are undoubtedly felt more by younger patients, who find the constraints more burdensome. It is normal for people in their 20s and 30s to be fully occupied with jobs, courtship and marriage, families and the fulfilment of ambitions. For the young person with renal failure, life had lain ahead of them, and that life plan has been brutally altered without the provision of an acceptable alternative. The only chance of re-establishing the course of events lies in the uncertain hope of receiving a good transplant. Sadly, this is not a planned event with a time scale within which to work (unless a living related donor is contemplated). Life for most of the young patients is, therefore, perceived as being 'on hold', and the longer the wait for a transplant, the more frustrated and downhearted they can become.

The young person

Many young patients find it hard to form relationships with the opposite sex, feeling that they have little to offer a prospective partner, and those who have a boyfriend or girlfriend often find their fears justified when relationships break up under the strain of the situation. Research such as the Oxford–Manchester study (Auer 1990a) suggests that younger patients, and particularly young men, find dependence on dialysis particularly frustrating, perhaps because society expects men to be more active, aggressive and ambitious in forging a role in life. It is certainly evident to those working in renal units that young male patients express more dissatisfaction, and are more likely to show this in non-compliant, self-destructive and despairing behaviour.

The middle–aged person

Middle-aged patients have usually established a role for themselves, and have achieved a number of their goals, such as marriage, family, a career and a home. From this base they are often, but not always, better able to adjust to limitations. For them, however, there is the fear of losing what has been achieved and being unable to carry out responsibilities to those who depend on them. Role changes within the family threaten the identity, pride and self-image of the patient, who does not wish to become a burden or liability. It is, however, comparatively rare for well-established relationships to break up in these circumstances. There is a taboo against leaving a sick partner that holds many couples together even in the most difficult situations. Marriages are, however, put under pressure, especially when sexual contact becomes diminished or non-existent.

The older person

Reasonably fit elderly people are in some ways the most satisfied group (Auer 1986, Westlie et al 1984). The attitude of many elderly patients is that they have already 'had a good life' and have reached an age when death would not be unlikely in any case. They have not been cheated of a normal lifespan by their illness. To be given the chance of a further few years due to dialysis is a bonus to those who still have an appetite for life. Those in their 70s and 80s probably do not want to pursue very strenuous activities, preferring a little gardening, cooking, and the company of friends and family. Those who live alone and feel isolated regard the trips to the hospital for treatment as a welcome social activity. A number who have never had help with daily living – home adaptations and home help, or meals from Social Services – receive this for the first time following contact with the hospital. Staff should, however, remain sensitive to the problems of elderly patients, particularly depression, and be aware that the patient may wish to discuss the option of withdrawal from treatment. If patients know that this is an option and understand that the unit would support them and their families following such a decision, this knowledge is often enough to provide them with the will to carry on. Knowing that one is in control of the situation, rather than trapped in a system, is reassuring. (See section on withdrawal from dialysis, on p. 93)

HOME HAEMODIALYSIS

A number of patients, especially those for whom an early transplant is unlikely and who wish to continue full-time work, opt to perform haemodialysis at home. Although the numbers entering home haemodialysis programmes are declining overall, this is still a good option for those who have strong motivation and good reasons for wanting the flexibility of this type of dialysis (Courts 2000). It is rarely the best treatment for very frail elderly patients, especially if assisted by an elderly spouse who may find the treatment stressful to learn and to supervise. From the psychological point of view, it is essential to offer good back-up to home patients, including respite treatment in hospital to give the spouse or assistant a break from time to time. It is also advisable, wherever possible, to ensure that at least two home assistants are available in case one is ill or wishes to be away at a certain time. As was stated earlier, patients may be far more negative and demanding towards family members than is evident in the unit, and one should not underestimate the burden that the spouse may be carrying.

Early research comparing quality of life on different types of renal replacement therapy suggested that home haemodialysis offers the greatest scope for pursuing normal life, including employment, with quality-of-life scores comparable to those of transplanted patients. More recently, Lunts (1999) describes how home haemodialysis is a viable and often optimal therapy for many patients.

PERITONEAL DIALYSIS

Those on PD usually experience the same phases of psychological adjustment as haemodialysis patients, that is, an initial honeymoon period, followed by a depressive phase that may last for weeks or months. The chief difference between the two treatment patterns is that the patient on PD is performing dialysis at home, rather than being in regular contact with nurses in the unit. The depression is, therefore, less likely to be noticed or openly discussed with staff. Patients, and spouses or carers, often suffer in silence during this period of adjustment. The problems are greatly reduced if the unit has community nurses able to do regular home visits.

PD training

The greatest dilemma in teaching the techniques of CAPD and other PD therapies is to strike a balance between promoting a consistent, safe and meticulous technique, while encouraging enough flexibility and latitude to enable the patient to explore the potential for freedom that the treatment allows. Younger patients who opt for PD in order to carry on with full-time employment are likely to use the possibilities fully, after a short period of 'feeling their way'. Most take holidays away from home, go away for weekends, and can tell stories of unlikely places in which they have successfully performed an exchange. It is harder to encourage elderly patients to do the same. Many feel that it is unsafe to attempt an exchange in unfamiliar surroundings and develop an almost superstitious fear of altering the circumstances of the exchange in any way. Some say that performing the four daily exchanges has become a way of life in itself rather than a means to an end.

Patients who are doing well on PD and making the treatment work for them may show this by devising compact travelling exchange kits, with ingenious ways of warming and hanging the bags, and portable surfaces that can be kept clean, such as a large plastic table mat. Such patients will be proud to show staff how they have found ways of solving problems. They also display confidence in the way they dress, finding flattering but convenient clothing, and taking trouble with grooming. In contrast, patients who are doing less well, and may benefit from advice and counselling, take little pride in their appearance, seldom or never travel with the treatment, and become housebound and isolated. Extrovert characteristics seem to be a great benefit, since such patients are not too shy or inhibited to perform exchanges in places where they may be seen by others. A few patients are so shy that they would rather not be seen dialysing even by family members, particularly children and grandchildren. Because they regard the exchange as an excretory function (which is, in many respects, true), they feel that it should be performed in private. (Those on haemodialysis may not see the treatment as excretory, even though the same process of waste removal is taking place.) The PD nurse who is sensitive to signs of good or poor adjustment to treatment is able to reinforce and encourage sensible and flexible use of this type of dialysis.

The individual and intensive training needed to prepare a patient to perform PD safely at home allows the formation of a strong supportive bond with the nurse, probably a closer relationship than that formed in the haemodialysis unit. In a recent survey of 65 patients (33 on PD and 32 on haemodialysis) who started treatment in the last year in the author's unit, the question 'Do you feel that you receive enough information about your treatment?' received a 'Yes' from 94% of PD patients and 69% of haemodialysis patients. Similarly, the question 'Do you feel you receive enough support?' received a 'Yes' from 85% of PD patients and only 63% of haemodialysis patients. This probably reflects good initial contacts with PD staff and a sense of continued support via phone calls to the unit whenever required. This 'accessibility' of the PD nurse is important, because patients discharged home on PD might otherwise feel more isolated and unsupported by the unit than those attending for regular haemodialysis. Visits from a community nephrology nurse are a regular procedure in some units, and are much appreciated by patients and spouses. At the very least, a visit to the patient's home is desirable before PD therapy starts. The equipment takes up a lot of space and it may be impossible to store a month's supply of fluids at a time. Such initial assessment visits should ideally be made by the social worker, occupational therapist and a community renal nurse together, so that advice can be given on performing exchanges, possible adaptations to the home if needed and any community support that may be available.

Automated peritoneal dialysis (APD) is now offered to most patients who want to keep the day free, though some, especially men and heavier patients generally, need to do a manual exchange around teatime to supplement the overnight treatment. From the social and psychological point of view, there are both benefits and disadvantages. There is increased freedom during the day, but at night the noise of the machine and its alarms can cause disturbance to the partner, and inhibit spontaneous lovemaking. Most spouses get used to the background noise, but a few opt to move into a separate room, which cuts down the physical contact and reassurance between the partners (Auer 2005).

GENERAL PROBLEMS AFFECTING PSYCHOLOGICAL WELL-BEING

SEXUAL PROBLEMS AND LOW FERTILITY

Renal failure affects both sexual desire and the ability to engage in sexual intercourse. Estimates of the problem are likely to be inaccurate owing to unwillingness to discuss this symptom – more often on the part of the staff than the patients; however, it is generally accepted that 70% of male patients suffer from a degree of impotence, and a similar proportion of female patients have problems with arousal and reaching orgasm. The reasons for this are likely to be multifactorial.

Physical causes may include the following factors:

- hormone imbalance
- anaemia leading to tiredness
- the effect of drugs, especially some antihypertensive medication
- vascular problems affecting blood flow to the genital area
- neuropathy, especially in those with diabetes, lowering sensitivity to sexual stimuli.

Psychological causes often compound and contribute to the problem:

- depression
- poor self-image/body image
- role changes, leading to dependence and lack of confidence in sexual identity
- sense of guilt towards the partner.

When sexual relations are rare or absent, affectionate touching and cuddling frequently stop as well, leading to further impoverishment of the physical relationship.

Physical problems leading to impotence in men can often be successfully treated. Efficient dialysis and treatment of anaemia with erythropoietin may be enough to restore sexual function. If there are still problems with achieving or maintaining an erection, there are several possible approaches to treatment. These include vacuum devices, insertion of prostaglandin pellets into the penis, injections into the base of the penis, and the drug sildenafil (Viagra), which is now licensed for the treatment of male renal patients. It is important that men with sexual problems are referred for help, because the effect of impotence on confidence and identity, let alone relationships with the spouse or partner, seriously affects well-being and happiness (Case study 3.1).

Treatment of loss of desire in women has received far less attention. There are currently trials of sildenafil to study whether increased blood supply to the genital area improves sexual response and lubrication, but in 2001 the drug is not yet licensed for treatment of female sexual problems. If female patients feel able to engage in intercourse, it is possible to maintain the physical bond with their partner, even if they do not themselves experience sexual satisfaction (Case study 3.2). Artificial lubrication may be necessary to prevent discomfort.

In women, the major issue affecting self-image is loss of fertility (irregular or absent ovulation and menstruation, and the knowledge that, while on dialysis, conception is unlikely and a successful pregnancy even more so).

Psychological problems leading to difficulties in sexual relationships are often much improved following discussion with a counsellor. This should preferably involve both partners, to achieve communication between the couple. It is often very reassuring for the fit partner to receive confirmation that it is the illness, rather than a decrease in affection, that is the cause of reduced or absent sexual interest. If affectionate touching has ceased it can be encouraged, strengthening the physical bond, and in some cases, occasional successful love-making results, with or without penetration.

Most of the problems described here are improved or eliminated following a successful transplant, although vascular problems and neuropathy associated with diabetes may continue to compromise sexual activity.

Case study 3.1

The 40-year-old wife of a long-standing haemodialysis patient contacted the renal sexual counsellor, owing to her extreme frustration. She explained that they had not had intercourse for over 2 years. She felt angry and irritable, both with her husband and her children. She also felt guilty, because it was not her husband's fault that he had kidney failure and no longer showed any interest in sexual relations.

During discussion with the couple, the counsellor asked the patient if he ever had an erection. He replied that he occasionally had a partial erection, in the early hours of the morning. The patient's wife was astonished, and asked why he had not told her about this. The patient pointed out that she had been taking sleeping pills for a long time, and was hard to wake, let alone sexually arouse, at 5 or 6 o'clock in the morning! The patient's wife immediately stopped taking the sleeping pills and the couple were able to report successful love-making a week later.

It is often useful for patients and their spouses to talk to a counsellor, because they start to communicate about their problem, which may be easy to improve or solve with simple adjustment in behaviour.

Case study 3.2

In conversation with the renal counsellor, a female haemodialysis patient, aged 45, mentioned that her husband was 'very good and caring' towards her, and never asked for sexual relations. The counsellor suggested that, if she felt able to do so, the patient should initiate love-making herself, even though she was no longer able to get aroused. This would be a way of reassuring her husband of her love, and thanking him for his care and consideration. The patient was sceptical about this, but a few months later called into the office. She said that she had taken the advice and just wanted to say 'thank you', because the effect upon the relationship had been very beneficial. 'He was so thrilled', she said, 'it has really brought our marriage to life again'.

It is also possible that it prevented this husband from getting so frustrated that he looked elsewhere for the physical warmth he needed.

BODY IMAGE

Both dialysis treatment and transplantation affect body image, making patients feel different, unattractive and ill at ease within their own bodies.

Access surgery often results in multiple scarring, involving the arms, chest and abdomen. A fistula, which is regarded as 'very good' by nursing staff, can be seen as a horrible disfigurement by the patient, who may try to conceal it from friends and the curious stares of strangers. Staff become so used to central lines that they forget the response to these outside the hospital. Patients with fistulae and grafts have even been thought to be drug addicts by the public, owing to the effects of multiple cannulation.

The Tenckhoff catheter is less evident to outsiders, but patients may be convinced that they look strange and that everybody is aware of this. Many feel embarrassed in front of their partners and feel that nobody could find them attractive any more. Some even imagine that the catheter smells offensive and that others are repelled. Most of these problems are subjective and reflect the patients' own attitude to and disgust with their own body.

Following transplantation, the immunosuppressive drugs, especially steroids, change the face, so that patients may feel they no longer recognise their image in the mirror as being the person they knew (Case study 3.3). In addition, the texture of the skin and hair changes, and hair grows in unwanted places, such as the eyebrows and cheeks. It is important to reassure patients that, as a general rule, these effects become less obvious as the drugs are reduced. However, in those cases where appearance remains changed, ongoing support and advice may be necessary.

Confidence and a sense of our own identity depend on a clear image of how we appear, both to ourselves and to others. If the integrity of this self-image is violated in some way, by drugs, surgery or even the distortions we mistakenly apply to ourselves, it can lead to severe psychological damage.

Case study 3.3

Following a transplant, a middle-aged man chose to grow a beard. When complimented on this, he replied that he had been forced into the decision, because he was unable to bear seeing his reflection in the mirror when shaving.

'It is no longer me that I see. I cannot recognise the face in the mirror and this frightens me', he said. After a year, when the effects of the immunosuppressive drugs had decreased, he was able to shave off his beard.

It is common to assume that women are more affected than men by their body image, but this is by no means always the case.

AWARENESS OF EARLY DEATH

Those who have a life-threatening illness such as renal failure live on 'the edge', maintained on a life-support system. Such patients are bound to be more than usually aware of the fragility of life and the possibility of early death. Although there are some who spend many decades on dialysis or with a transplant, and approach a normal span of life, statistically these are the exception. For the young patient, the diagnosis is more devastating than for someone in their 70s or 80s, who could expect to die within a decade in any case. Most patients cope by putting the thought out of their minds as far as possible, but there are gloomy reminders on visits to hospital, when friends or acquaintances are found to have suffered complications or died. Most wonder whether they will be next. Dialysis patients form a close community who know, better than most, 'not to ask for whom the bell tolls, for it tolls for thee'.

This predicament can lead to mental conflict – whether to make hay while the sun shines, by living life to the full and risking the consequences, or to live a restricted life observing all the rules, which may offer a longer life, but without the fun or range of experiences that others can enjoy. The most successful patients seem to be those who find a coping mechanism by balancing between the two extremes. Sadly, patients cannot control everything that happens, even if they try to follow all advice. The condition is 'perverse' and frustrating (Hooper 1994). More than most of us, those with renal failure have to learn to live with uncertainty about the future.

The young patient with no ties or emotional attachments is often considered to be at a disadvantage but, paradoxically, the happiness of marriage and children carries its own price in suffering – there is so much more to lose (Case study 3.4).

FAILURE TO TAKE MEDICAL/NURSING ADVICE – NON-ADHERENCE

Few patients take all the advice that is given by medical and nursing staff, or follow instructions all the time. This probably represents a healthy

Case study 3.4

A man of 38, who had been on haemodialysis since the age of 14, was referred during an admission for a hip replacement. He had been very active and had always managed to stay in employment as well as doing voluntary work. Bone disease had made him increasingly disabled and he had recently started to use a wheelchair. A few years ago he had married, and he and his wife had had a child by donor insemination. He was thrilled at the birth of the child – a little boy, now aged three – and was a devoted father. Now, with time on his hands owing to his hospital admission, he had become acutely aware of the possibility – in fact, the likelihood – of early death, which would prevent him seeing this child grow to adulthood. He wanted to care for his wife and son over the span of a normal marriage, but the illness had denied him this natural expectation. 'It was bad enough', he said, 'when I only had myself to worry about. When I got married, I had my wife's needs and feelings to take into account. She would suffer by my death. Now that I have a child, it is the greatest joy of my life, but he is so little and vulnerable. How can he understand about my illness? The thought that I will not be there to protect him and see him grow up is absolutely unbearable'.

There is no answer or true comfort to offer in this situation. The counsellor suggested that he should write letters to his son, to be kept for the future, saying the things he would like the child to know. These could be tailored to different ages - perhaps a letter for a 5-year-old, a 10-year-old, and so on. In this way he could be sure that the boy was aware of his father's love and concern, even if he was no longer living.

and adaptive sign rather than otherwise, unless, of course, patients put themselves at serious risk. Those with renal failure have little chance of disguising the fact that they are failing to follow advice, because blood results, blood pressure and weight gain reveal underdialysis and diet and fluid abuses, as well as failure to take medication.

Within reason, such 'non-adherence' may be a good sign. Obsessional concern with the illness and treatment is not a desirable outcome. However, persistent non-adherence to a dangerous level, often for no discernible reason, is cause for serious investigation. The commonest causes appear to be the following.

- A lack of understanding, either of the instructions themselves, or of the implications of not following them. Much of the advice to renal patients takes into account that the condition is long-term. There is often no immediate perceived consequence of failure to take advice (e.g. drugs to protect the bones or antihypertensive medication). This can lead to the patient assuming that the drugs are having no effect. The long-term effects on the heart, produced by habitual fluid overload, are also hard to appreciate. The patient may feel that fluid abuse merely leads to a short lecture and a little longer on dialysis, and regard this as a worthwhile price to pay for a good night out. On an occasional basis, this may be a sensible attitude, but it easily becomes a habit.
- Depression – apathy about treatment and life in general. Since life is barely tolerable, it really does not matter greatly if one takes risks with it.
- A negative, and in some ways emotionally regressed sense of defiance, often directed against what is seen as 'nagging' by staff. Many adult patients will not have been 'told what to do' in a motherly or teacher-like fashion since they were children.

- Denial – underlying denial there is often desperation. The patient is aware of the reality of the situation but cannot bear to face it squarely. Acting as if the painful situation does not exist enables the patient to maintain a fantasy that is bearable. Denial is not always dysfunctional. It can be a useful coping mechanism. In dying patients, for example, those who maintain hope and act as if life is going to carry on may make things easier for themselves (and those around them), although there may be problems in realistic communication of feelings and planning for the future. Denial in the dialysis situation may, however, make it impossible for patients and relatives to discuss the illness on a realistic basis, and can become a threat if it leads to behaviour that is a risk to life (Case study 3.5).

One can only sympathise with both nurses and patients in the whole subject of non-adherence. Dialysis nurses are in a highly stressful job with a high technical component and limited time to interact with individual patients, yet have prolonged contact, over months or years. They are unable to 'cure' their patients and, therefore, have very specific target outcomes, gaining their satisfaction and measuring their own success by the efficiency and efficacy of the dialysis process. Nurses who have one or a number of patients who seem to be wilfully denying them that satisfaction are at high risk of engaging in a personal battle, which can culminate in frustration, anger and burn-out. One patient is often singled out as the nurse's personal crusade, waged, of course for the good of that patient and, therefore, utterly justified. Sadly, we do not like our 'failures' but cannot let go of them either! The struggle is likely to descend to the level of the school playground: 'Go on, kill yourself, see if I care!' becomes the nurse's unspoken response to the patient's 'One in the eye for the staff!'

Case study 3.5

A young man of 28 was referred owing to serious abuse of his fluid limits. He frequently attended for dialysis with 5–6 L of fluid weight gain, which was beginning to cause cardiac enlargement.

During discussion of the long-term effects of this, he said: 'It is as much as I can do to think about surviving from day to day. I cannot even *begin* to think about several years in the future. Whatever I do, I probably won't live that long in any case, so I might as well enjoy things today'. After further discussion of his attitudes to treatment and underlying feelings, he added: 'I hate the way the nurses nag me. I wonder how they would cope? They make me really angry. So now, when I come in with several kilos extra fluid, I think…'that's one in the eye for staff!'

If adherence becomes a battle between the patient and the staff, it is a battle that is already lost. Patients can only be told the consequences of their actions. After that, it is up to them to decide what to do.

The depressive reaction is most commonly seen in older patients, and defiance and denial are usually seen in younger patients. All these reactions seem to be indirect appeals for help and need to be treated as such. Anger from staff, threats of dire consequences or lectures on the behaviour expected of a dialysis patient are unlikely to be helpful. Naturally, patients need to be given a clear explanation of the reasons for the rules that are set, and the possible results and risks that they run in choosing to break those rules, but they also need to have their underlying motives and feelings explored and respected. Some of the causes for distress may be alleviated by counselling, changes in medication, adjustment of dialysis regime or other measures. It is always helpful to focus on what *can* rather than cannot be had or done.

WITHDRAWAL FROM DIALYSIS

This decision may be taken by a patient at any age, but is most frequent in elderly patients, who are sometimes very poorly adjusted to life on treatment. This may be due to depression following bereavement or experiencing additional medical problems, such as stroke, malignancies, amputations and ischaemic heart disease, which further restrict their quality of life. Such patients may wish to withdraw from dialysis, a subject that needs sympathetic exploration. If found to be a considered and serious wish rather than an expression of frustration or an oblique request for a particular problem to be recognised, such requests to withdraw from treatment should be supported and respected. Dialysis may prove to be an intolerable burden to those who have other reasons to feel that life no longer offers any opportunities and satisfactions. Some bitterly resent the limitations of the ageing process, cannot adjust to being a 'spectator' and wish only to turn back the clock. In a minority of cases, it is overwhelmingly the fear of dying rather than a wish to live that makes the patient continue with dialysis, making it hard to achieve any real life satisfaction.

It is common for renal unit staff to feel that the treatment of very frail older people, especially those with multiple medical problems, by means of a scarce and expensive resource such as hospital haemodialysis, is unjustified. If little or no subjective quality of life results, it would be hard to disagree. It is very important that we explore the attitudes of elderly patients, and do not carry on with treatment that is giving no quality of life, remembering, however, that quality of life is a subjective matter, and only the person concerned can tell whether life is worth living. One can be surprised both by the apparently full life that is unacceptable to one patient, and by the apparently burdensome life that is regarded as worthwhile by another. Respecting these views can be difficult, especially in the case of the patient who seems to have a good life, yet wishes to discontinue treatment. Kaplan De Nour (1994) concludes that the answer to the question 'Is it all worth the effort – is machine-dependent life worth living?' lies in the psychological condition of the patient rather than any objective quality of life.

SPECIAL PROBLEMS OF PEOPLE FROM ETHNIC MINORITIES

Members of Asian and Afro-Caribbean ethnic groups have a higher incidence of renal failure than the Caucasian UK population (Bradley 2000). This seems to be connected to the greater prevalence of diabetes in the Asian community, especially in those past the age of 40, and a higher incidence of hypertension in the Afro-Caribbean population.

In order to allow patients from cultural backgrounds other than the UK to obtain equal benefits from the healthcare system, it is important to be aware of factors that could affect the situation. These include:

- language and understanding
- dietary differences
- attitudes to illness
- family relationships.

It is difficult enough for members of the multidisciplinary team to communicate fully and effectively with those of the same cultural background and language, let alone those who have language problems and different cultural concepts. It is necessary to remain sensitive to the effects of ethnicity, both on understanding and attitudes to illness and treatment (Allison et al 1983).

LANGUAGE

The most obvious of these is language. Elderly Indian, Pakistani and Chinese patients, for example, often rely on younger family members for the translation of interviews with medical and nursing staff, and to relay information on symptoms and feelings. Medical advice and information are also given via a third party and may suffer in translation. It is advisable to have a qualified interpreter for any sensitive and important communication, since family members may be too involved to give an impartial and accurate interpretation, relaying nuances of meaning.

All patient information material needs to be available in translation, but it is necessary to check reading ability rather than assuming that by giving a leaflet one has imparted the information.

DIET

Diet, which plays a major role in the management of renal disease, can be a source of considerable problems. Most renal diets are based on native UK eating habits, and are hard to adjust to the religious and cultural requirements of other countries. Many Asian patients prefer to have food brought in by the family during hospital admissions. Those on PD who are vegetarian have a greater need to maintain adequate protein intake, and sometimes find it hard to do so when pulses are their major source of dietary protein. Specialist dietetic advice is necessary to achieve good serum albumin levels in such diets (see Ch. 11).

ATTITUDES TO ILLNESS

It is usual for Asian families to take a major part in the everyday care of a sick family member (whether at home or in hospital), and for a number of relatives, both young and old, to spend a lot of time at the bedside. Staff used to the less involved attitude of many native UK families may find this unusual or inconvenient, especially if there is a lack of space and facilities on the ward.

Attitudes to illness, and even the conceptual understanding of disease and treatment, may differ from culture to culture, needing the sensitive understanding of the nurse. Cause and effect may be differently perceived. Religious acceptance of illness as a predestined fate to be accepted without attempts to change matters is a further concept that may cause misunderstandings. Culturally acceptable responses to illness may also differ from country to country. An Asian patient will often cover the whole body, including the head, with a blanket, making some staff and other patients uneasy and puzzled. Accepted responses to pain may also differ from one ethnic group to another, leading to an overestimation or underestimation of the subjective suffering involved.

Some ethnic groups may have religious or cultural beliefs about cadaver or living related grafts. Even if these problems do not apply, the likelihood of a well-matched graft is reduced for patients from an ethnic minority, whose tissue type may be uncommon in the UK. There are major initiatives by the Department of Health to promote both cadaver and living related donation of kidneys in the ethnic minority population, in the hope of increasing transplantation rates in these groups – the fastest-growing section of the transplant waiting list in the UK.

It is important that all members of the team remain sensitive, both to the needs of the patients and families and to their own attitudes.

FAMILY RELATIONSHIPS

The family structure and hierarchy should also be taken into account, since some cultures regard any major decision as traditionally the preserve of the senior male member of the family present, leading to unwillingness on the part of a female patient to determine her own preference or accept responsibility without consultation with a husband, father, uncle or son.

It can be difficult to understand Asian family structure and relationships since, in many families, anyone with a family connection tends to be designated 'a cousin', even, in some cases, where there is no relationship. (In native UK culture the same pattern leads us to call close family friends 'uncles' and 'aunties', without explaining that the title is 'honorary'.) Many patients have relatives, including spouses, in their country of origin and like to visit them every few years. It can, therefore, be very traumatic to have an illness that precludes travel owing to lack of medical facilities at home. If elderly parents die, and the patient is unable to return for the funeral, there can be great distress, not only because of the natural pain of bereavement, but because of the religious implications of duty and respect, which carry greater significance than in Western culture.

TRANSPLANTATION

From what has already been said about the stresses of life on dialysis, it is obvious that, for many patients, dialysis is a period of 'marking time' while awaiting transplantation. Almost every study of quality of life so far has shown that successful transplantation offers the best chance of leading a near-normal life, and is associated with the highest perceived life satisfaction. Objectively, the quality (although, contrary to the belief of some patients, not the quantity) of life is greatly increased. Successful transplantation is associated with a number of benefits, including:

- higher chance of employment
- greater energy
- improved mental alertness and concentration
- freedom from a restrictive diet
- the return, in most cases, of sexual capacity
- the possibility of child-bearing.

It would, however, be misleading to regard even successful transplantation as a panacea. Following transplantation, the patient with ERF needs to feel that life is wonderful. A successful transplant is, after all, the nearest to normality that the patient will ever achieve, and has often been the long-awaited 'answer' to the patient's problems; so, from a psychological point of view the patient has a need to feel that life has been transformed. The reality is sometimes rather different. Those who want to return to employment find that, although declared fit by the doctor, the view of prospective employers is less enthusiastic. Many find it hard to get a job in competition with others. Therefore, the financial position is worse than on dialysis in the UK because disability benefits are often withdrawn and the patient can only claim basic unemployment benefit. Relationships sometimes become strained, because less tolerance is now shown by spouses and families. The individual requiring dialysis has every right to claim that life is a burden, but gradually and subtly, sympathy is withdrawn from the transplant patient, who should after all be 'grateful for the gift of life', which, whether this is actually stated or not, is seen to have been won at the cost of the death of a cadaveric donor or through the sacrifice of a living relative. This can be a hard gift to accept, carrying with it a burden of responsibility to make the suffering of others worthwhile. Patients who lose their grafts quite often feel that they have let down not only the team caring for them, but also the donor and donor family.

Immediately post-transplant, provided all goes well, there is usually a euphoric phase, possibly accentuated by steroid immunosuppression, and the sudden 'clearing of the mind' reported by many patients, which has never been fully explained. This is mixed with anxiety that rejection will occur and the graft will be lost. One of the hardest aspects of this stage is the sudden removal of conscious control. Dialysis patients have been conditioned to be very much in control of their health through adherence to diet and fluid restrictions, a regular treatment regime, scrupulous care of access, and weight and blood pressure measurement. After a transplant, the situation changes dramatically. Apart from regularly taking immunosuppressive medication and attending for follow-up, patients' contribution to the survival of the graft is minimal. They are, as it were, at the mercy of factors beyond conscious control – their own immune response and the effects of the foreign body, which now needs to become accepted as part of the self. It is no wonder that many patients become acutely superstitious (the natural human response to forces that cannot be influenced by reason or action). Anxiety can reach almost obsessional levels and may become displaced from the transplant itself to attach to other health concerns.

The side-effects of immunosuppression for some may cause little distress, but for others have a considerable psychological effect and, in a very few, produce a psychotic response. The commonest effects are upon body image. Cushingoid changes in the appearance are distressing to both sexes. Facial hair and changes in hair texture are more distressing to women. Many men choose to grow a beard following transplant, chiefly to disguise the 'moon face'. Weight gain as a result of appetite increase on steroids compounds the body-image problem. Ciclosporin has many advantages as an immunosuppressive agent but patients can be very distressed by the tremor sometimes associated with this drug.

A good counselling programme should be provided, including access to advice on facial hair removal, treatment for changes in skin texture and advice on skin care to help avoid malignant changes stimulated by exposure to sun. The creation of a positive body image after transplantation is every bit as important as on dialysis.

Counselling may also be needed to help with emotional oversensitivity at this time. Both male and female patients who regarded themselves as previously emotionally controlled are sometimes surprised to find themselves liable to tearful episodes and mood swings, partly due to the drugs and partly due to the very considerable inner turmoil created by the experience of transplantation. The need for sympathetic reassurance and support from the transplant team in the early stages cannot be overestimated.

It is comparatively common for young women who are keen to have children to become pregnant soon after having a transplant. Often they are unmarried and unsupported. It seems that the desire to have a baby overrides all other considerations for these women, and that rational arguments and advice are unlikely to have any part to play against such an imperative. Fear of losing the graft, damaging their own health, risking stillbirth or a seriously premature child, let alone the problems of trying to care for a baby without the security of a permanent relationship, seem completely unimportant. Grafts can be lost due to the strain of pregnancy, especially when undertaken less than a year after transplantation. While it is essential to counsel young women on the risks, advise on birth control and advocate a reasonable delay before becoming pregnant, it seems unlikely that this will prevent some of them from seizing what they see as their only chance of having a child, regardless of the consequences. It is a further way of ratifying their 'normality' following the very artificial and restricted life on dialysis. In the few cases where termination is performed, the feelings of ambivalence are likely to be severe, and may even be directed against the graft itself, whose survival has been protected at the expense of the child.

GRAFT LOSS

The patient whose graft is rapidly rejected experiences an acute disappointment, but is in many ways better able to recover and come to terms with the situation than the patient who has several months of unsatisfactory graft function before finally returning to dialysis. In such cases, there may have been heavy courses of methylprednisolone or monoclonal antibodies, numerous biopsies and possibly further surgery to no avail, resulting in a state of physical debility and mental anguish far worse than before the operation. Such patients often say at the time that they regret ever having tried transplantation, yet the great majority return to the transplant list within a few months.

PATIENTS WITH MULTIPLE PATHOLOGY

There are increasing numbers of patients now receiving dialysis for whom renal failure is the most treatable aspect of a serious systemic illness, such as diabetes, scleroderma, primary amyloid or myeloma. A further large patient group consists of those with generalised vascular disease. The complications of these underlying conditions are responsible for many long hospital admissions, and a great deal of the morbidity and mortality of patients on dialysis programmes.

The patient with diabetes can be particularly hard to counsel and distressing to nurse. As the disease reaches its late phases, one has no sooner supported a patient through the loss of one limb, when the next becomes problematic. Eyesight may already have been poor, only to be followed by total blindness. Autonomic neuropathy may then lead to diarrhoea and incontinence, and inability to maintain blood pressure when changing position.

As with all those on renal replacement therapy, there are two important aspects for nursing and other staff to consider: the psychological impact of the illness and the practical arrangements that may be necessary to enable the patient to spend time at home. Patients who are aware that their underlying condition is fatal, and that dialysis is a means of prolonging life in the short term, need every help to spend as little time in hospital as possible. This entails involving community nursing, occupational therapists, physiotherapists and care managers from Social Services to provide a package of care. This may involve visits from home-care staff several times a day, the provision of meals, day-centre attendance, respite care in nursing homes and the provision of equipment such as stair lifts, rails and ramps for wheelchair access.

There is occasionally some conflict with community nurses and carers, who express the opinion that the patient is not well enough to be out of hospital, and that it is 'too risky' for the patient to be at home. In their opinion, the patient might fall, sustain fractures, succumb to a massive haemorrhage or a cardiovascular crisis, or have some other medical emergency. This is, of course, true, but the philosophy of renal units can be at odds with the 'normal' world. Our patients would all have perished without renal replacement. They are alive against the odds and, for them, a degree of risk is an acceptable price to pay for seizing the chance to experience life outside the hospital. A more lengthy admission is unlikely to reduce the chance of sudden and maybe fatal complications. If patients are happy to take that risk, they need our support.

The strain on spouses and family members is considerable. Many will have jobs and family responsibilities, and may feel guilty if they do not put the patient's needs above their own. Support needs to be given to relatives in this situation, to reduce guilt wherever possible. This entails allowing opportunities for the expression of feelings and encouraging relatives to set aside time for themselves. Some will, for example, visit daily from long distances during the patient's admissions to hospital – a time when there is the chance for carers to recharge their own batteries, take much-needed relaxation or catch up with other tasks. This is also a time when unfinished business may need to be resolved. This may be in the form of reconciling old family differences and feuds to secure the future for those who will be left when the patient has died. Another aspect of this may be the desire of common-law partners to marry.

Staff need to be aware of the patient's state of mind, and ready to hear the message that the patient has had enough. It is not unreasonable to choose death from uraemia in preference to a short period of further suffering before succumbing to a more distressing end to life. Some, it is true, are never able to let go, but others may wish to do so while they are still capable of determining their own destiny through rational decision. It may, however, be hard to express this to staff who are unwilling to hear.

ACUTE RENAL FAILURE AND ACUTE PRESENTATION IN ESTABLISHED RENAL FAILURE

Patients with acute renal failure often come to the renal ward via intensive therapy units, following overwhelming illnesses. Illness severe enough to cause acute renal failure requiring dialysis or haemofiltration is always a crisis for patient and relatives, attended by high levels of anxiety. This is justified, since the mortality in such patients is very high. Once the precipitating illness is controlled and the patient's condition is stable, concern is transferred to the renal failure, and whether the kidneys will recover. During this period, patient and relatives often need emotional support from staff, and reassurance that renal function is expected to return in spite of the need for dialysis over several weeks. From the psychological point of view, it is important to help the spouse to visit as often as possible, both for the sake of the patient and the partner.

Providing support

It is always recognised that children need a parent to be with them, and that recovery is helped by the security this offers. It is seldom realised how lonely and frightened adults, especially if elderly, can become when seriously ill and separated from their partner and environment.

The patient is often admitted to a unit many miles from home, making visiting expensive. Help with transport costs should be sought from the Department of Social Security or charitable funding if hardship is suspected. It is not uncommon for the family of a critically ill patient, admitted for 3–4 weeks, to incur £300–£400 in visiting costs. Staff need to explore the possibilities for inexpensive accommodation in or near the hospital for relatives of such patients. When the patient is finally ready to leave hospital, it is important for a care manager to assess the home circumstances, since the illness may have had permanent debilitating effects. Preparation for this may help to mitigate the emotional blow of returning home, and finding that, while home is the same as ever, the person who left it a few weeks ago has changed. Following leg amputations, patients may show a reluctance to go on a visit home to assess future ability to cope. The 'safe and familiar place' has lost its ability to reassure, because it now contains challenges and hazards. Sensitivity, honesty and understanding are needed to build the confidence of patients who feel, rightly, that they will 'never be the same again'.

Despite attempts to improve early referral rates, through liaison with GP practices, many patients are still seen in a renal unit for the first time when at the point of needing renal replacement therapy. For these patients, the adjustment process is condensed into a very short period. Both responses to the diagnosis and adjustment to treatment itself are experienced concurrently, leading to greater problems with acceptance. In a retrospective study of those starting dialysis during the previous year in a large UK renal unit, higher current levels of depression and anxiety were reported by patients who had started treatment acutely, without time for psychological preparation (Auer et al 1995).

SUMMARY

The care of those with renal disease is a highly specialised area of nursing, with unique satisfactions and unique stresses. There is no other field of hospital nursing that involves such intensive involvement with patients over such long periods. High technology may appear to predominate but in spite of, or because of, the dependence of the patient on complicated artificial life-support systems, it is the quality of the human relationships created between the patient and the professional team that determines the success of the whole undertaking. Clinical skills are not enough to give the patient on dialysis the chance to live to the best potential. The commitment of both patient and team is, quite simply, lifelong. As a result, it is an unusually close relationship with all the benefits and disadvantages that this implies. Those who work in renal units have in common a sense of belonging to an extended family group. This is not to say that they are free of conflict, stresses and frustration, rather the reverse. Staff as well as patients need support, and many units recognise this and have good support systems, some formal, some informal.

It is not possible for the renal nurse to avoid a degree of personal involvement. Total detachment from a patient with whom the fight for survival is shared over months, years or even decades is scarcely a realistic proposition. Hospital staff cannot help but admire the tenacity and courage of patients and their spouses , feel frustrated by them and for them, and experience anger, exhausted patience, great sadness at battles lost and great happiness at battles won.

References

Abram HS, Moore GL, Westevelt FB. Suicidal behaviour in chronic dialysis patients. Am J Psychiatry 1971; 127: 1199–1204.

Abram HS. Survival by machine: the psychological stress of chronic haemodialysis. Psychiatr Med 1970; 1: 37.

Abram HS. The psychiatrist, the treatment of chronic renal failure and the prolongation of life. Am J Psychiatry 1969; 126: 57.

Allison M, Gregg D, Randell E et al. Social work with patients suffering from kidney disease and with their families. Birmingham: British Association of Social Workers, 1983.

Auer J, Charters V, Brownson A et al. Support and counselling pre-dialysis and on dialysis – need and outcome. Paper presented at EDTNA/ERCA Conference, Athens, 1995.

Auer J. Living well with kidney failure. London: Class Publishing, 2005: 87–88.

Auer J. Psychological aspects of elderly renal patients. In: Stevens E, Monkhouse P (eds) Aspects of renal care, Vol. 1. Eastbourne: Baillière Tindall, 1986: 200–208.

Auer J. Psychological problems in chronic illness. In: Badawi M, Biamonti B (eds) Social work practice in health care. Cambridge: Woodhead Faulkner, 1990b.

Auer J. The Oxford–Manchester study of dialysis patients: age, risk factors and treatment method in relation to quality of life. Scand J Urol Nephrol 1990a; 131(Suppl.): 31–37.

Binik YM, Devins GM, Barre PE et al. Live and learn: patient education delays the need to initiate renal replacement therapy in end stage renal disease. J Nerv Ment Dis 1993; 181: 371–376.

Bradley C, McGee H. Improving quality of life in renal failure: ways forward. In: McGee H, C. Bradley (eds) Quality of life following renal failure. Chur: Harwood Academic Publishers, 1994: 275–299.

Bradley J. Ethnic susceptibility to renal disease. Br J Renal Med 2000; 5: 4.

Chandra SM, Schulz J, Lawrence C, Greenwood RN, Farrington K. Is there a rationale for rationing chronic dialysis? A hospital based cohort study of factors affecting survival and morbidity? Br Med J 1999; 318: 217–223.

Courts NF. Psychosocial adjustment of patients on home hemodialysis and their dialysis partners. Clin Nurs Res 2000; 9:177–190.

Department of Health: The expert patient: a new approach to chronic disease management for the 21st century. London: Department of Health, 2001.

Gudex C. QALYs and their use by the health services. Discussion paper 20. York: University of York Centre for Health Economics, 1986.

Hooper G. Psychological care of patients in the renal unit. In: McGee H, Bradley C (eds) Quality of life following renal failure. Chur: Harwood Academic Publishers, 1994: 181–196.

Kaplan De Nour A, Czackes, JW. Emotional problems and reactions of the medical team in a chronic hemodialysis unit. Lancet 1968; ii: 987.

Kaplan De Nour A. Staff–patient interactions. In: NB Levy (ed.) Psychonephrology, Vol. 2. New York: Plenum, 1983.

Kaplan De Nour, A. Psychological social and vocational impact of renal failure. In: McGee H, Bradley C (eds) Quality of life following renal failure. Chur: Harwood Academic Publications, 1994: 33–42.

Klang B, Bjorvell H, Clyne N. Predialysis education helps patients choose dialysis modality and increases disease-specific knowledge. J Adv Nursing 1999; 29: 869–876.

Kline SA, Burton HJ, Akhtar M. The elderly patient on dialysis – psychosocial considerations. In: Oreopoulos DG (ed.) Geriatric nephrology. Boston: Nijhoff, 1986.

Kubler Ross E. On death and dying. London: Tavistock, 1970.

Kutner NG. Is there bias in treatment for renal failure? In: McGee H, Bradley C (eds) Quality of life following renal failure. Chur: Harwood Academic Publications, 1994: 161.

Levy JB, Chambers EJ, Brown EA. Supportive care for the renal patient. Nephrol Dial Transplant 2004; 19: 1357–1360.

Loomes G, McKenzie L. The use of QALYs in health care decision making. Soc Sci Med 1989; 28: 299–308.

Lunts P. Rediscovering home haemodialysis. Returning choice to patients. EDTNA/ERCA J 1999; XXV: 40–41.

Neu S, Kjellstrand CM. Stopping long-term dialysis. N Engl J Med 1986; 314: 14–20.

Quarello F, Piccoli GB, Bonello F et al. Dialysis in the elderly: ten year experience in a large population. Geriatr Nephrol Urol 1992; 2: 190–191.

Shambaugh P, Kanter S. Spouses under stress: group meetings with spouses of patients on haemodialysis. Am J Psychiatry 1969; 125: 7.

Smith C, daSilva-Gare M, Chandra S. Choosing not to dialyse: evaluation of planned non-dialytic management in a cohort of patients with end-stage renal failure. Nephron Clin Pract 2003; 95: c40–c6.

Stanton J. The cost of living: kidney dialysis, rationing and health economics in Britain, 1965–1996. Soc Sci Med 1999; 49: 1169–1182.

Stout JP, Auer J, Kincey J. Sexual and marital relationships and dialysis patients. Perit Dial Bull 1985; 7: 97–99.

Westlie L, Umen A, Nestrud S et al. Mortality, morbidity and life satisfaction in the very old dialysis patient. Trans Am Soc Art Intern Organs 1984; 30: 21–31.

Williams A. Economics of coronary artery bypass grafting. Br Med J 1985; 291: 326–329.

Further reading

McGee HM, Bradley C. Quality of life following renal failure. Chur: Harwood Academic Publishers, 1994.

Stein A, Wild J (eds) Kidney failure at your fingertips. London: Class Publishing, 2001.

Auer J. Living well with kidney failure. London: Class Publishing, 2005.

Chapter 4

Acute renal failure

Natasha McIntyre

CHAPTER CONTENTS

■ To understand the different types and causes of acute renal failure (ARF)
■ To help and support the patient and family during an episode of ARF
■ To describe the signs and symptoms of ARF
■ To analyse the nutritional requirements of those with ARF
■ To evaluate the various treatment options for ARF

**LEARNING OUTCOMES
FOR THIS CHAPTER**

INTRODUCTION

Since the kidney has multiple functions, the patient with acute renal failure (ARF), also referred to as acute renal injury (ARI), will often present the nurse with a complex scenario (Sinert et al 2001). Despite the availability of various dialysis treatments and different drug therapies, these patients face a mortality rate of up to 50% and, for those who are critically ill, up to 85% (Chen et al 2001).

Acute renal failure has often been defined as a sudden deterioration in renal function that results in the inability to excrete the products of metabolism. In turn, this produces a rise in blood urea and other nitrogen waste products (Dauguirdas 2000). Depending on its severity and duration, ARF is often transient in nature and, with careful nursing care, the patient can regain normal renal function. However, without appropriate specialised treatment, the patient may be denied the opportunity to make a full recovery and a precipitation of further impairment may lead to chronic or established renal failure (ERF).

The aim of this chapter is to emphasise the vital role the nurse plays in the delivery of care for the patient in ARF. The importance of the nurse–patient role is vital to the well-being of the patient, whereby the nurse can monitor the patient for complications, participate in emergency renal replacement therapy, assess the patient's progress and response to treatment, and provide physical and emotional support. In this central role, the nurse can maintain close links with the patient's family, which can be instrumental to a family-centred approach to the patient's treatment. The alliance between the patient, the family and the nurse is paramount in keeping the family informed of the patient's condition, assisting them to understand treatments and providing psychological support. Figure 4.1 gives an overview of the signs and symptoms of ARF.

However, in recent years, the intensive care nurse has taken over from the renal nurse in caring for those requiring continuous renal replacement therapy (CRRT). Specific nursing activities for CRRT are, therefore, beyond the scope of this book, but further reading can be found at the end of this chapter.

MORTALITY

It is important for nurses and carers to be able to understand that ARF is a serious condition that should never be underestimated. Constant improvements in dialysis technology, combined with a growing chronic kidney disease population and limited funds, have put clinicians under pressure to try and predict the outcomes of treatment. Whilst improvements in technology have enabled there to be greater comfort and survival, there are greater monetary costs (Peeters & Rublee 2000). A number of attempts have been made to predict the outcome of ARF but, owing to its complex and erratic nature, this has been difficult to predict (Levy et al 1996).

However, it can be seen that there are a number of patient groups in whom ARF has a particularly high mortality rate. For example, the

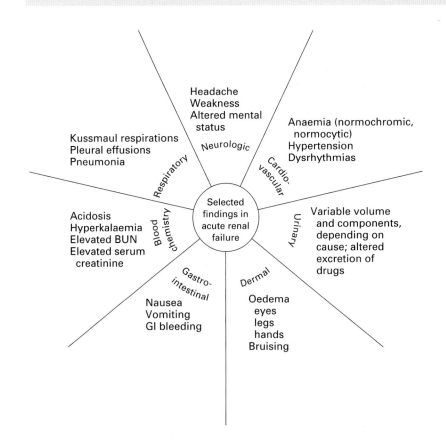

Figure 4.1
Signs and symptoms of acute renal failure. BUN, blood urea nitrogen; GI, gastrointestinal. (From Brundage D. Renal disorders. Mosby, 1992, with permission from Mosby.)

mortality rate of those patients whose ARF is caused by burns can be as high as 96% (Cantarovich & Verho 1996). The need for rapid identification of the cause of ARF and those patients at highest risk is essential so that the current course of treatment can be adopted (Du Bose et al 1997). Therefore it is vital for the nurse to play a major role in assisting physicians in the treatment options available for this fragile group of patients.

CLASSIFICATION

Acute renal failure may be divided into three major categories, in which each category has a physiological location of the insult (Table 4.1):

- prerenal – relates to the ineffective perfusion of the kidneys, which are structurally normal
- renal (intrinsic) – damage to the renal parenchyma, sometimes secondary to prerenal problems
- postrenal – disordered urinary drainage of both kidneys or of a single functioning kidney.

In addition, an acute impairment may present in the patient with existing chronic kidney disease, which may lead to further structural damage; this presentation is often referred to as acute-on-chronic renal failure.

Table 4.1   Acute renal failure: major causes and aetiology

Stage	Major causes	Aetiology
Prerenal	Cardiovascular	Congestive cardiac failure
		Myocardial infarction
		Cardiogenic shock
		Cardiac tamponade
		Pulmonary embolism
	Vasodilation	Sepsis
		Anaphylaxis
	Hypovolaemia	Haemorrhage, including blood loss due to surgery
		Burns
		Gastrointestinal loss
		Renal loss
Renal (intrinsic)	Glomerulonephritis	Poststreptococcal infection
		Systemic lupus erythematosus
		Haemolytic–uraemic syndrome
		Wegener's granulomatosis
		Goodpasture's syndrome
	Vascular	Vasculitis
		Hypertension
		Eclampsia of pregnancy
		Renal artery stenosis
		Renal vein thrombosis
	Intratubular	
	Pigment	Myoglobin (see rhabdomyolysis)
	Proteins	Myeloma
	Crystals	Nephrotoxins (see nephrotoxicity)
Postrenal	Obstruction of lower urinary tract	Prostatic hypertrophy
	Obstruction of upper urinary tract	Ureteric obstruction (clots, extrinsic compression, calculi)

PRERENAL ACUTE RENAL FAILURE

Prerenal causes of ARF are directly related to hypoperfusion states or a decline in the blood supply to the kidneys. The structure of the kidneys is normal. However, when the renal blood supply is restricted, glomerular filtration is reduced, causing decreased perfusion of the kidneys. The net effect is a decreased blood flow to the glomeruli, which therefore leads to ineffective filtration because of inadequate blood flow. Without an effective renal plasma flow rate the glomeruli are unable to filter waste from the blood but the structure of the renal tubules remains intact (Fig. 4.2).

In this prerenal state, urine osmolarity is high and sodium low, which is consistent with renal hypoperfusion and well-preserved renal function. If at this state renal blood flow can be restored, then normal renal function will return. However, if the prerenal state is prolonged, then this

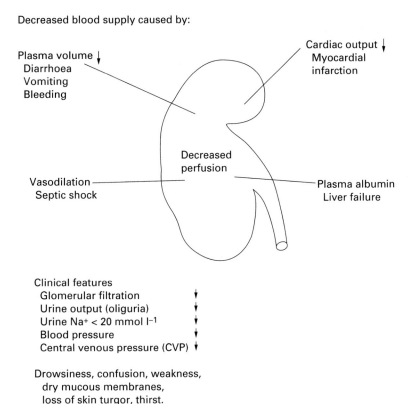

Decreased blood supply caused by:

Plasma volume ↓
  Diarrhoea
  Vomiting
  Bleeding

Cardiac output ↓
  Myocardial
  infarction

Decreased
perfusion

Vasodilation
  Septic shock

Plasma albumin
  Liver failure

Clinical features
  Glomerular filtration   ↓
  Urine output (oliguria)   ↓
  Urine Na+ < 20 mmol l−1   ↓
  Blood pressure   ↓
  Central venous pressure (CVP) ↓

Drowsiness, confusion, weakness,
  dry mucous membranes,
  loss of skin turgor, thirst.

Figure 4.2
Prerenal failure.

may lead to ischaemic damage due to poor perfusion, which in turn may lead to acute tubular necrosis (Sinert et al 2001).

The importance of early recognition, diagnosis and treatment is vital in prerenal failure, in order to prevent the condition progressing to renal failure with a degree of parenchymal damage.

RENAL (INTRINSIC) FAILURE

This cause is sometimes referred to as intrinsic or intrarenal failure, and is associated with structural damage to the glomeruli and renal tubules. The difference between pre- and postrenal failure and intrinsic failure is that, in intrinsic failure, the correction of the aetiology will not guarantee the complete recovery of renal function because of damage to the nephron itself. Here the episode of ARF may run a lengthy duration and can often lead to ERF.

The clinical course of intrinsic renal failure is often complex and, depending upon underlying disorders, the recovery may be prolonged for up to 6 weeks. As illustrated in Table 4.1, there are a wide variety of causes for intrinsic renal failure that may involve multisystem disease or originate from a primary renal disorder, but often involve complicating severe illness that causes vasomotor nephropathy.

Some specific causes are now discussed.

Acute interstitial nephritis

This condition often follows exposure to drugs in the form of antibiotics, analgesics and non-steroidal anti-inflammatory agents. Infections can cause a very similar clinical and pathological picture, and these include *Salmonella*, *Streptococcus*, *Meningococcus*, leptospirosis and many viral disorders.

Other categories of interstitial nephritis are caused by systemic disease, such as systemic lupus erythematosus and sarcoidosis, or present as the primary disease.

Clinical features

Fever, rash, arthralgia, back pain and eosinophilia are clinical features of acute interstitial nephritis. ARF may not develop for some weeks but, in some cases, renal dysfunction may occur within a few hours after exposure to a causative drug.

Rhabdomyolysis

A major cause of ARF is toxic in nature. Rhabdomyolysis occurs as a result of the release of muscle contents, including myoglobin, into the plasma and is often caused by trauma, for example, a crush injury or pressure-induced muscle necrosis. This causes damage to muscle that allows the pigment myoglobin to be released into the plasma. Myoglobin is a red respiratory agent and in high plasma levels becomes nephrotoxic.

Clinical features

The urine is often brown or coffee-coloured owing to the presence of myoglobin. Patients often present with acute illness with fever, weakness, pain, and nausea and vomiting.

Renal failure and liver disease

Acute renal failure is often associated with acute liver injury that may result from:

- paracetamol overdose
- circulatory shock
- severe leptospirosis sepsis.

It may also be seen in surgery on the biliary tract.

For the patient with advanced liver disease, the onset of renal failure is often referred to as the hepatorenal syndrome. Septicaemia, fluid and electrolyte imbalance, or hypovolaemia from gastrointestinal haemorrhage are common causes of the syndrome. These patients often require intensive care and the appropriate choice of therapy is of utmost importance (Rialp et al 1996).

Cortical necrosis

Cortical necrosis may follow any course of intensive or prolonged ischaemia. The condition is also associated with sepsis, shock, transfusion reactions and burns.

Renal biopsy reveals pathology or patchy necrosis of the glomeruli, tubules and small vessels of the renal cortex. The renal medulla remains intact, but the renal cortex becomes infarcted and calcifies, and this may be seen on plain abdominal X-ray.

The return of renal function is often slow, but if cortical necrosis is extensive, recovery is unlikely and the patient may become dialysis-dependent.

Acute tubular necrosis

Acute renal failure owing to ischaemic changes or toxic renal injury presents a clinical syndrome that is often referred to as acute tubular necrosis. It is a very common cause of ARF and has a high mortality rate of around 50%. It causes damage to the tubular portion of the nephron. Unfortunately, despite 35 years of haemodialysis, little progress has been made in altering the outcome for acute tubular necrosis (Lieberthal & Nigam 2000).

Although the aetiology of acute tubular necrosis can vary, the common factor is that there is a reduction of oxygen and nutrients to the active tubular cells, which results in a lack of cell function and patchy necrosis. The tubular cells will regenerate at the basement membrane level. The aim is to keep the patient alive and well during this regeneration phase. An almost full recovery can be made provided the appropriate and timely treatment is undertaken (Pusnani & Hazra 1997). Most intrinsic renal failure is caused by ischaemia through exposure to toxic agents, such as drugs or bacterial endotoxins.

In any patient with ARF, particularly acute tubular necrosis, a potential causative effect could be a therapeutic agent. Therapeutic agents can affect the kidney in any of the three categories listed, as illustrated in Table 4.2 (Coffman 1998).

Ischaemic acute tubular necrosis is often associated with inadequate perfusion to the kidney, in that the efferent and afferent arterioles are unable to maintain their autoregulatory function, and this leads to a fall in the glomerular filtration rate. This interruption in blood flow to the kidney may be due to surgical intervention, e.g. aortic repair, and is quite likely to cause ischaemia (Weldon & Monk 2000).

POSTRENAL FAILURE

Postrenal conditions obstruct the flow of urine. Obstruction will not cause renal failure except for in those with a solitary kidney; therefore,

---

Table 4.2 Therapeutic agents that can affect the kidney

Clinical syndrome	Causative agents
Prerenal	Ciclosporin, radiocontrast, amphotericin B, ACE inhibitors, NSAIDs
Intrinsic: acute tubular necrosis	Aminoglycosides, amphotericin B, cephalosporins
Acute interstitial nephritis	Penicillins, cephalosporins, sulphonamides, rifampicin, NSAIDs, interferon, interleukin-2
Postrenal	Aciclovir, analgesic abuse
	Other heavy metals, including gold, lithium, mercury, silver

ACE, angiotensin-converting enzyme; NSAIDs, non-steroidal anti-inflammatory drugs.

the obstruction has to be bilateral in order to cause failure. The rapidity of recovery will depend on the duration and completeness of the obstruction.

The urinary tract may be obstructed by three mechanisms:

- obstruction from within (e.g. ureteric stones)
- disease of the wall
- obstruction from outside.

As with all types of renal failure, it is important to find the cause and start treatment as soon as possible since, in theory, all postrenal failure is reversible (Barrat 2000).

MANAGEMENT OF ACUTE RENAL FAILURE

Since the normal kidney is essential to homeostasis of the body, particularly with regard to volume, electrolyte balance, acid–base balance and excretion of nitrogenous waste products, loss of these functions can lead to hyperkalaemia, volume overload, acidosis and uraemia.

The first step in good management is to detect any degree of renal failure. It is important to screen fully those patients at risk from renal failure prior to any invasive event (Alkhunaizi 1996).

HYPERKALAEMIA

Hyperkalaemia is often a fatal complication in ARF. The failing kidney is unable to excrete potassium effectively when the patient is oliguric ($< 400 \, \text{mL urine day}^{-1}$) or, worse, anuric (no urine). It is further complicated by the very complex treatment of an individual who is often infected, hypoxic, and requiring blood transfusions and potassium-containing drugs.

Haemodialysis is the most efficient treatment for hyperkalaemia but this may take time if vascular access is required. Other alternatives available are listed below.

- Oral or rectal potassium exchange agents in the form of calcium resonium.
- The administration of intravenous insulin and dextrose will help move potassium ions back into the intracellular compartment and away from the extracellular compartment. It is important to monitor the patient's blood sugar, since hypo-hyperglycaemia can occur.

VOLUME OVERLOAD

Successful volume homeostasis permits maintenance of a constant internal circulatory and extracellular volume despite consumption of varying quantities of water and salt, and variable invisible losses of water.

The presence of oedema may be seen in the feet, legs and sacral area. This is often pitted in nature. The skin is particularly at risk at this stage and extra care must be taken. Shortness of breath and especially orthopnoea are indicative of pulmonary oedema.

Each patient in ARF should have an individual prescription for fluid and sodium intake. As a generalisation, the fluid intake volume should equal the daily urine output plus 300–500 mL. Patients with a large insensible loss, as happens with burns, obviously need a larger fluid intake and special care should be taken. It is important that the patient and family are involved in accurate fluid balance.

METABOLIC ACIDOSIS

The presence of ARF must not lead the nurse to think that it is the only cause of acidosis until other causes have been eliminated, e.g. ketoacidosis, lactic acidosis.

Acidosis in renal failure occurs when the renal tubules fail to regenerate bicarbonate and secrete hydrogen ions into the urine. In turn this causes an acid–base imbalance.

It is possible, since most acid comes from the breakdown of dietary protein, to reduce the level of acidosis by limiting the level of intake of protein. Another alternative is to infuse sodium bicarbonate, but one has to be aware of fluid overload and hypernatraemia. The most efficient way of treating acute acidosis is bicarbonate haemodialysis.

URAEMIA

The accumulation of nitrogenous waste products will produce acute uraemia. Symptoms of uraemia often include nausea, vomiting, hiccups; bleeding risks; infection risks; neurological problems; irritability, confusion and twitching. As previously mentioned, it is necessary to begin appropriate dialysis.

DIALYSIS IN ACUTE RENAL FAILURE

The purpose of dialysis is to prevent morbidity and to support the kidney during its recovery phase. The amount and frequency of dialysis are dictated by the severity of the patient's condition (Dauguirdas 2000).

Indications for dialysis:

- uraemic symptoms, e.g. pericarditis
- volume overload
- hyperkalaemia
- metabolic acidosis
- 'space-making', e.g. nutrition, transfusions.

When prescribing acute dialysis, certain factors need to be considered and these include time on dialysis (possibly only 2h for the first treatment), frequency (daily dialysis may be required), potassium concentration of dialysate (3 mmol L^{-1} may be necessary), a biocompatible dialyser and good fluid balance control. For those patients who are too haemodynamically unstable for conventional haemodialysis, other forms of renal replacement therapy (RRT) may be appropriate and this is discussed later in the chapter.

THE CLINICAL COURSE OF ACUTE RENAL FAILURE

The clinical course of ARF can be divided into four stages or phases:

- initiating stage
- oliguric stage
- diuretic stage
- recovery stage.

Types of urine output can be found in Table 4.3.

INITIATING STAGE

This occurs when the kidneys are injured, and when diagnosis is made and treatment established. It can last anything from hours to days (Venkataraman & Kellum 2000).

OLIGURIC STAGE (FIG. 4.3)

This can last from 5 days to over 15 days. When ARF persists for weeks, endocrine problems, such as reduced erythropoietin production, are noticed. Functional renal changes occur, such as decreased tubular transport, reduced urine formation and lowered glomerular filtration. Renal healing will begin to occur, with the basement membrane being replaced with fibrous scar tissue and the nephron clogged with inflammatory products. The patient is particularly susceptible to bleeding and infection.

DIURETIC STAGE

With continued healing the kidney begins to regain most of its lost function, but this depends on the severity of the initial injury. The signs and symptoms of the original condition begin to disappear. Urine output can begin to increase back to normal levels of up to $3 \, L \, day^{-1}$.

Table 4.3 Types of urine output	
Anuria	**No urine output**
Oliguria	$< 400 \, mL \, day^{-1}$
Non-oliguria	$> 400 \, mL \, day^{-1}$
Polyuria	Normal or high urine output

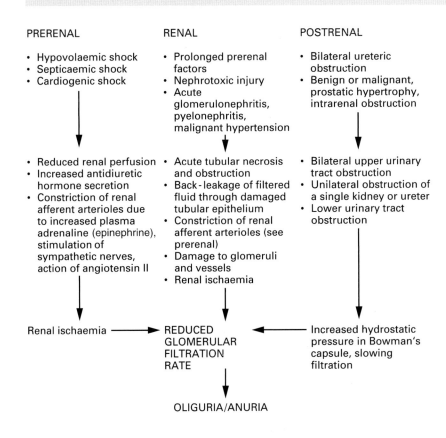

PRERENAL

- Hypovolaemic shock
- Septicaemic shock
- Cardiogenic shock

- Reduced renal perfusion
- Increased antidiuretic hormone secretion
- Constriction of renal afferent arterioles due to increased plasma adrenaline (epinephrine), stimulation of sympathetic nerves, action of angiotensin II

RENAL

- Prolonged prerenal factors
- Nephrotoxic injury
- Acute glomerulonephritis, pyelonephritis, malignant hypertension

- Acute tubular necrosis and obstruction
- Back-leakage of filtered fluid through damaged tubular epithelium
- Constriction of renal afferent arterioles (see prerenal)
- Damage to glomeruli and vessels
- Renal ischaemia

POSTRENAL

- Bilateral ureteric obstruction
- Benign or malignant, prostatic hypertrophy, intrarenal obstruction

- Bilateral upper urinary tract obstruction
- Unilateral obstruction of a single kidney or ureter
- Lower urinary tract obstruction

Renal ischaemia ⟶ REDUCED GLOMERULAR FILTRATION RATE ⟵ Increased hydrostatic pressure in Bowman's capsule, slowing filtration

OLIGURIA/ANURIA

Figure 4.3
Acute renal failure: mechanisms involved in the genesis of oliguria.

RECOVERY STAGE

The recovery stage can last from several months to over a year. The basement membrane is restored to its previous structure; scar tissue will remain but is not clinically significant. The kidneys respond in a regulatory excretory function to the body's needs.

As previously, the mortality rate for ARF is very high, and appropriate treatment and management are essential (Fiaccadori et al 2000).

NUTRITIONAL MANAGEMENT OF ACUTE RENAL FAILURE

Approximately 40% of patients with ARF have been reported to be malnourished (Fiaccadori et al 1999) and protein–calorie malnutrition has been implicated as one of the factors contributing to the high mortality rate seen in ARF (Brivet et al 1996, Mault et al 1983). However, feeding these patients can be a challenge because optimal nutritional therapy is hard to define and metabolic derangement is often present.

Acute renal failure is often associated with accelerated protein breakdown, which unfortunately may be difficult to suppress, even with adequate nutritional intake. The cause of this excessive protein catabolism is multifactorial – uraemic toxins, underlying disease, hormonal changes, metabolic acidosis, insulin resistance and nutrient losses during renal replacement therapy will all play a part (Druml 1998). Changes in water, electrolyte and acid–base metabolism are invariably complicated by alterations in protein, carbohydrate and lipid metabolism.

Hyperglycaemia is common due to a combination of insulin resistance and accelerated hepatic gluconeogenesis, resulting from the conversion of amino acids released during protein catabolism into glucose (Campbell 1999). In addition, lipid metabolism is altered, with an impaired ability to use free fatty acids and triglycerides owing to decreased activity of lipoprotein and hepatic tri-glyceride lipases (Druml et al 1992).

The aims of nutritional support are to:

- preserve lean body mass/prevent or minimise malnutrition
- stimulate immunocompetence
- repair tissue damage
- preserve organ function
- maintain biochemistry/fluid balance
- enhance recovery.

REQUIREMENTS

As patients with ARF are a heterogeneous population, nutrient requirements need to be calculated on an individual basis. It has been shown that renal failure does not have an influence on energy expenditure per se (Bouffart et al 1987, Schneeweiss et al 1990) and therefore requirements need to be determined by the underlying disease. The most common method involves calculation of the patient's basic metabolic rate (BMR) from standard equations, which are based on age, gender and weight (Schofield 1985). Modifications to cover stress, activity, the energy requirements of feeding and temperature can be added to the BMR (Elia 1990). To avoid overfeeding, the provision of carbohydrate energy during the dialysis therapy also needs to be taken into account. Dextrose absorption during renal replacement therapy varies with the type of dialysis therapy, from zero or very little in conventional intermittent haemodialysis, to the equivalent of approximately 500–900 kcal absorbed during continuous arteriovenous haemodialysis, with 1.5% and 2.5% dialysate solutions, respectively (Sigler & Teehan 1987). The rate of glucose oxidation is approximately $4\,\mathrm{mg\,kg^{-1}\,min^{-1}}$ (Wolfe et al 1979) and in critical illness this should not be exceeded. Glucose overload is more likely when fat-free total parenteral nutrition (TPN) solutions are administered or if the dextrose calories from the dialysate solutions are not accounted for. If TPN has been instigated, then the changes in lipid metabolism associated with renal failure should not prevent the use of lipid emulsions.

The optimal requirement for protein is more influenced by the illness causing the ARF, the associated complications, extent of protein catabolism and the type and frequency of dialysis. Patients may range from being in a non-catabolic state to being critically ill and hypercatabolic, and protein requirements will range from 1.2 to $1.5\,\mathrm{g\,kg^{-1}\,day^{-1}}$ (Campbell 1999). Account should also be taken of the losses of amino acids during renal replacement therapy.

The electrolyte content of the nutritional prescription should be adjusted based on each individual patient and whether the patient is on renal replacement therapy. Sodium should not be greatly restricted unless oedema is present. If the patient is being dialysed, then sodium will be removed from the patient, enabling a balance to be achieved.

Serum levels of potassium, magnesium and phosphorus are generally elevated in patients with ARF, but can decrease as a result of intracellular shifts associated with carbohydrate delivery and losses incurred during treatment with continuous renal replacement therapy. Frequent monitoring to assess the need for supplementation is essential.

The requirements for micronutrients are not well documented in ARF. Many of the recommendations are extrapolated from work conducted with patients with chronic kidney disease. There is a potential, in patients with chronic kidney disease, for toxicity of some fat-soluble vitamins and minerals which are renally excreted. However, one study involving eight patients with ARF demonstrated, with the exception of vitamin K, deficiencies of fat-soluble vitamins (Druml 1998). Most centres will supplement fat-soluble vitamins with caution. Owing to dialysis losses, there is a potential for deficiency of water-soluble vitamins (B vitamins and folic acid) with the exception of vitamin C. Large doses of vitamin C have resulted in oxalate deposition, and supplementation of no greater than $200\,mg\,day^{-1}$ is recommended (Druml 2001). The requirements for trace elements in ARF are not well defined.

Patients with ARF are frequently anuric, hence monitoring of fluid balance and restriction of intake is often necessary. The development of continuous renal replacement therapy has allowed fluid to be more easily managed without the need for the reduced fluid allowances that previously meant having to limit nutritional support.

ROUTE OF FEEDING

The enteral route for feeding is generally considered to be cheaper, safer and more physiological than feeding intravenously, and is therefore the feeding method of choice. However, in the critically ill patient it may not be possible to feed enterally, and either TPN or a combination of both methods may be considered.

The development of concentrated low-electrolyte feeds has proven invaluable in allowing delivery of optimal protein and calories with the minimum of fluid and electrolytes. However, these special feeds are not normally needed if the patient is receiving continuous renal replacement therapy.

NOVEL SUBSTRATES

The use of novel substrates in acute illness to modulate the stress response is an area of research that is expanding. Glutamine, recognised as a conditionally essential amino acid, has many functions. One of its major roles is as an oxidative substrate for rapidly replicating cells, such as the gastrointestinal mucosal cells and immune cells – lymphocytes and macrophages. Glutamine may play a vital role in the maintenance of intestinal integrity and function and has been shown to reduce infectious complications (Houdijk et al 1998). Arginine, nucleotides and omega fatty acids, thought to aid the immune system, are now available in specialised enteral feeds but the evidence for their benefit has been mixed (Beale et al 1999, Mendez et al 1997). What is apparent is that the outcome of using novel substrates in patients with ARF needs further research.

CONTINUOUS RENAL REPLACEMENT THERAPY

The use of CRRT has developed enormously during recent years and involves either dialysis (solute removal using diffusion) or filtration (solute and water removal using convection) treatments. The first therapy of this type was continuous arteriovenous haemofiltration, described by Kramer et al in 1982. This became a popular method of managing the fluid and electrolyte balance of patients in intensive care with ARF. The advantage of continuous therapy is the slower rate of fluid or solute removal, thus making it better tolerated by critically ill patients. Patients who required more efficient fluid and electrolyte clearance remained dependent on intermittent haemodialysis treatments performed by renal nurses.

The 1990s witnessed both an evolution of the treatments and a concomitant devolution of the responsibility of prescribing and monitoring renal replacement therapy. The nurses in the intensive care unit have developed their skills, taking on additional responsibilities that were once the domain of the renal nurse. It is recognised that intermittent haemodialysis may be contraindicated in patients with ARF who are critically ill.

Complications such as cardiovascular instability, sepsis and multiorgan failure make conventional treatments difficult. There are a large variety of treatment options available and choice will depend on physician preference, nurse expertise and availability of the appropriate equipment.

Today the options fall broadly into three categories: continuous haemofiltration, continuous haemodiafiltration and continuous haemodialysis. When performed continuously over long periods of time, they allow optimal values to be obtained for urea and fluid exchange control, and electrolyte and acid–base balance.

CONTINUOUS HAEMOFILTRATION

Continuous arteriovenous haemofiltration

Continuous arteriovenous haemofiltration has been performed in intensive care since the early 1980s (Kramer et al 1982). This procedure provides a simple method of removing fluid from the patient and, at the same time, convective removal of solutes. It is rarely used today as more advanced techniques have been developed, but its main benefit is that it is relatively simple to use and does not require a mechanical blood pump, relying on the patient's blood pressure.

Continuous haemofiltration with the aid of a blood pump provides solute removal by convection. It offers high-volume ultrafiltration using replacement fluid, which can be administered in a variety of concentrations according to the patient's biochemistry. The pump guarantees adequate blood flow to maintain required ultrafiltration rates. This method can be performed using several litres of replacement fluid each hour. The addition of a blood pump to the circuit removes the necessity for arterial access, and provides a more reliable and controllable method of delivering treatment (Fig. 4.4).

CONTINUOUS HAEMODIAFILTRATION

To increase the efficiency of small-molecule clearance, a dialysis solution is continuously pumped through the filter in a countercurrent direction to the blood. Small-molecule (urea) clearance by diffusion is more efficient. It is possible to use a standard blood monitor for the extracorporeal circuit and then use infusion pumps to administer dialysate and replacement fluid (Fig. 4.5).

This method incorporates the same principles as intermittent haemodialysis but operates at a greatly reduced rate. From the nursing perspective, the use of fully automated systems provides a reliable

Continuous venovenous haemofiltration (CVVH)

Continuous venovenous haemodiafiltration (CVVHDF)

Continuous venovenous haemodialysis (CVVHD)

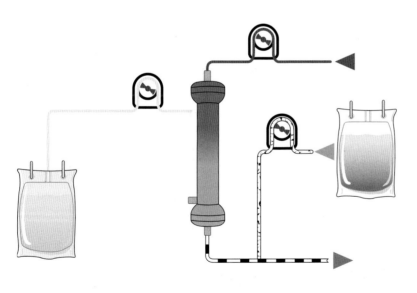

Figure 4.4
Continuous venovenous haemofiltration. (With permission from Gambro Hospal Ltd, UK.)

—————— Access line

⊳————⊲ Return line

⊸⊸⊸⊸ Replacement fluid

—————— Dialysate fluid

··········· Filtrate

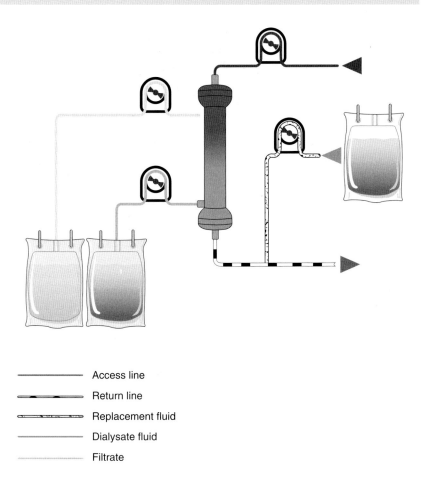

Figure 4.5
Continuous venovenous haemodiafiltration. (With permission from Gambro Hospal Ltd, UK.)

———————————— Access line

———————————— Return line

———————————— Replacement fluid

———————————— Dialysate fluid

·························· Filtrate

and easy method of monitoring the fluid balance of patients who are critically ill. This allows nurses more time to dedicate to direct patient care. An example of an integrated system for continuous fluid management and automated renal replacement therapy is the Prisma machine (Fig. 4.6).

The machine comprises a basic blood module with blood pump, venous and arterial pressure monitoring and an air detector. The fluid monitor has two integral pumps – one to remove fluid from the filter and the second to pump replacement fluid to the patient. The replacement fluid and the ultra filtrate are suspended on a weigh scale, which calculates and controls a linear patient weight.

With such accurate fluid control, the nurse does not need constantly to measure and record fluid loss and replacement as with previous methods. The ultrafiltration rate and physiological solutions are prescribed by the physician based on available clinical data (fluid state, biochemistry).

Nursing interventions for CRRT can be found in the further reading section at the end of this chapter.

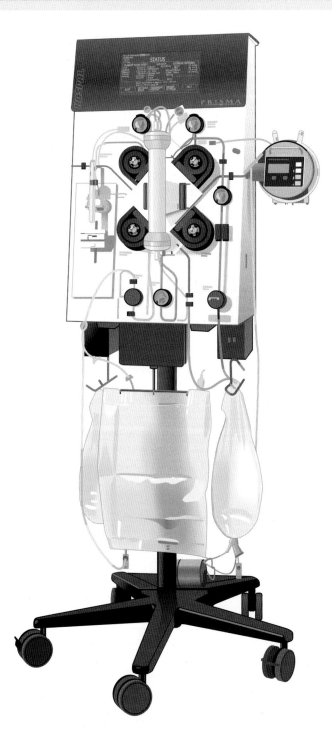

Figure 4.6
Prisma machine. (With
permission from Gambro Hospal
Ltd, UK.)

SLOW LOW-EFFICIENCY OR EXTENDED DAILY DIALYSIS (SLEDD OR EDD)

Although not continuous regimens, these therapies have been developed to have aims in common with the other forms of CRRT, including lower solute clearances that are maintained over longer periods of time. In comparison to conventional dialysis, SLEDD uses a lower blood flow and dialysate flow rate, and elongates the time on dialysis, usually between 6 and 8 hours (Kumar et al 2000, Marshall et al 2001). It has been shown to be safe for patients, providing good control of electrolytes and ultrafiltration is well tolerated. However, as with other continuous therapies, owing to the lower blood flow rates, special attention must be made to anticoagulation of the circuit to prevent clotting.

Another advantage of SLEDD is that, because of its similarity to conventional dialysis, it makes it much easier for training staff.

INTERMITTENT HAEMODIAFILTRATION

Intermittent haemodiafiltration can be a therapy option for both patients with acute and established renal failure. The principle is the same as described in CVVHDF, but lasts for shorter periods of time. As it combines the advantages of diffusion (dialysis) with convection (haemofiltration), it is suitable for use in patients with cardiovascular instability, especially those with fluid overload. It has superior small solute clearance over haemofiltration. Blood flow rates are higher than those of CVVHDF and it requires an HDF membrane that is more permeable than a normal haemofilter. However, owing to the efficiency of small molecule clearance, this would not be a treatment of choice for the severely uraemic patient at risk of disequilibrium.

PLASMA EXCHANGE

Therapeutic plasma exchange (TPE) is an extracorporeal blood purification technique, designed for the removal of large-molecular-weight substances from the plasma (Fridley & Kaplan 2002). Most TPE procedures are performed for neurological, immunological or haematological diseases; including anti-GBM disease, thrombotic thrombocytopenic purpura (TTP), Guillain–Barré syndrome, systemic vasculitis, acute renal failure secondary to myeloma of the kidney and the haemolytic–uraemic syndrome (HUS).

Plasma is separated from whole blood and then a replacement fluid is infused in equal volumes to the plasma that has been removed. It is a non-specific therapy, removing all circulating substances within the plasma. A plasma filter is used to separate the plasma from all other cellular elements, using a semipermeable membrane. As TPE removes all circulating substances in the plasma, care should be taken to avoid disturbances with clotting factors, calcium and magnesium levels, and any other substances that may be depleted as a result.

The fluid volume removed by TPE must be replaced to prevent marked volume depletion. Fresh-frozen plasma (FFP), and albumin alone, or with normal saline, can be used. The optimum choice depends on the disease being treated, e.g. saline and albumin for hyperviscosity, and FFP for TTP.

Albumin has the advantage that there is no risk of viral transmission and minimal risk of anaphalaxis.

Albumin

When colloid and crystalloid solutions are used in combination, the amount of colloid should not be less than 50% of the total infusion. General recommendations are one-third saline to two-thirds albumin (UK Blood Transfusion Guidelines 2005).

Albumin–saline combination

Fresh-frozen plasma replaces the normal proteins that have been removed, therefore there is no depletion of coagulation factors or immunoglobulins. However, FFP can produce many complications, including anaphalaxis, muscle cramps and urticaria. FFP is the fluid of choice for TTP, since it may provide a protein that diminishes platelet aggregation.

Fresh-frozen plasma

Regimes for plasma exchange vary greatly depending on physician preference and clinical need.

SUMMARY

The impact of ARF on patients and families is often unexpected and, despite new technology, it remains a serious disease with a high mortality rate. Unlike most patients who have had renal failure for some time, the patient with ARF and who requires RRT will not have had the opportunity to have had counselling and the chance to evaluate their condition. The key aim of care is to balance humanistic caring skills with the technological and clinical expertise required to optimise the patient's survival and quality of life.

All patients require nutritional support to maintain protein stores. In ARF it is not renal insufficiency per se that determines the need for nutritional support but the type and severity of the underlying disease and the degree of associated hypercatabolism. Understanding the nutritional requirements, careful interpretation of nutritional assessment and familiarity with the various forms of renal replacement therapy will greatly improve the success of nutritional therapy, although the optimal nutritional regimen has not yet been defined.

The renal nurse now has much less of a role in the care of the acutely ill person with ARF, as many patients are managed in the intensive care unit. However, it is imperative that renal nurses keep up to date with new technologies, as they may often act in a supportive role for those intensive care nurses who are new to filtration therapies.

ACKNOWLEGEMENT

With grateful thanks to Tim Armstrong who was the original author of this chapter, and to Gemma Bircher who wrote the section on nutrition.

References

Alkhunaizi AM. Management of acute renal failure: new perspectives. Am J Kidney Dis 1996; 28: 315–328.

Barrat J. Outcome of acute renal failure following surgical repair of ruptured abdominal aortic aneurysms. Eur J Vasc Endovasc Surg 2000; 20: 163–168.

Beale RJ, Bryg DJ, Bihari DJ. Immunonutrition in the critically ill: a systematic review of clinical outcome. Crit Care Med 1999; 27: 2799–2805.

Bouffart Y, Viuale JP, Annat GM et al. Energy expenditure in the acute renal failure patient mechanically ventilated. Intens Care Med 1987; 13: 401–404.

Brivet FG, Kleinknecht DJ, Loirat P et al. Acute renal failure in intensive care units – causes, outcome, and prognostic factors of hospital mortality: a prospective, multicentre study. Crit Care Med 1996; 24: 192–198.

Campbell IT. Limitations of nutrient intake. The effect of stressors: trauma, sepsis and multiple organ failure. Eur J Clin Nutr 1999; 53(Suppl. 1): S143–S147.

Cantarovich F, Verho MT. A simple prognostic index for patients with acute renal failure requiring dialysis. Renal Failure 1996; 18: 585–592.

Chen YC, Hsu HH, Kao KC et al. Outcomes and APACHE II predictions for critically ill patients with acute renal failure. Renal Failure 2001; 23: 61–70.

Coffman TM. Primer on kidney disease. 2nd edn. USA: National Kidney Foundation, 1998.

Dauguirdas JT. The handbook of dialysis. 3rd edn. Philadelphia: Lippincott Williams & Wilkins, 2000.

Davies SP, Reaveley DA, Brown EA et al. Amino acid losses in patients with acute renal failure. Crit Care Med 1991; 19: 1510–1515.

Druml MD. Nutritional management of acute renal failure. Am J Kidney Dis 2001; 37(Suppl. 2): S89–S94.

Druml W, Fischer M, Sertl S et al. Fat elimination in acute renal failure: long-chain vs short-chain triglycerides. Am J Clin Nutr 1992; 55: 468–472.

Druml W. Protein metabolism in acute renal failure. Mineral Electrolyte Metab 1998; 24: 47–54.

Du Bose TD, Warnock DG, Mehta RL et al. Acute renal failure in the 21st century: recommendations for management and outcomes assessment. Am J Kidney Dis 1997; 29: 793–799.

Elia M. Artificial nutritional support. Med Int 1990; 82: 3392–3396.

Fiaccadori E, Lombardi M, Leonardi S et al. Prevalence and clinical outcome associated with preexisting malnutrition in acute renal failure: a prospective cohort study. J Am Soc Nephrol 1999; 10: 581–593.

Fiaccadori E, Maggiore U, Lombardi M et al. Predicting patient outcome from acute renal failure comparing three general severity of illness scoring systems. Kidney Int 2000; 58: 283–292.

Fridley J, Kaplan A. Prescription and technique of therapeutic plasma exchange. www.uptodate.com 2002; 10: 1.

Houdijk APJ, Rijnsberger ER, Janse J et al. Randomised trial of glutamine-enriched enteral nutrition on infectious mortality in patients with multiple trauma. Lancet 1998; 352: 772–776.

Kramer P, Bohler J, Kehr A et al. Intensive care potential of CAVH. Trans Am Soc Artif Organs 1982; 28: 28.

Kumar VA, Craig M, Depner TA, Yeun JY. Extended daily dialysis: a new approach to renal replacement therapy for acute renal failure in the intensive care unit. Am J Kidney Dis 2000; 36: 294–300.

Levy EM, Viscoli CM, Horwitz EI. The affect of acute renal failure on mortality. A cohort analysis. JAMA 1996; 275: 1489–1494.

Lieberthal W, Nigam SK. Acute renal failure II. Experimental models of acute renal failure: experimental but indispensable. Am J Physiol Renal Physiol 2000; 278: F1–F12.

Marshall MR, Thomas AG, Shaver MJ, Alam MG, Chatoth DK. Sustained low-efficiency dialysis for critically ill patients requiring renal replacement therapy. Kidney Int 2001; 60: 777–785.

Mault JR, Dechert RE, Clark, SF et al. Starvation: a major contribution to mortality in acute renal failure. Trans Am Soc Artif Intern Organs 1983; 29: 390–395.

Mehta, RL. Continuous renal replacement therapy in the critically ill patient. Kidney Int 2005; 67: 781.

Mendez C, Jurkovich GJ, Garcial I et al. Effects of an immune-enhancing diet in critically injured patients. J Trauma 1997; 42: 933–940.

Peeters P, Rublee D. Analysis and interpretation of cost data in dialysis: review of western European literature. Health Policy 2000; 54: 209–227.

Pusnani ML, Hazra DK. Early haemodialysis in acute tubular necrosis. J Assoc Physicians India 1997; 45: 850–852.

Rialp G, Roglan A, Betbese AJ et al. Prognostic indexes and mortality in critically ill patients with acute renal failure treated with different dialytic techniques. Renal Failure 1996; 18: 667–675.

Schneeweiss B, Graninger W, Stockenhuber F et al. Energy metabolism in acute and chronic renal failure. Am J Clin Nutr 1990; 52: 596–601.

Schofield WN. Predicting basal metabolic rate. New standards and review of previous work. Hum Nutr Clin Nutr 1985; 44: 1–19.

Sigler, MH, Teehan BP. Solute transport in continuous hemodialysis. A new treatment for acute renal failure. Kidney Int 1987; 32: 562–571.

Sinert R, Salomone JA, Talavera F et al. Renal failure, acute. EMed J 2001; 2: 5.

UK Blood Transfusion Guidelines. www.transfusionguidelines.org.uk/docs/pdfs/uk_btg_edition_7_full.pdf (2005).

Venkataraman R, Kellum JA. Novel approaches to the treatment of acute renal failure. Expert Opin Invest Drugs 2000; 9: 2579–2592.

Weldon BC, Monk TG. The patient at risk for acute renal failure. Recognition, prevention and preoperative optimisation. Anaesthesiol Clin North Am 2000; 1: 705–717.

Wolfe RR, Allsop JR, Burke JF. Glucose metabolism in man: responses to intravenous glucose infusions. Metabolism 1979; 28: 210–220.

Further reading

Adam SK, Osbourne S. Critical care nursing: science and practice. Oxford: Oxford University Press, 1997.

Baker LRI, Hurst MJ, Rudge CJ et al. Practical procedures in nephrology. London: Arnold, 2000.

Grassmann A, Uhlenbusch-Körwer I, Bonnie-Schorn E et al. Good dialysis practice: composition and management of hemodialysis fluids. Lengerich: Pabst Science, 2000.

Jacobs C, Kjellstrand CM, Koch KM et al. Replacement of renal function by dialysis. 4th edn. Dordrecht: Kluwer Academic, 1996.

Levy J, Morgan J, Brown E. Oxford handbook of dialysis. Oxford: Oxford University Press, 2001.

Neilson EG. Immunologic renal diseases. Philadelphia: Lippincott, Williams & Wilkins, 2001.

Vander AF. Renal physiology. 5th edn. New York: McGraw-Hill, 1995.

Whitworth JA, Lawrence JR. Textbook of renal disease. 2nd edn. Edinburgh: Churchill Livingstone, 1994.

Useful websites

DOQI guidelines: www.kidney.org/professionals/doqi/

European Dialysis and Transplant Nurses Association/ European Renal Care Association: www.edtna-erca.org

Hypertension, Dialysis and Clinical Nephrology: www.hdcn.com

National Kidney Foundation: www.kidney.org/

Renal Association: www.renal.org/

Renal Registry: www.renalreg.org/

Renal Web: www.renalweb.com/

US Renal Data System: www.usrds.org/

Acute Dialysis Quality Initiative: www.ADQI.net

Chapter 5

Chronic kidney disease and predialysis care

Judith Hurst and Nicola Thomas

**LEARNING OUTCOMES
FOR THIS CHAPTER**

- To review the National Service Framework for Renal Services (2005)
- To understand the classification of chronic kidney disease (CKD)
- To debate the scope of practice of primary care practitioners in managing CKD
- To review the care and management of patients with early CKD
- To evaluate emerging research into management of CKD
- To evaluate best practice guidelines and strategies for predialysis care

INTRODUCTION

This chapter will investigate the care of those with early kidney disease before renal replacement therapy (RRT) is required. Renal nurses are often involved with the technical, monitoring and evaluative aspects of RRT for those with established renal failure (ERF). However, many people may experience reduced renal function for years before needing RRT. This chapter will describe recent initiatives to manage the group of people who have early kidney disease, and will discuss the published practice guidelines and strategies to guide care for this group. New healthcare roles are developing in this area of care and so the potential for renal nurses to expand their scope of practice will be discussed. The final section will discuss ideas for future clinical management of chronic kidney disease.

CHRONIC KIDNEY DISEASE

Chronic kidney disease (CKD) is now recognised as a major health problem. Studies have been carried out both in the United States (US) and the United Kingdom (UK) to investigate the prevalence, progression and referral rates of CKD in the general adult population. The prevalence of CKD in the US was shown to be 11% (19.2 million) from data analysed from a sample of 15 625 adults aged 20 years and over extracted from the Third National Health and Nutrition Examination Survey (NHANES III) (Coresh et al 2003). Older age was strongly associated with moderate or severely decreased function as well as diabetes and hypertension. In the UK study (John et al 2004), the prevalence of CKD was 5554 per million population, identified from a population of 688 193 in East Kent, who were unknown to renal services and been subject to a serum creatinine measurement by non-renal clinicians.

THE NATIONAL SERVICE FRAMEWORK AND EARLY CKD

The National Service Framework (NSF) for Renal Services (Part Two) was published in February 2005. It identifies four quality requirements covering chronic kidney disease, acute renal failure and end of life care. Nephrology teams are familiar with caring for and managing patients with acute renal failure (see Ch. 4) and are developing strategies to care for patients who have withdrawn from, or do not wish to have, dialysis (see Ch. 9). However, the management of patients with early CKD is a relatively new remit for health care professionals in nephrology.

The two quality requirements of the NSF (Part Two) that relate to CKD are as follows.

- *Quality requirement one: prevention and early detection of chronic kidney disease*. People at increased risk of developing or having undiagnosed chronic kidney disease, especially people with diabetes or hypertension, are identified, assessed and their condition managed to preserve their kidney function.
- *Quality requirement two: minimising the progression and consequences of chronic kidney disease*. People with a diagnosis of chronic kidney disease receive timely, appropriate and effective investigation, treatment and follow-up to reduce the risk of progression and complications.

One of the specific recommendations within the NSF has made a huge change to the way in which kidney function is measured and this change in practice will now be described.

KIDNEY FUNCTION AND ESTIMATED GLOMERULAR FILTRATION RATE

Traditionally kidney function has been assessed by measurement of serum creatinine. Serum creatinine is determined by the rate of production of creatinine, which is dependent on muscle mass, as well as the rate at which the kidney excretes it. Because of the wide variation in patients' body size, weight and muscle mass, serum creatinine is an inaccurate measure of kidney function. It is now recommended that kidney function should be assessed by an estimation of glomerular filtration rate (eGFR).

The NSF for Renal Services recommends the use of the four-variable Modification of Diet in Renal Disease (MDRD) formula to estimate glomerular filtration rate (GFR). Laboratories will work out the eGFR on the results of the serum creatinine, plus the gender and age of the patient. Once the eGFR is reported back to primary care or the renal clinic, an adjustment must be made if the patient is African–Caribbean (not mixed race). If the patient is African–Caribbean, then the eGFR result must be multiplied by 1.21. Assumption of Caucasian ethnicity can be made when using MDRD if ethnicity is unknown. It was recommended that hospital laboratories should report eGFR alongside serum creatinine from April 2006. Online calculators (http://www.renal.org/eGFRcalc/GFR.pl) can also be utilised.

The use of eGFR enables healthcare professionals to evaluate kidney function within the accepted staging of CKD. It is important to note that an eGFR of 60–89 mL min^{-1} is only indicative of CKD in the presence of other laboratory or clinical indicators. This reduces the possibility of inappropriately labelling people as having CKD.

However, there are some cautionary notes to interpreting eGFR results. The following cautions are adapted from Renal Association (2006) guidance (http://www.renal.org/eGFR/about.html).

1. *eGFR is only an estimate and a significant error is possible*: eGFR is most likely to be inaccurate in people at extremes of body type, for example, people who are malnourished. It is not valid in pregnant women or in children. A total of 90% of patients will have a measured GFR within 30% of their estimated GFR.
2. *Race:* Some racial minorities may not fit the MDRD equation well. It was originally validated for US white and black patients. For African–Caribbean black patients, eGFR was 21% higher for any given creatinine in the MDRD study. So if race was not included in the estimate, it should be increased by approximately 20% for a black patient. In the UK white population, and probably in South Asians living in the UK, the equation seems to work quite well.
3. *Not so good near normal:* The MDRD equation tends to underestimate normal or near-normal function, so slightly low values should not be overinterpreted. Furthermore, laboratory differences in creatinine estimations may make significant differences. *Routine reporting of eGFR values > 90 is not recommended.*
4. *Creatinine level must be stable:* eGFR calculations assume that the level of creatinine in the blood is stable over days or longer. They are not valid if it is changing.
5. *Different equations:* from April 2006 in the UK, most local laboratories calculate eGFR on all samples sent for creatinine measurement. The equation they use will take into account local variations in accuracy of creatinine assays, so *eGFR values obtained in this way should be a little more accurate* than those generated by any of the online calculators.

In summary, a normal range for serum creatinine should no longer be given and management of the patient needs to be based on eGFR. The widespread use of eGFR will greatly improve recognition of, and appropriate care of, individuals with CKD.

STAGING OF CKD

There is now worldwide acceptance of numerical stages of CKD, based on the Kidney Disease Quality Outcomes Initiative (KDOQI) classification (KDOQI 2005). Table 5.1 shows the KDOQI stages of chronic kidney disease. It is useful to stage CKD in this way as it allows renal teams to give specific advice to patients and primary care teams within local clinical guidelines (see later section on this).

MANAGEMENT OF EARLY KIDNEY DISEASE

Understanding the prevalence of CKD means that strategies for identification, assessment and management need to be developed to help reduce the health burden that CKD poses in the UK. Around 5% of the population may have CKD stages 3–5 (Anandarajah et al 2005), but not all patients with CKD need to be referred to or managed by nephrologists, although input from renal specialist nurses may be appropriate in some

Table 5.1 KDOQI stages of chronic kidney disease. Adapted from Renal Association guidance (www.renal.org/eGFR/about.html)

Stage	GFR	Description	Treatment stage
1	90+	Normal kidney function but urine findings or structural abnormalities or genetic trait point to kidney disease	Observation, control of blood pressure
2	60–89	Mildly reduced kidney function, and other findings (as for stage 1) point to kidney disease	Observation, control of blood pressure and risk factors
3	30–59	Moderately reduced kidney function	Observation, control of blood pressure and risk factors
4	15–29	Severely reduced kidney function	Referral to nephrology and planning for established renal failure
5	< 15	Very severe, or established renal failure	Dialysis, transplant or conservative management (end of life care)

GFR, glomerular filtration rate; KDOQI, Kidney Disease Quality Outcomes Initiative

cases. These patients are at high risk of cardiovascular death and should be managed appropriately irrespective of referral to a nephrologist. The development of local guidelines enables progressive CKD and associated complications, such as cardiovascular risk and anaemia, to be managed in the community or general medical clinics and aims to ensure appropriate referrals to renal services. Referral of all patients with CKD stages 3–5 would overwhelm renal services and is not necessary. Anecdotal evidence suggests that referral rates to renal teams from primary care have at least doubled since introduction of eGFR reporting and a variety of methods to manage the increased numbers are being evaluated. Examples include employment of specialist renal nurses, or computerised systems to identify patients most at risk.

NATIONAL AND LOCAL CLINICAL GUIDELINES FOR CKD

Early diagnosis and prompt treatment of kidney damage may prevent progression to ERF and the need for RRT. Co-morbidities are reduced and the prognosis and quality of life on RRT are improved (Vora et al 2000). However, this is only possible with prompt referral to a nephrologist or joint management of the individual by the general practitioner (GP) and the nephrologist/specialist renal nurse. The Renal Association's Guidance on Chronic Kidney Disease (2006) noted that, although ERF is not common, the treatment required (e.g. dialysis) when a person reaches such a stage of renal dysfunction is very expensive (around £25 000 per person per year). Therefore, strategies that make *any* improvement in early kidney dysfunction are highly desirable. So, for the multidisciplinary renal community, it is important to note the following.

- CKD increases in prevalence exponentially with age; the most common identifiable causes being diabetes and vascular disease.
- ERF is more common in ethnic minority populations.
- Late referral of patients with established renal failure requiring renal replacement therapy to specialist renal services is associated with significant extra cost and poor clinical outcomes.
- The great majority of patients starting RRT have progressed from earlier stages of CKD, and many could have been identified and referred earlier.
- The great majority of patients with early CKD do not progress to ERF but do have increased risks of cardiovascular disease; the risk of death outweighs the risk of progression.
- Progression is associated with proteinuria and uncontrolled hypertension.
- Optimal management of the risk factors for cardiovascular disease also reduces the risk of progression from early CKD to ERF (adapted from Renal Association 2006).

Renal Association and Royal College of GPs comprehensive guidance for CKD was published in 2006. The document gives information for specialist referral based on estimated GFR, and then goes on to identify the types of information required for that referral, the pre-referral management required in order to reach a diagnosis of the stage of renal dysfunction, and the rationale for intervention. The identification and management of certain conditions that may influence the progression to CKD are detailed (diabetes mellitus, atherosclerosis, acute renal failure). Some of this guidance will be discussed in more detail below. In 2006, the Scottish Intercollegiate Guidelines Network (SIGN) also developed draft guidance for management of CKD and the final document is expected in Autumn 2007.

However, for GPs and non-specialist healthcare providers to engage effectively with these sorts of publications, consideration must be made of the context of primary care and the current political and financial influences that affect care management. For example, information technology (IT) issues still need to be resolved to facilitate an interface between biochemistry laboratories and GP surgeries, and to ensure adequate support for the GPs.

GENERAL MEDICAL SERVICES (GMS) CONTRACT

A new contract for GPs in 2004 enabled GPs to be awarded points (related to income) if their surgery achieved specific indicators within a quality and outcomes framework (QOF). With the advent of the coronary heart disease (CHD), Diabetes and Renal NSFs and this new General Medical Services (nGMS) contract, it is important that work undertaken to improve the outcomes for patients with CKD is carried out in conjunction with primary and secondary care. Many of the QOF points concerning early detection and prevention of CKD are common to all three NSFs and the nGMS

Table 5.2   The chronic kidney disease quality and outcomes framework in the new General Medical Services contract (2006). From www.nhsemployers.org/primary/primary-656.cfm#NHS-26771-3 (accessed 28.03.06)

Indicator	Points	Payment stages (%)
CKD 1: The practice can produce a register of patients aged 18 years and over with CKD (US National Kidney Foundation: Stage 3–5 CKD)	6	
CKD 2: The percentage of patients on the CKD register whose notes have a record of blood pressure in the previous 15 months	6	40–90
CKD 3: The percentage of patients on the CKD register in whom the last blood pressure reading, measured in the previous 15 months, is 140/85 mmHg or less	11	40–70
CKD 4: The percentage of patients on the CKD register who are treated with an angiotensin-converting enzyme inhibitor (ACE-I) or angiotensin receptor blocker (ARB) (unless a contraindication or side effects are recorded)	4	40–80

contract. These include protection strategies for blood pressure, urine testing for microalbuminuria, glycaemia and lipid control and, therefore, do not add dramatically to the work already being undertaken.

The implementation of the nGMS contract in 2004 coincided with the drive to implement measures in primary and secondary care for early detection and prevention of the progression of CKD. The inclusion of tests in the Diabetes QOF, such as measurement of microalbuminuria and annual testing of creatinine for people with diabetes, has increased the quality of screening and documentation, potentially allowing easier identification for those people with varying stages of CKD caused by diabetes.

The QOF for CKD was introduced in April 2006, and comprises four indicators as shown in Table 5.2.

It is hoped that the Renal QOF will indeed see better identification of patients with CKD which in turn will enable better blood pressure control and slowing down of renal dysfunction.

INTERNATIONAL GUIDANCE ON CKD

The Renal Association CKD guidelines (2006) can be compared with CKD guidance published in other parts of the world, in order that the evidence base for CKD care delivery is considered in the *context of the individual* with renal dysfunction, and not just the context of healthcare delivery specific to certain countries.

In the USA, the K/DOQI (2005) publication on CKD states:

Unfortunately, chronic kidney disease is 'under-diagnosed' and 'under-treated'…, resulting in lost opportunities for prevention. One reason is the lack of agreement on a definition and classification of stages in the progression of chronic kidney disease. A clinically applicable classification would be based on laboratory evaluation of the severity of kidney disease, association of level of kidney function with complications, and stratification of risks for loss of kidney function and development of cardiovascular disease.

In the UK, much is being done to move to prevention and early management of CKD, but it was early days in 2006, and the challenge of managing and caring for large numbers of patients (up to a few hundred in an average GP practice of 10 000 patients) has to be realised.

For the general renal nurse, or the community-based practice nurse, local guidelines for CKD may seem unrealistic, medically orientated and beyond their scope of professional influence. However, it is important for all those involved in caring for those with some form of renal dysfunction to understand what these parameters are, particularly the significance of urinalysis and control of blood pressure. Being able to share knowledge with those performing these tasks in other areas of care delivery can only enhance knowledge, and may prompt further investigation when abnormal results are found. Guidelines and protocols must not be considered the panacea of future CKD care, but can provide one way of supporting non-specialist practitioners involved in caring for those with renal dysfunction.

OUTREACH AND JOINT CLINICS

The kidney is involved in hypertensive disease and diabetes mellitus so good collaboration amongst those who care for these individuals may be able to halt the progression to ERF. The kidney may also be involved in other systemic immunological disorders, such as vasculitis and systemic lupus erythematosus, often later on in the disease progression. Monitoring the use of nephrotoxic agents, such as non-steroidal anti-inflammatory drugs, and the use of contrast media in individuals who have reduced renal function or who are at high risk of ERF is important. Again, collaboration between nephrologists and those delivering care for these individuals can assist in the review of care delivery, often in joint clinics.

Joint clinics may occur frequently, as in the case of diabetes and hypertensive care, but may be less regular in rheumatology, and antenatal clinics, for example. Since the recommendation from the Renal Association in 1997, these joint clinics are slowly evolving in some renal units, but in the renal care community overall it can be argued that there is still room for much more improvement in interdisciplinary and interspecialty renal care. There is a definite role for the experienced renal nurse to be involved in these formal structures, and also to assist other nursing colleagues to identify renal complications and precursors.

ACCESS TO RENAL SERVICES

It is necessary to be mindful of the access the general population has to renal services. A number of recent studies have evaluated acceptance rates to renal services assessing geographical, gender and ethnic variations. In the UK, Roderick et al (1999) found that age was a major determinate of acceptance, with a seven-fold higher rate in males over 64 years compared to younger men, and acceptance rates in females were much lower again. Amongst Asian and African–Caribbean groups, acceptance rates were high, but generally there was an inverse relation of acceptance with distance to the main renal unit. Roderick et al (1999) concluded that local need and supply factors influenced service use, and pressure to expand renal services needed to be aimed at areas with large ethnic minority populations and those living long distances from existing renal units.

CARE AND MANAGEMENT OF EARLY KIDNEY DISEASE

DIABETES MELLITUS

Good blood glucose control in individuals with Type 1 diabetes mellitus has been shown to prevent or slow down the progression of renal failure (Diabetes Control and Complications Trial Research Group; DCCT 1993). For example, a reduction in HbA1c (glycated haemoglobin) from 9.0% to 7.0% was associated with a 39% reduction in the occurrence of microalbuminuria and a 54% reduction in the occurrence of proteinuria over 6.5 years in patients with Type 1 diabetes (DCCT 1993).

More recent research in Type 2 diabetes has indicated that tight blood pressure control is also crucial (United Kingdom Prospective Diabetes Study Group 1998). The American Diabetes Association (2006) has published a revised position statement on diabetic nephropathy, which recommends protein intake should be limited to the recommended dietary allowance (RDA; i.e. $0.8\,g\,kg^{-1}$) in those with any degree of CKD, and that serum creatinine should be measured at least annually for the estimation of GFR in all adults with diabetes regardless of the degree of urine albumin excretion.

Lifestyle advice that is culturally sensitive, including and encouraging cardiovascular exercise, has been identified as a necessary strategy for ultimate success in blood pressure control (Box 5.1). Use of specific medication (angiotensin-converting enzyme (ACE) inhibitors for microalbuminuria) and the pursuit of tight glycaemic control for those with diabetes (Hood & Gennari 1996) are important. Exercise that encourages cardiovascular fitness is particularly recommended for those with diabetes mellitus (Diabetes UK 2005).

Box 5.1   Discussion point: Stages of Chronic Kidney Disease

Greenhalgh et al (1998) interviewed older people with diabetes about their understanding of their diabetes and their adherence to the treatment prescribed. One elderly Muslim man could not understand why his doctor kept asking him to 'do more exercise'. 'But I do ... I pray five times a day'. What the diabetes care team had failed to understand was that in this man's culture and language, 'exercise' meant spiritual exercise, and to create a sweat with cardiovascular exercise was considered unseemly. Sweat was for manual labourers. This paper also highlighted that women who are restricted in their dress code and their ability to go out and about unaccompanied need very careful consideration to interpret the general lifestyle recommendations that are published.

The Scottish Intercollegiate Guidelines Network (2001) details risk factors for the development of diabetic nephropathy as:

- raised blood pressure
- hyperglycaemia
- microalbumin excretion
- increasing age
- duration of diabetes
- presence of retinopathy
- smoking
- genetic factors
- raised cholesterol and triglyceride levels
- male sex.

CONTROL OF BLOOD PRESSURE

The control of systemic hypertension and the primary disease are the only interventions proven to prevent the progression of renal failure (Williams et al 2004; Box 5.2). Again, lifestyle advice must be part of the care, as it is well known that to continue smoking whilst receiving hypertensive treatment obliterates any cardiovascular morbidity effect-sthat the treatment is trying to achieve. Blood pressure targets can be as low as 125/75 mmHg for patients with diabetes and proteinuria.

MONITORING AND CONTROL OF CHOLESTEROL AND LIPID LEVELS

This may require medication as well as dietary intervention. These levels may not directly affect the progression of renal function, but may exacerbate the cardiovascular disease (CVD) as a co-morbidity. The current recommendations are that statin therapy is indicated up to age 70 years when serum cholesterol is $\geq 5.0 \, \text{mmol} \, L^{-1}$, and for secondary prevention (when there is already evidence of CVD) when cholesterol levels are $> 5.0 \, \text{mmol} \, L^{-1}$, and the 10-year coronary heart disease risk is ≥ 30 (SIGN 1999).

Box 5.2 Diabetes and blood pressure control

Whilst a treatment target blood pressure is 140/85 mmHg for all ages, it is thought that those with diabetes may need blood pressure to be lower (130/80 mmHg) to achieve the same clinical benefits (Williams et al 2004). There is evidence that the use of angiotensin-converting enzyme inhibitors or angiotensin receptor blockers may prevent diabetic nephropathy or slow its progression (National Institute for Health and Clinical Excellence 2002, United Kingdom Prospective Diabetes Study Group 1998).

COMPLICATIONS AFFECTING THE EYES AND FEET

Whilst this may not be directly related to renal function, complications may indicate reduced microvascular and macrovascular competency, which also affects the kidneys (United Kingdom Prospective Diabetes Study Group 1998).

MONITORING AND TREATMENT OF MICROALBUMINURIA

As renal insufficiency progresses, protein in the form of microalbuminuria ($30–300\,mg\,24\,h^{-1}$) may be found. Microalbuminuria can be detected by an abnormal albumin–creatinine ratio (ACR) test result, which should be undertaken annually, preferably by an early-morning urine (EMU). An ACR $> 2.5\,mg\,mmol^{-1}$ in men and $> 3.5\,mg\,mmol^{-1}$ in women is abnormal (National Institute for Clinical Excellence 2002). When this occurs, it is regarded as the earliest sign of diabetic nephropathy and predicts increased total mortality, cardiovascular mortality and morbidity, and can progress to ERF. Debate continues as to the cost and long-term benefit outcome when testing for microalbuminuria.

The National Institute for Health and Clinical Excellence (National Institute for Health and Clinical Excellence; 2002) recommends the following renal care for all people with Type 2 diabetes.

- Arrange recall and annual review for people with diabetes.
- Review complications and risk factors at diagnosis and at least annually thereafter.
- Measure urinary ACR (early morning urine sample preferred).
- If microalbuminuria or proteinuria is present, repeat twice more (within 1 month where possible).
- Measure serum creatinine and eGFR annually.
- Classify albumin excretion annually as:
  – lower risk (absence of microalbuminuria or proteinuria) or
  – higher risk.

Proactive management is provided for the non-specialist, as well as guidance on some treatment options (e.g. use of ACE inhibitors), and when to refer to a nephrologist.

PREVENTION OF DETERIORATION OF KIDNEY FUNCTION

CONTROL OF SYSTEMIC HYPERTENSION

In CKD hypertension may also be the result of increased cardiac output because of sodium retention and fluid overload, or as a complication of severe anaemia. Vasopressor functions of the kidney and the production of renin can also play a major role in the development of hypertension.

Generally the blood pressure management aims are:

- the threshold for drug treatment is 140/90 mmHg
- the target is 130/80 mmHg (125/75 mmHg, if proteinuria $>100\,mg\,mmol^{-1}$)

- use ACE inhibitor or angiotensin receptor blocker, if microalbuminuria/ proteinuria/heart failure
- refer to the renal unit if > 150/90 mmHg despite three complementary hypotensive agents.

OPTIMAL DIETETIC MANAGEMENT OF PROTEIN AND CALORIE INTAKE

Management of nutrition, especially the controversial issue of reducing protein intake in CKD, is discussed in Ch. 11.

CONTROL OF SERUM BICARBONATE WITHIN NORMAL LEVELS

As an individual becomes more uraemic, the pH balance in the internal environment starts to become more acidic. The body's natural response to this is to produce bicarbonate, metabolised from the liver and activated by the kidney, which acts as a buffer to return the pH to more neutral levels. However, if the kidney is defective, this process is thwarted and supplementary bicarbonate may be administered. The nurse must be aware that administering bicarbonate may result in plasma volume expansion and hypertension, which should be reported. The safest way to control bicarbonate balance is with dialysis. Hence, if this condition is not adequately controlled, then commencement of dialysis may be indicated (see later for further discussion of acid–base balance).

CONTROL OF CARDIOVASCULAR DISORDERS

Left ventricular heart failure is seen in many people with CKD and may be the result of chronic anaemia, hypertension and volume overload. However, studies into cardiovascular function by Amann et al (1999) indicate that left ventricular hypertrophy in renal failure is independent of the long-term complications associated with ERF. There appears to be another aspect of the renal disease process that causes these cardiac effects.

Whilst there is thought to be little influence of lipid levels on the progression of renal failure, recommendations centre around cholesterol concentrations, as in the non-renal population. From a holistic point of view, cardiac health and prevention of CVD as a complication and co-morbidity for people with CKD is paramount.

MANAGEMENT OF BONE DISEASE

Renal failure causes an abnormality of vitamin D metabolism, causing deficient calcium levels, skeletal damage and bone pain. (See Ch. 2 for further information on the underlying physiological processes.) The aim of care is to keep calcium and phosphate levels within normal ranges, preventing hyperparathyroidism. After correcting the acidosis, plasma phosphate and calcium levels can be controlled with oral phosphate binders, calcium supplements and dietary changes.

Significant disturbance of calcium or phosphate in CKD should usually lead to nephrological referral or advice. The aim in stage 3–5 CKD is to keep serum calcium normal, serum phosphate below $1.8\,mmol\,L^{-1}$ and PTH below twice the upper limit of normal. Calcium is commonly low-normal or low in CKD. High parathyroid hormone (PTH) is a physiological response to low calcium. Phosphate is retained in CKD and high phosphate is a physiological stimulus to PTH release. Often dietary advice and phosphate binders taken with food are needed to keep phosphate within acceptable limits (Renal Association CKD guidelines 2006).

CONTROL OF ANAEMIA

Anaemia in chronic renal failure is usually normocytic and normochromic, and due to primary causes such as reduced production of erythropoietin, uraemic toxins inhibiting erythropoiesis and haemolysis, owing to uraemic changes to the red cell membrane.

The individual will become more anaemic as renal failure progresses, as three types of cells in the blood are affected:

- erythrocytes – causing anaemia
- leukocytes – causing immunosuppression
- platelets – causing bleeding tendencies.

It is now recommended that early treatment with erythropoietin should commence in the early stages of CKD. The European Best Practice Guideline for the Management of Anaemia (Locatelli et al 2004) states that:

All patients with chronic anaemia associated with chronic kidney disease should be investigated for possible treatment, *irrespective* of the stage of kidney disease and requirement for renal replacement therapy.

In general, patients with CKD should maintain a target haemoglobin (Hb) concentration of $>11\,g\,dL^{-1}$ or reach this target within 4 months of starting treatment (Locatelli et al 2004). If anaemia is corrected, the lethargic and cardiac complications are managed. However, until recently, erythropoietin has not been used extensively before the established phase of renal failure, largely due to the high costs of supplying this hormone. Of course, the costs of supply must be compared with the costs of caring for a person with the side-effects of chronic anaemia. The increased mortality and morbidity rates of those with a haemoglobin level of $< 10\,g\,dL^{-1}$ are well documented (KDOQI 1997). Treatment of anaemia must also include correcting contributing factors to anaemia, e.g. gastrointestinal bleeding, iron and vitamin B12 deficiency, and maintaining adequate calorie intake and nutritional status. Persistent anaemia may be indicative that the individual needs to start RRT.

Over the last 5 years developments in renal anaemia management have also been influenced by the introduction of new erythropoiesis-stimulating agents (ESAs), and the emergence of adverse events, such as pure red cell aplasia (PRCA), readjustment of the definitions of CKD and ERF through eGFR (as detailed earlier), and the stages of CKD (also detailed earlier). The European Best Practice Guidelines (Locatelli et al

2004) detail other care of anaemia including evaluation, diagnosis, targets and investigations to non-response. (See the complete guidance details for further information: www.ndt-educational.org/guidelines.asp.)

CONTROL OF GASTROINTESTINAL DISORDERS

These disorders are common in CKD, especially as the individual approaches ERF. The person may experience anorexia, nausea and vomiting, hiccups, a metallic taste in the mouth and, for those with diabetes, exacerbation of gut complications presenting as episodes of diarrhoea. Bleeding from the gut may be seen in the advanced stages of CKD causing haematemesis or melaena. Urea is excreted in the gut, and broken down, releasing ammonia, which acts as an irritant. Some medications may give unpleasant side-effects, e.g. heartburn with phosphate binders and oral iron supplementation. Constipation can be common in ERF as fluid intake is reduced, as is the residue in the diet as part of reducing potassium intake. Generally, the person with renal disease is less physically active owing to the effects of a chronic illness causing lethargy and tiredness.

TREATMENT OF DERMATOLOGICAL DISORDERS

Generalised uraemic pruritus is a distressing symptom in persons with CKD, with often little relief from drugs. Deposits of calcium and phosphorus in the skin and sweat glands excreting urea are thought to be the causative factors of pruritus, but dry skin and drug allergies must not be overlooked as causes. Platelet defects and capillary permeability, both complications of renal failure, can cause bleeding and bruising of the skin, especially if there is continued scratching. Many persons with advanced renal failure have a yellow tinge to their skin that is a combined result of hypermelanosis and the deposition of pigments in the skin (urochrome and carotene) that are usually excreted by the kidneys. Although medications may be of some help, commencement of dialysis may be the only long-term relief.

CONTROL OF VOLUME DISORDERS

During the progression of kidney disease, some nephrons remain intact whilst others continue to be destroyed. The remaining undamaged nephrons hypertrophy and produce an increased volume of filtrate with increased tubular reabsorption, even though there is a reduction in the glomerular filtration rate. This process allows the kidney to continue to function until three-quarters of the nephrons are destroyed. In persons with CKD with blood urea levels above $40\,\mathrm{mmol\,L^{-1}}$, the solute load becomes greater than can be reabsorbed, producing an osmotic diuresis accompanied by polyuria of up to $3\,\mathrm{L}$ in a 24-h period. The kidney's ability to concentrate urine is lost, so the urine is dilute and the person will have nocturia. As more nephrons are destroyed, oliguria with the retention of waste products is evident. The individual develops a wide range of biochemical, haematological and endocrine disorders, and the clinical features of fluid overload.

Changes in fluid allowance may be required in association with diuretics. Loop diuretics, such as frusemide, will increase sodium excretion from the kidney and so prevent sodium retention. During episodes of polyuria, volume replacement should be administered to prevent further reduction in renal perfusion and worsening of kidney function. When volume overload is unresponsive to treatment, the commencement of dialysis is indicated.

CONTROL OF POTASSIUM DISORDERS

Excess potassium is normally removed by renal excretion, but as CKD progresses, excretion of urinary potassium decreases because of a reduced glomerular filtration rate caused by tubular defects in diseases such as diabetes mellitus, ultimately resulting in hyperkalaemia. Hyperkalaemia (indicated as a potassium level above $6.0 \, \text{mmol} \, L^{-1}$) can occur in CKD following episodes of acute illness, infection or non-adherence to dietary restrictions. Chronic metabolic acidosis also causes potassium to shift out of the cells and into the extracelluar fluid, giving rise to hyperkaleamia.

If metabolic acidosis is present, this should be corrected first, and this will then help to reduce the serum potassium to within safe limits. If chronic hyperkalaemia is present, dietary advice may be indicated, so high-potassium foods are avoided. Potassium-sparing diuretics should be discontinued, as these drugs block the distal potassium transfer so that potassium is retained. If hyperkalaemia persists, this should be monitored very closely and managed in one of two ways – either conservatively or with dialysis. Conservative management of hyperkalaemia may involve the use of exchange resins (e.g. calcium resonium). Oral resins are not absorbed but exchange potassium for calcium or sodium from the gastrointestinal tract. The choice of calcium or sodium depends on the level of hypercalcaemia or fluid overload in the individual. Serum calcium should be monitored in CKD, and exchange resin therapy discontinued when the serum potassium falls to $5 \, \text{mmol} \, L^{-1}$.

Acute hyperkalaemia may be managed using a glucose and insulin infusion where insulin shifts potassium back into the cells and glucose prevents hypoglycaemia. The effect of reducing potassium can last up to 2h, so it is a short-term measure, but may be life-saving. Intravenous calcium gluconate may be used to reduce the cardiotoxic effects of potassium, protecting cardiac muscle and preventing arrhythmias. Intravenous infusion of sodium bicarbonate will temporarily reduce serum potassium, especially in persons with acidosis, but it should only be given when no fluid overload is present. Essentially dialysis is the safest and most efficient way of removing potassium from the body, so the above measures may be used if a dialysis facility is not possible, or is not possible immediately. Dialysis can be repeated often if the potassium levels require it (e.g. in rhabdomyolysis) and side-effects associated with the conservative treatment can be avoided.

CONTROL OF ACID–BASE BALANCE

In normal health, acid–base balance is maintained by the excretion into the renal tubules of excess acid (hydrogen or H+ ions) where the following processes then take place.

- Filtered bicarbonate is reabsorbed.
- There is increased production of ammonia that combines with H+ ions and is then excreted in the form of ammonium salts.
- A titratable acid is formed.
- Tubular fluid pH is reduced.

In CKD, a mild metabolic acidosis may be present as normal renal tissue is not sufficient to perform the above functions efficiently. Metabolic acidosis may also be worse in persons who have renal tubular acidosis.
The individual will present with the following.

- A blood pH of less than 7.35.
- Hyperkalaemia, as metabolic acidosis shifts potassium from the cells into the extracellular fluid.
- Signs of renal bone disease, as metabolic acidosis reduces the bone carbonate buffers, allowing calcium to be lost from the bones: calcium is more soluble in an acid environment.
- Gasping for breath caused by acidosis as the person attempts to breathe off the excess acid through expired carbon dioxide.

Intravenous sodium bicarbonate may correct acidosis but the sodium may cause hypernatraemia, leading to fluid retention and hypertension. Essentially, metabolic acidosis can indicate terminal chronic renal failure, and the most efficient and safest way to treat it is with dialysis.

DISORDERS OF THE CENTRAL NERVOUS SYSTEM

In CKD, nervous system dysfunction can cause numerous mental disabilities such as poor memory function, loss of concentration and slower mental ability. Physical disabilities result in peripheral neuropathies affecting the legs and feet, and may result in 'restless legs' and paraesthesia. More serious neurological problems may rarely be seen, where there is fluid overload and hypertension in advanced renal failure, in the form of convulsions and cerebral oedema. A 'uraemic flap' may be seen in very toxic patients, where the hands involuntarily flap from the wrists. Other electrolyte disorders, e.g. hypercalcaemia/hypocalcaemia, also cause shaking or an involuntary reflex when nerve points are stimulated. All these symptoms and complications can be avoided with the introduction of early dialysis.

SEXUAL FUNCTION

In women, the loss of sexual function may take the form of infertility due to amenorrhoea and other menstrual abnormalities. Loss of libido may be present. If pregnancy does occur, there is a high risk of miscarriage due to the effects of uraemia (Levy et al 1998). There is also risk to the mother's health as it is possible that renal failure will accelerate because of the extra workload on damaged kidneys.

In men, the incidence of infertility and impotence increases with age and the advancement of CKD. There are multiple causes of impotence, which include poor nutrition, anxiety, side-effects of antihypertensive drugs and reduced plasma testosterone. The individual and partner should be given ample opportunity to express fears and talk about symptoms that are causes for concern.

With the wider use of erythropoietin to correct anaemia, fewer women with decreased renal function are experiencing loss of fertility and amenorrhoea. Successful pregnancy for couples where at least one partner has a degree of renal failure is becoming more common and requires careful planning and monitoring for a successful outcome (Giatras et al 1998). In some cases, storage of sperm or eggs may be possible until such time as the renal failure is stabilised and a successful pregnancy is possible. Collaboration with obstetric medical and nursing colleagues cares for both the mother and the unborn child in these unusual medical circumstances (Jungers & Chauveau 1997).

EDUCATION IN THE PREDIALYSIS PHASE

The need for good education and preparation of the individual and the family at all stages of CKD, potentially heading towards ERF, cannot be underestimated (King 1998). The psychological aspects of dealing with this chronic illness have been dealt with in Ch. 3, but it is worth reiterating the importance of education and information as part of the preparation process. It is essential that the person and renal staff work in collaboration, not only to ensure the best care possible for the person, but also for the renal team to understand the patient and family perspective. In Canada, a nationally agreed core curriculum for education in the predialysis period has been developed (Porter 1998). For some, it is very important to be able to continue in their present employment, and so education about RRT modalities must include consideration of how that dialysis is to be performed. For example, peritoneal dialysis that individuals can perform for themselves, or some form of home dialysis programme would be key to maintaining employment status. In this instance, the employers need information and support to ensure that prejudices and fallacies about renal failure are dispelled, and that the individual is not discriminated against in the work environment.

For some, the thought of attempting to understand any aspect of the RRT process is daunting and overwhelming. This may be due to the immediacy of the circumstances in which they commenced RRT, or indeed their sense of control and unique personal characteristics can allow them to assume that healthcare professionals should take the lead in directing care. This in no way means that the individual absolves responsibility or plays no part in any of the decision-making processes about care and treatment. But it does mean that a greater understanding of the individual's psychological and personality profiles will enable a good working relationship to develop, and mutually agreed expectations to be identified (Brun 1997).

For predialysis preparation to be effective, influences on learning, such as cultural and religious beliefs about the context of CKD, have to be taken into consideration. Indeed, misunderstanding and misinterpretation by the individual and their family may have more to do with the way information is presented (e.g. the jargon used) by healthcare professionals. For many patients, the cultural and religious contexts of health are crucial in shaping how far healthcare advice is accepted. The renal unit is a confusing place where the individual has to make sense of their symptoms and proposed treatment plan. Patients also have to work through the stages of grief of losing an old life, and also have to realign the new (renal) life with personal ideology and life goals.

The ultimate skill any renal healthcare professional can hope to achieve in the care of those approaching RRT is to be able to gain an understanding of each individual. That person is unique as regards the personal hopes and aspirations held for the future, the ability to understand the care and treatment strategies that lie ahead, and how he or she wishes to be involved in that care delivery. All too often, renal professionals of all kinds can be very focused on the pathological and technical aspects that dominate their understanding of their role as a renal practitioner. For the individual approaching RRT, the priorities may be quite different, so information-giving should start very early on, at least one year before dialysis is required. Patients have reported that they do not mind who gives them the information, but it is vital that they have a trusting and ongoing relationship with that person, and that the information should not be censored, even though it may be hard to accept at times (O'Donnel & Tucker 1999). The emphasis seems to be on the quality of the relationship, rather than what information is given when and how. An approach that is flexible in terms of media, clear in terms of language and communication strategies, and realistic to the individuals needs and life goals, will go some way to enhancing the support and information offered to individuals and their families along the renal life trajectory.

There may also be those for whom initiation of dialysis may not be feasible. The option of not commencing dialysis at all is discussed in detail in Ch 9.

PREDIALYSIS EDUCATION PROGRAMMES

There are many benefits to running a structured predialysis education programme (PDEP). Many units run group education sessions for patients, and the content of the programmes may include introductions to haemodialysis, peritoneal dialysis and transplantation plus other issues, such as nutrition and the social/psychological support available. PDEPs should enable patients to make informed choices about dialysis and, indeed, Goovaerts et al (2005) found that a high percentage of patients exposed to a structured PDEP often choose a self-care modality, such as home haemodialysis.

A large audit of predialysis care run by the Pan Thames Renal Audit Group (PTRAG 2006) explored the predialysis care of more than 600 patients. Following the audit, the PTRAG recommended that units without predialysis group education implement this type of education within one year of the report, and that all patients who start dialysis in an unplanned way be offered group education and a review of their dialysis type within 6 months of commencing dialysis. The full report and related material are available under Definition 11 Specialist Renal Services on the UK NHS website (can only be accessed from an NHS computer): nwww.esussex.nhs.uk/aiau. Clearly there are benefits to patients if education in groups is offered alongside more traditional one-to-one education with specialist nurses or nephrologists.

WHEN SHOULD DIALYSIS COMMENCE?

The optimal time at which the individual concerned can benefit most from commencing RRT is controversial. Indeed, for some individuals, pre-emptive transplantation may be possible. What is not disputed is the fact that the later in the progression of renal failure and the later the person starts RRT, the poorer the outcome in terms of mortality and morbidity rates and quality of life experienced during this period (Jungers et al 2000). The issues concerning when a person is referred to the renal care team are not just medical, but may have more to do with access to services and resources available nearby. So, what benefits are there from referring an individual to the nephrologist early? In some instances, the rate of decreasing renal function may be slowed or halted. However, Jungers et al (2000) found that the prevalence of cardiovascular disease was nearly twice as high in persons who were referred less than 6 months before starting RRT than in those who had benefited from effective nephrological care for more than 3 years in the predialysis period. Considering that CVD is the major cause of death in ERF, this is a significant finding.

Sesso & Belasco (1996) also found health benefits for those who had an early referral. Indeed, mortality rates were higher (2.77%) in persons who were referred to a nephrologist within the 6 months before commencing than those who had had an earlier referral. Most of these deaths were of cardiac origin which 'could have been prevented with dialysis care'. Levin (2000) and Roubicek et al (2000) also found more access problems and reduced therapeutic options open for individuals who had had a late referral, indicating that their quality of life on dialysis must be compromised; the persons experienced more short-term morbidity, and presented with severe hypertension.

But how early is early? National guidance (Renal Association 2006) suggests that patients in stage 4 CKD (eGFR < 30) should be referred to or at least discussed with the renal team. This should allow at least one year in the predialysis phase as recommended by the NSF (Department of Health 2004). Table 5.3 shows the management of patients in stages 4–5 CKD as recommended by the Renal Association (2006).

Table 5.3   Management of patients in stages 4–5 chronic kidney disease (CKD)

Planning of management	Renal replacement therapy or conservative/palliative care. Includes timely placement of vascular access or peritoneal dialysis catheter, and planning of pre-emptive transplantation
Blood tests	3 monthly estimation of: – Creatinine and calcium/phosphate: oral phosphate binders will often be necessary – Haemoglobin: if Hb < 110 g dL^{-1} and no other cause found, consider management with intravenous iron and erythropoeitin – Cholesterol
Blood pressure	Meticulous control, to 130/80 mmHg max, or 125/75 mmHg in patients with urinary protein/creatinine > 100 mg mmol (approx. equivalent to 2+ or greater on dipstick test)
Correction of acidosis	Oral bicarbonate
Cardiovascular risk	Advice on smoking, exercise and lifestyle
Immunisation	Hepatitis B is added for patients in stages 4 and 5 CKD, in addition to influenza and pneumococcal immunisation
Medication review	Regular review of medication to minimise nephrotoxic drugs (particularly non-steroidal anti-inflammatory drugs) and ensure doses of others appropriate to renal function

Tattersall et al (1995) showed why such high rates of early morbidity and poor quality of life in terms of being able to return to employment after diagnosis of renal failure exist. In the UK, he showed that persons starting dialysis had a weekly Kt/V of 1.05 (see Chapter 7). Comparing this with the KDOQI guidelines (1997) and the Canada–USA (CANUSA) study (1996), which recommend a prescribed Kt/V of 2.0, it can be seen that, at the start of dialysis in the UK, patients could be functioning on half the Kt/V of what is considered optimal for dialysis. This picture is repeated in the USA and Canada, where patients studied were seen to have a Kt/V of about one-third optimal dialysis (CANUSA 1996). So a rather bizarre situation occurs where persons are started on dialysis treatment at an endogenous Kt/V level that is lower than is expected to be optimal for persons who are already on dialysis.

Other benefits of starting dialysis early may also be seen in people who have been in contact with the renal care team for a lengthy period before commencing dialysis. Education and preparation for the treatment ahead was seen to serve the individual better in a longer pre-dialysis period than in a short predialysis and early dialysis periods. Hayslip & Suttle (1995) demonstrated the benefit of early education not only in assisting the person to adapt to a new way of life, but also in the outcomes of adherence to predialysis treatments. Whilst it has been discussed above how certain medical interventions may slow the progression of renal failure, it is important that the involvement and incorporation of the person in the treatment process are understood to be just as important a component as all the scientific treatment that can be done (Brun 1997). Informed choice and timely access creation, and maturation

---

Box 5.3   What is a nephrology assessment?

Essentially the nephrology care team is concerned about the present cause of renal insufficiency and its cause. All members of the multiprofessional team are involved to give a holistic approach to care. The aim is to delay the progression towards established renal failure and dialysis. Investigations into renal function include:

- estimation of glomerular filtration rate (eGFR) and stage of chronic kidney disease (CKD)
- treatment of the underlying cause of the renal insufficiency (e.g. exacerbation of an acute illness, complication of a chronic illness, use of nephrotoxic agents, congenital abnormalities, etc.)
- blood pressure control (see discussion earlier)
- avoidance of nephrotoxic agents such as contrast media and non-steroidal anti-inflammatory drugs

- possible dietary restriction of protein (see discussion earlier)
- imaging and assessing renal function
- assessment of vascular competency generally and for potential access for haemodialysis
- X-ray and scans to view the kidney size and shape, and possible bone scans to assess the state of the skeletal structure for the effects of renal bone disease
- a sample of kidney tissue may be taken by biopsy to identify the underlying cause of renal failure and the state of the disease process. However, interpretation and accuracy of the results depend on the skill of the expert and are usually only carried out when access to a renal histopathology service is available and results are expected to inform treatment.

---

and assessment of the most appropriate treatment modalities are essential for quality of life on RRT. The renal care team needs to rethink its ideas about the commencement of early dialysis, and consider further a 'healthy start' to RRT (Box 5.3).

CONCLUSION

Having reviewed the guidelines and strategies for supporting the individual with CKD, it can be seen there is an evolution in this area of care encompassing many of the biomedical parameters individuals with CKD face in terms of symptoms and prevention of longer term complications. Whilst these efforts are in no way to be underestimated in terms of the impact on clinical practice, and the individual's experience, it could perhaps be argued that future developments of CKD practice need to incorporate a more patient-centred 'life-wide' approach to interdisciplinary CKD care.

Primary care practitioners and non-specialist healthcare professionals are now increasingly expected and encouraged to be involved in CKD care delivery. There have been developments in the management of CKD anaemia, nutrition, eGFR and patient education. Recently there have been global, national and local approaches to prevention of CKD. Literature is emerging about the importance of the cessation of smoking and exercise for individuals with CKD (Clyne 2004, Diabetes UK 2005), and there is a substantial body of literature on the psychological adaptation and adjustments these individuals and their families need to make.

Future development of approaches to CKD need to include racial, cultural and religious considerations when these areas of a person's life clearly impact on the presenting biomedical symptoms, as well as psychological adaptation and coping strategies. Nurses in particular have many professional skills that could be harnessed within guidelines to address these issues.

SUMMARY

This chapter has discussed epidemiological, medical and therapeutic methods of screening for and preventing ERF. Strategies must address renal care both within the acute hospital setting and in the communities within which levels of renal insufficiency are a major cause for concern. Clearly a healthy start on to RRT can only be initiated if early contact is made with the renal care team. It is in this area that the specialist renal nurse can play an important role. Outreach, collaborative working, education, research and specialist clinical skills of the renal nurse can assist in the promotion of renal health. By collaborating with primary care, the renal care team will not only prevent more individuals reaching ERF with complex co-morbidities, but essentially stop them ever needing the scarce resources of RRT.

References

Amann K, Munter K, Wagner J et al. Treatment of cardiovascular changes in renal failure – ACE inhibition, endothelin receptor blockade or a combination of both strategies? Nephrol Dialysis Transplant 1999; 14(Suppl 4): 43–44.

American Diabetes Association. Summary of revisions for the 2006 clinical practice recommendations. Diabetes Care 2006; 29: S3.

Anandarajah S, Tai T, de Lusignan S, Stevens P, O'Donoghue D, Walker M, Hilton S. The validity of searching routinely collected general practice computer data to identify patients with chronic kidney disease (CKD): a manual review of 500 medical records. Nephrol Dialysis Transplant 2005; Oct 20(10): 2089–2096.

Brun R. Preparation for dialysis treatment using the psychologist. Eur Dialysis Transplant Nurses Assoc Eur Renal Care Assoc (EDTNA-ERCA) J 1997; 13: 31–35.

Canada-USA (CANUSA) Peritoneal Dialysis Study Group. Adequacy of dialysis and nutrition in continuous peritoneal dialysis: association with clinical outcomes. Canada-USA (CANUSA) peritoneal study group. J Am Soc Nephrol 1996; 7: 198–207.

Clyne N. The importance of exercise training in predialysis patients with chronic kidney disease. Clin Nephrol 2004 May; 61 Suppl 1: S10–3.

Coresh J, Astor BC, Greene T, Eknoyan G, Levey A. Prevalence of chronic kidney disease and decreased kidney function in the adult US population: Third National Health and Nutrition Examination Survey. Am J Kidney Dis 2003; 41: 1–12.

Department of Health. The Quality and Outcomes Framework (QOF), General Medical Services Contract for General Practices, 2004. www.dh.gov.uk/policyandguidance/ (accessed 06/09/2006).

Diabetes Control and Complications Trial Research Group. The effect of intensive treatment of diabetes on the development and progression of long-term complications in insulin-dependant diabetes mellitus. N Engl J Med 1993; 329: 977–986.

Diabetes UK. Structured care, Part Three of Diabetes Updates; 'Delivering better diabetes care' series, 2005. www.diabetes.org.uk/home.htm (accessed 27/04/2005).

Giatras L, Levy DP, Malone FD et al. Pregnancy during dialysis: case report and specific management guidelines. Nephrol Dialysis Transplant 1998; 13: 3266–3272.

Goovaerts T, Jadoul, M, Goffin E. Influence of a pre-dialysis education programme (PDEP) on the mode of renal replacement therapy. Nephrol Dial Transplant 2005; 20: 1842–1847.

Greenhalgh T, Helman C, Chowdhury AM. Health beliefs and folk models of diabetes in British Bangladeshis: a qualitative study. Br Med J 1998; 7136: 316.

Hayslip DM, Suttle D. Pre-ESRD person education: a review of the literature. Adv Renal Replace Ther 1995; 3: 217–226.

Hood VL, Gennari FJ. Established renal disease. Measures to prevent or slow its progression. Postgrad Med 1996; 11: 163–166.

John R, Webb M, Young A, Stevens PE. Unreferred chronic kidney disease: a longitudinal study. Am J Kidney Dis 2004; 43: 825–835.

Joint Specialty Committee on Renal Medicine of the Royal College of Physicians and the Renal Association, and the Royal College of General Practitioners. *Chronic kidney disease in adults: UK guidelines for identification, management and referral.* London: Royal College of Physicians, 2006.

Jungers P, Chauveau D. Pregnancy in renal disease. Kidney Int 1997; 52: 871–885.

Jungers P, Chokroun G, Robino C et al. Epidemiology of established renal disease in the Ile-de-France area: a prospective study in 1998. Nephrol Dialysis Transplant 2000; 12: 2000–2006.

KDOQI Clinical Practice Guidelines for Chronic Kidney Disease: Evaluation, Classification, and Stratification (2002). American Journal Kidney Diseases 2002; 39, (2 Supp 1) S1-266.

Kidney Dialysis Outcome Quality Initiative (KDOQI). Development of methodology for clinical practice guidelines. Nephrol Dialysis Transplant 1997; 10: 2060–2063.

Kidney Disease Outcome Quality Initiative (K/DOQI). K/DOQI Clinical practice guidelines for chronic kidney disease: evaluation, classification, and stratification 2005. www.kidney.org/professionals/kdoqi/guidelines_ckd/toc.htm (accessed 08/09/2006).

King K. Education factors affecting modality selection: a National Kidney Foundation study. Eur Dialysis Transplant Nurses Assoc Eur Renal Care Assoc (EDTNA-ERCA) J 1998; 14: 27–29.

Levin A. Consequences of late referral on person outcomes. Nephrol Dialysis Transplant 2000; 15(Suppl 3): 8–13.

Levy D, Giatras L, Jungers P. Pregnancy and established renal disease-past experience and new insights. Nephrol Dialysis Transplant 1998; 13: 3005–3007.

Locatelli F, Aljama P, Barany P et al (European Best Practice Guidelines Working Group). Revised European best practice guidelines for the management of anaemia in patients with chronic renal failure. Nephrol Dial Transplant 2004; 19(Suppl 2): ii, 1–47.

National Institute for Clinical Excellence. Management of Type 2 diabetes: Renal disease – prevention and early management, 2002. www.nice.org.uk (accessed 01/09/2006).

O'Donnel A, Tucker L. Predialysis education: a change in clinical practice. How effective is it? Eur Dialysis Transplant Nurses Assoc Eur Renal Care Assoc (EDTNA-ERCA) J 1999; 15: 29–31.

Pan Thames Renal Audit Group 2006. Audit of pre-dialysis care, Accessed from nww.esussex.nhs.uk/aiau (can only be accessed from an NHS computer).

Porter E. Predialysis initiatives in Canada. Nephrol News Issues 1998; 11: 15–16.

Ramsay LE, Williams B, Johnston DG et al. Guidelines for the management of hypertension: report of the third working party of the BHS. J Hum Hypertens 1999; 13: 569–592.

Renal Association. Treatment of adult persons with renal failure. Recommended standards and audit measures. London: Royal College of Physicians, 1997.

Renal Association. Identification, management and referral of adults with chronic kidney disease: concise guidelines 2006. www.renal.org/CKDguide/full/Conciseguid141205.pdf (accessed 01/09/2006).

Roderick P, Clements S, Stone N et al. What determines geographical variation in rates of acceptance on to renal replacement therapy in England? J Health Service Res Policy 1999; 7: 139–146.

Roubicek C, Brunet P, Huiart L et al. Timing of nephrology referral: influence on mortality and morbidity. Am J Kidney Dis 2000; 7: 35–41.

Scottish Intercollegiate Guidelines Network (SIGN). Lipids and the primary prevention of coronary heart disease. SIGN Publication No. 40, 1999 (www.sign.ac.uk).

Scottish Intercollegiate Guidelines Network (SIGN). Management of diabetes. SIGN Publication No. 55, 2001 (www.sign.ac.uk).

Scottish Intercollegiate Guidelines Network. Draft guidance on CKD (www.sign.ac.uk).

Sesso R, Belasco AG. Late diagnosis of chronic renal failure and mortality on maintenance dialysis. Nephrol Dialysis Transplant 1996; 12: 2417–2420.

Tattersall J, Greenwood R, Farrington K. Urea kinetics and when to commence dialysis. Am J Nephrol 1995; 15: 283–289.

United Kingdom Prospective Diabetes Study Group (UKPDS). Tight blood pressure control and risk of macrovasular and microvascular complications in type 2 diabetes: UKPDS 38. Br Med J 1998; 317: 703–713.

Vora JP, Ibrahim HA, Bakris GL. Responding to the challenge of diabetic nephropathy: the history of detection, prevention and management. J Hum Hypertens 2000; 10: 667–685.

Williams B, Poulter NR, Brown MJ et al. The BHS Guidelines Working Party Guidelines for Management of Hypertension: Report of the Fourth Working Party of the British Hypertension Society, 2004 – BHS IV. J Human Hypertens 2004; 18: 139–185.

Chapter 6

Renal investigations

Althea Mahon

LEARNING OUTCOMES
FOR THIS CHAPTER

- To explain the procedures commonly undertaken in the diagnosis of acute and chronic kidney disease
- To evaluate the nurses' role in postprocedure care
- To gain knowledge and understanding of the investigations required in the diagnosis of renal impairment
- To provide a rationale for the use of those investigations and procedures

INTRODUCTION

Patients referred to a nephrologist are subjected to a bewildering array of diagnostic tests and procedures. Nurses working in this area should familiarise themselves with these investigations in order to be able to explain these procedures to the patient adequately, and consent will then be truly 'informed'. The tests covered in this chapter include those involving blood and urine, invasive diagnostic investigations, X-rays, scans, isotope studies and methods of evaluating glomerular filtration rate. Investigations that are carried out prior to erythropoietin therapy are discussed, as well as those used in cases of diminished or non-response to erythropoietin therapy.

Some patients who have progressive renal disease show no specific signs or symptoms, and do not feel unwell until the disease is well advanced. Abnormal results of blood and urine tests carried out at routine medical examinations, whether they be pre-employment, pre-life insurance or preoperative, or during visits to a general practitioner for other reasons, may warrant referral. Patients in acute renal failure (see Ch. 4) for whatever cause, also come under the remit of a nephrologist, and urgent diagnosis and treatment in this potentially life-threatening situation are vital. Sometimes only a large number of investigations will help make the diagnosis.

Nurses are responsible for the correct procedure of many investigations, so an understanding of the nature of these tests is vital, as is the ability to recognise abnormal results.

An individual with established renal failure (ERF) is subjected to constant investigations to monitor the effectiveness of renal replacement therapy (RRT), with the objective of giving the patient maximum benefit from treatment with the minimum of side-effects, in order to maintain a reasonable quality of life.

VENEPUNCTURE

Traditionally, venepuncture has not been regarded as a procedure routinely performed by nurses in the UK; the exception was those nurses who were carrying out what was known as an 'extended role'.

Collecting blood samples was considered to be the job of the medical staff and phlebotomists. However, in 1994, the UK Department of Health recommended that, while redefining nurses' activities, venepuncture should now be considered a routine nursing procedure, to be shared with the medical staff in the absence of a phlebotomist (Greenhalgh Report 1994). In the renal field, as urgent blood test results can be vital to successful treatment, nurses who can demonstrate competency have extended their scope of practice to include venepuncture (United Kingdom Central Council for Nursing, Midwifery and Health Visiting (UKCC) 1992).

Before embarking on the collection of blood samples there are several factors that should be considered:

- the safety of healthcare personnel
- the safety and comfort of the patient
- the correct collection system.

SAFETY OF HEALTH CARE PERSONNEL

In order to keep the danger of blood-borne infection to a minimum, universal precautions should be observed at all times; that is, all patients' body fluids should be assumed to be carriers of infective organisms (Department of Health 1998). Disposable gloves (also aprons and eye shields in some situations) should be worn as appropriate and attention paid to proper hand-washing before and after each procedure.

Needlestick and sharps injuries account for 17% of reported accidents in the UK. Hepatitis B, C and Human immunodeficiency virus (HIV) are among the 20 dangerous blood-borne pathogens that can be transmitted via contaminated needles.

Many new safety devices have been developed, such as closed blood collection system, shielded and retractable needles, safety lancets, blunt needles and needle-free systems with recommended systems available on The NHS Purchasing and Supply Agency website (www.pasa.nhs.uk).

Closed systems avoid the need to transfer blood from syringe to laboratory sample tube, as the blood collection device fulfils both functions. Decanting blood from syringe to blood tube should only be carried out when absolutely necessary. Local protocol may demand that samples from patients known to be infected with HIV, or hepatitis B or C and other contagious organisms should be identified with internationally recognised yellow biohazard labels and be processed at the end of a laboratory run. On completion of the procedure, no attempt should be made to resheathe the needle; it should immediately be discarded at the point of use in a suitable sharps container (Department of Health, 2005).

CHOICE OF VEIN

When carrying out venepuncture on a patient with chronic kidney disease (CKD), great care must be taken of veins as they may be needed in the future for fistula formation for haemodialysis. For this reason the cephalic vein in the forearm must be avoided for both venepuncture and intravenous infusion. The veins of the antecubital fossa should be used for venepuncture whenever possible, with the veins of the upper aspect of the hand as second choice, although this can be a painful site for the patient (Fig. 6.1). It is best to avoid the antecubital veins in those with diabetes due to difficulties with access formation. Arteriovenous fistulae sites should not be cannulated except for dialysis purposes, to exclude the slight danger of infection or haematoma, which may render the fistula unsuitable for dialysis in either the short or long term.

Figure 6.1
Veins of the arm.

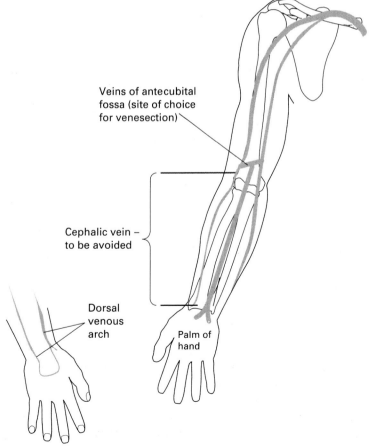

Veins of antecubital fossa (site of choice for venesection)

Cephalic vein – to be avoided

Dorsal venous arch

Palm of hand

Alternative site for venesection

THE CORRECT COLLECTION PROCEDURE

Before attempting venepuncture, the correct method of collection according to local policy should be ascertained and all necessary equipment assembled. There are many designated tubes available; if blood is sent to the laboratory in the wrong tube, it cannot be processed, time and money are wasted and unnecessary discomfort is caused to the patient in repeating the procedure. Check unfamiliar tests with the laboratory before commencing.

If difficulties arise in collecting a blood sample from a patient, it is advisable that only two attempts should be made before calling for assistance from a more experienced member of staff. Factors that can cause difficulties locating a vein include dehydration, hypotension, obesity and fragile veins.

POINTS FOR CONSIDERATION

If difficulty is encountered in locating a suitable vein:

- Gently tap the chosen site.
- Ask the patient to open and close the fist several times.
- Inflate a sphygmomanometer cuff to a pressure between the patient's systolic and diastolic blood pressure proximal to the venepuncture site.
- Hang the arm down towards the floor for a few minutes.
- In cold weather, keep clothing intact until the last moment, or immerse the chosen arm in warm water to encourage peripheral circulation.

Haematoma formation can be prevented by applying adequate pressure to the puncture site until clotting occurs.

Blood samples from dialysis access needles or lines must be free of saline and anticoagulants (e.g. heparin), and of clotted material, must be of blood directly from the patient and not the machine, and must not be recirculated blood. Blood for any clotting tests should be taken pre-dialysis from another site such as the back of the hand or antecubital fossa, as any heparin contamination will falsify the result.

Haemodialysis samples should all have 'pre-, mid- or postdialysis sample' clearly marked on the request form to avoid confusion.

The following items are important:

- Always check that the correct collection tube and request form are to hand.
- Know whether the sample has to be delivered immediately to the laboratory, or can be stored at room temperature, in a fridge or on ice.
- Check whether the patient should be fasting.
- Use minimum pressure with a tourniquet to avoid haemolysis, and also to minimise bruising of the patient.
- Ensure the sample is correctly labelled.
- Use biohazard labels for known contaminated samples (as per local protocol). However, all samples should be treated as potentially hazardous.

BIOCHEMICAL BLOOD TESTS

NORMAL VALUES

These are listed in Table 6.1. They may vary locally and may be expressed in alternative units of measurement. Paediatric normal values should always be checked, as these vary with age.

Monitoring blood biochemistry of patients with chronic kidney disease is central to their diagnosis and ongoing care, as this reflects the kidneys' function in excreting the waste products of metabolism. Serum or heparinised plasma samples are suitable for most biochemistry investigations.

Blood to be separated for serum samples is collected in a plain clotting tube (no additives) or in a tube containing beads treated with a clotting activator. Blood to be separated for plasma samples is collected in a tube containing lithium heparin or beads treated with lithium heparin. The beads form a layer between the blood clot and serum or plasma after centrifugation, which allows serum to be withdrawn by pipette (by mechanised or manual methods) for the appropriate analysis. Some tubes contain a gel for the same purpose to act as a barrier between cells and plasma or serum.

RENAL PROFILE

The following tests (urea, creatinine, sodium, potassium, corrected calcium, phosphate, bicarbonate and albumin) are often requested together. The result is generated from one 5-mL blood sample in a plain or lithium heparin tube. Some centres may include other tests under this profile.

It is important to mention here that creatinine levels may not show a significant increase until there is a 50% loss of kidney function. Therefore, serum creatinine is not a sensitive test for early renal disease. Estimated GFR is now recommended (see Ch. 5).

Table 6.1
Analysis of a normal blood sample

Urea (blood urea nitrogen)	Adult 2.5–6.4 mmol L^{-1}
	Child 1.1–6.4 mmol L^{-1}
Creatinine	Adult 70–120 µmol L^{-1}
	Child (increasing with age)
	27–88 µmol L^{-1}
Sodium	135–147 mmol L^{-1}
Potassium	3.5–5 mmol L^{-1}
Calcium	2.2–2.6 mmol L^{-1}
Phosphate	0.8–1.5 mmol L^{-1}
Bicarbonate	22–30 mmol L^{-1}
Cholesterol	3.5–5.7 mmol L^{-1}
Total protein	60–80 g L^{-1}
Albumin	35–50 g L^{-1}
Glucose (fasting)	3.6–5.8 mmol L^{-1}

Urea is one of the principal end-products of protein metabolism. Urea is formed in the liver, carried by the blood and excreted by the kidneys in the urine. Raised blood urea indicates failure of the kidneys and usually increases in tandem with creatinine levels in chronic kidney disease and established renal failure. However, serum urea levels may remain within normal limits whilst serum creatinine levels increase.

Urea can rise dramatically in previously healthy individuals who experience overwhelming infection or major crush injuries and are admitted to hospital in acute renal failure. A slight rise in urea may be seen if a very-high-protein diet is consumed, and in low-protein diets a lower level of blood urea may be observed. Certain drugs, such as corticosteroids and tetracycline, can cause a sudden rise in blood urea, especially if the patient already has chronic kidney disease.

- High-protein diet
- Chronic malnutrition – increased protein metabolism
- Gastrointestinal bleeds – increased protein absorption
- Dehydration – increased urea reabsorption.

A normal or low urea level is not necessarily indicative of adequate dialysis if a patient is malnourished with a low protein intake.

Urea

Non-renal causes of increased urea levels

Creatinine is produced by the breakdown of creatine phosphate in muscle by catabolism and is excreted by the kidney. Raised creatinine can reliably be used as a specific indicator of kidney malfunction, as it is fairly constant from day to day and rises steadily with progressive renal impairment. A higher level of serum creatinine may be expected with higher body weight, in males, and in those of Afro–Caribbean ethnicity.

Creatinine levels in patients with progressive renal failure may eventually rise to a level where it is considered expedient to commence dialysis. This may be in the region of $500–1000\,\mu mol\,L^{-1}$ but varies with each patient, the symptoms experienced by the patient, and the policy of the renal unit. Patients with diabetes are usually commenced on dialysis earlier, sometimes with creatinine levels of $400–500\,\mu mol\,L^{-1}$. Creatinine levels can be plotted on a log graph at regular intervals over a period of time, and used as a predictor of the time when renal replacement therapy is likely to be necessary.

It was recommended in the National Service Framework for Renal Services (Part Two) (2005) that from April 2006 all hospital laboratories should report the value of estimated glomerular filtration rate (eGFR), alongside serum creatinine. Further discussion about the limitations of reporting serum creatinine alone and ways in which eGFR can be calculated can be found later in this chapter and also in Ch. 5.

Creatinine

Sodium is the principal electrolyte (Na^+) of the extracellular fluid of the blood, maintaining osmotic pressure, and is involved in acid–base balance and the transmission of nerve impulses. Sodium is taken into the body with the diet and is conserved or excreted by the kidneys. Hyponatraemia ($< 135\,mmol\,L^{-1}$) can be an indication of excess body fluid, and is also often present in burns, diarrhoea, vomiting, nephritis, neoplasms and diabetic acidosis.

Sodium

Hypernatraemia (> 148 mmol L^{-1}) can be an indication of dehydration and insufficient water intake, multiple myeloma, diabetes insipidus, metabolic acidosis or excessive intravenous isotonic fluids in renal failure. Patients may be proportionally hypernatraemic or hyponatraemic without an altered fluid state.

Potassium

Potassium is the principal electrolyte (K$^+$) of the intracellular fluid, with only low concentrations (2%) circulating in the extracellular fluid. Potassium is provided by the diet and excreted mainly by the kidneys, where regulation of the body potassium content occurs – a small amount is also lost in the faeces. Potassium is necessary to maintain nerve conduction and plays a major role in control of cardiac output. Potassium levels usually remain normal if a urine output in excess of 1500 mL day^{-1} can be maintained. Hypokalaemia (< 3.5 mmol L^{-1}) may be found in cases of diarrhoea, vomiting, renal tubular acidosis, diuretic usage, intravenous fluid administration without added potassium, and when excess insulin causes an increase in the cellular uptake of potassium. Hypokalaemia can cause cardiac arrhythmias.

Hyperkalaemia (> 5.5 mmol L^{-1}) may be seen in renal failure, burns, insulin deficiency, post-traumatic conditions (including surgery), disseminated intravascular coagulation or when potassium-sparing diuretics are used with Slow-K, and any condition where cell damage has occurred, causing leakage of intracellular potassium into the extracellular fluid. In patients with renal failure, a potassium level > 6.5 mmol L^{-1} may be a medical emergency requiring immediate instigation of dialysis or other treatments. If left unattended, the patient may suffer cardiac arrest caused by the arrhythmic effect of potassium build-up. Blood samples for accurate potassium analysis should be delivered swiftly to the laboratory or, if this is impossible, separated and stored, to prevent leaching of intracellular potassium into the serum, which results in a falsely raised level. (See Ch. 4 for hyperkalaemia treatments.)

Calcium

Calcium (normal range total Ca^{2+} 2.2–2.6 mmol L^{-1}) is provided by the diet and is excreted by the kidneys. Most body calcium is found in the skeleton but a small proportion is circulated in the blood. About 50% of serum calcium is protein-bound and 50% is ionised. Ionised serum calcium is responsible for muscle contraction, cardiac function and blood clotting. Corrected calcium estimates the total concentration of calcium as if the albumin concentration was normal (i.e estimates the free calcium) and is calculated as follows:

Corrected calcium (mmol L^{-1}) = Calcium + [40 – albumin (g L^{-1})] × 0.02

In the healthy individual, calcium homeostasis is controlled by parathyroid hormone, vitamin D and the hormone calcitonin.

Hypocalcaemia is found in chronic kidney disease where phosphate retention is present (calcium carbonate is given to alleviate this; see Ch. 9). Chronic hypocalcaemia causes an excess of parathyroid hormone to be excreted into the blood stream, which in turn releases calcium from the bone, resulting in the renal bone disease often seen in conjunction with vitamin D deficiency in renal patients. In nephrotic syndrome, low levels of calcium will be found due to albumin leaking into the urine, taking bound calcium with it. In the nephrotic patient, the ratio of protein-bound and ionised calcium will remain the same. The acidosis of renal failure is an added cause of loss of bone calcium. Hypercalcaemia may be an indication of hyperparathyroidism, sarcoidosis or malignancy. High levels of calcium can cause renal stones and renal tubular disease.

Phosphate

Phosphorus is found in the diet. Phosphate (normal value PO_4^{3-} 0.8–1.5 mmol L^{-1}) is mainly combined with calcium in the skeletal bone. It is controlled, with calcium, by parathyroid hormone and, apart from its skeletal function, has a role in the metabolism of glucose and lipids. Phosphates are excreted by the kidney. When phosphate is increased, calcium is lowered and vice versa.

Hypophosphataemia may be found in the patient with renal tubular disease who loses phosphate, possibly leading to osteomalacia. Hyperphosphataemia will often be found in conjunction with hypocalcaemia.

OTHER BIOCHEMICAL BLOOD TESTS

Uric acid

Uric acid (normal values: female 200–350 μmol L^{-1}; male 260–500 μmol L^{-1}) is an end-product of purine metabolism and is excreted mainly by the kidney, but in part by the bowel. In gout, excess uric acid crystallises in joints. Patients in renal failure have an impaired ability to excrete uric acid and a high serum level may be found in association with raised urea and creatinine. Increased serum uric acid is also found in pre-eclampsia of pregnancy, leukaemia, multiple myeloma, various cancers and in acute shock.

Bicarbonate

The normal value of bicarbonate (HCO_3^-) is 22–30 mmol L^{-1}. Low plasma HCO_3^- indicates metabolic acidosis caused by CKD with an inability to excrete hydrogen ions adequately.

Glucose

The normal value of fasting serum glucose is 3.6–5.8 mmol L^{-1}. Blood glucose levels are maintained by the liver, which absorbs and stores glucose as glycogen, and releases it into the circulation in response to the demands of the body. Glucose is regulated by insulin, which is synthesised by the beta cells in the islets of Langerhans in the pancreas.

Plasma total proteins

The normal value of plasma total proteins is 60–80 g L^{-1}.

Hypoproteinaemia associated with low albumin (normal value 35–55 g L^{-1}) levels may be found in the many conditions associated with nephrotic syndrome, where protein leakage occurs from the kidney into the urine. Also, decreased total protein in conjunction with low albumin may be found in liver disease, burns and haemorrhage.

Hyperproteinaemia (increase of total plasma protein) with a normal albumin–globulin ratio may occur in dehydration. If total protein increases with a falling albumin–globulin ratio (i.e. a raised globulin), this may indicate autoimmune disease, such as systemic lupus erythematosus, or shock, chronic infection or myeloma.

Albumin

The normal value of albumin is 35–50 g L^{-1}.

Albumin levels can be elevated in patients with dehydration. Low albumin levels are common in CKD owing to protein loss through peritoneal dialysate, poor dietary intake and nephrotic syndrome. Other causes of low albumin levels are decreased absorption in liver disease and increased breakdown in malignancy.

Serum protein electrophoresis

This test measures specific proteins in the blood, which helps to diagnose certain renal diseases, such as multiple myelomas. Serum protein electrophoresis uses an electrical field to separate out the proteins in the serum as the proteins carry a positive or electrical charge.

Lipids

The normal values are: total cholesterol 3.5–5.7 mmol L^{-1}; triglycerides 0.45–2.0 mmol L^{-1}. A major cause of morbidity and mortality in patients with kidney disease can be attributed to cardiovascular events, one of the main risk factors of which is hyperlipidaemia. Hyperlipidaemia is often found in those with CKD, especially those with nephrotic syndrome and in transplanted patients.

Parathyroid hormone

See below in the section on erythropoietin.

SEROLOGY

Serological tests are frequently required as renal impairment is often only one manifestation of a systemic disease. Many renal disorders arise from immune dysfunction and serology will often, therefore, provide an exact diagnosis. Antineutrophil cytoplasmic antibodies (ANCA) are present in collagen or autoimmune diseases, and they are an important diagnostic marker. The test itself will identify whether antibodies are present using the technique of immunofluorescence. A positive ANCA test is found in disease states, such as systemic and renal vasculitis. Anti-glomerular basement membrane (anti-GBM) is an antibody detected in Goodpasture's syndrome. Other tests include those for immunoglobulins that are found in autoimmune diseases.

COMPLEMENT

The most common complement studies performed are for C3 and C4. These levels rise during an acute inflammatory state. However, there are many other specialised complement studies that can be undertaken in order to diagnose a particular disease process.

HAEMATOLOGY

Haematological tests give information about anaemia, haematological malignancies and clotting disorders. Infections, inflammatory disease and other conditions can be indicated by changes in total and differential white cell counts. Normal values are shown in Table 6.2 (note that there may be slight local variations, especially in the paediatric normal range).

Full blood count (FBC)

This test provides information regarding the platelets and the red and white blood cells, often providing evidence of renal anaemia in the patient with CKD. It may be appropriate to investigate further those values falling outside normal parameters (further information is given in the erythropoietin section below).

Values for mean corpuscular volume (MCV) reflect the size, and those for mean corpuscular haemoglobin (MCH) and mean corpuscular haemoglobin concentration (MCHC) reflect the haemoglobin concentration of individual cells (normal ranges: MCV, 76–96 fL; MCH, 27–32 pg; and MCHC, 30–36 g dL^{-1}). These red blood cell indices are useful in the diagnosis of types of anaemia.

Anaemias are classified on the basis of cell size (MCV) as microcytic, normocytic or macrocytic, and on the basis of the amount of haemoglobin (MCH) as microchromic, normochromic or macrochromic. They can therefore be classified as follows.

- Normocytic/normochromic anaemia: from acute blood loss, prosthetic heart valves, sepsis, tumour or aplastic anaemia.
- Microcytic/hypochromic anaemia: from chronic blood loss, iron deficiency, lead poisoning or thalassaemia.
- Microcytic/normochromic anaemia: erythropoietin deficiency in chronic kidney disease.
- Macrocytic/normochromic anaemia: from chemotherapy, folate deficiency, or vitamin B12 deficiency.

White blood cell count and differential

White blood cells are the cells in the body that fight against infections, allergies, etc. There are five types of white blood cells, which can be split into two groups: granulocytes and agranulocytes. The granulocytes include neutrophils, eosinophils and basophils, and have granules in the

Haemoglobin	Male 13.5–18 g dL^{-1}
	Female 11.5–16.5 g dL^{-1}
Haematocrit	Male 40–55%
	Female 35–45%
Platelets	150–350 × 10^9 L^{-1}
Leukocytes (white blood cells)	5–10 g L^{-1}

Table 6.2
Normal values:
haematological tests

cytoplasm of their cells and also have a multilobed nucleus. Agranuloctye white blood cells, lymphocytes and monocytes do not have granules and have non-lobular nuclei. They are sometimes referred to as mononuclear leukocytes.

The normal range for total white blood cell count is $4–11\times10^9$ g/L. A low white cell count is referred to as leukopenia and a high white cell count as leukocytosis. Leukocytosis is usually due to an increase in one of the five types of white blood cells and is given the name of the cell that shows the primary increase (i.e. neutrophilia, eosinophilia, basophilia, lymphocytosis and monocytosis).

Leuckocytosis may be indicative of an infection, inflammation or a haematologic malignancy and leukopenia may be due to bone suppression or replacement, hypersplenism or deficiences of cobalamin or folate.

Differential (or relative value)

This is a count of the five different types of white blood cell expressed as a percentage of the total white cell count (rather than their absolute value).

- *Neutrophils:* 50–70% relative value (2500–7000 absolute value). An increase may indicate infection and is called neutrophilia. A decrease is called neutropenia and may be due to chemotherapy.
- *Eosinophils:* 1–3% relative value (100–300 absolute value). An increase may indicate infections or allergies.
- *Basophils:* 0.4–1% relative value (40–100 absolute value). Basophilia is an uncommon cause of leukocytosis but can be caused by infections or inflammatory conditions, such as inflammatory bowel disease and chronic airway inflammation.
- *Lymphocytes:* 25–35% relative value (1700–3500 absolute value). Absolute lymphocytosis may be caused by acute infections (cytomegalovirus, Epstein–Barr virus, pertussis, hepatitis, toxoplasmosis), chronic infections (tuberculosis, brucellosis) or lymphoid malignancies (chronic lymphocytic leukaemia). Relative lymphocytosis is seen in the acute phase of several viral illnesses, in connective tissue diseases, thyrotoxicosis, Addison's disease and splenomegaly with splenic sequestration.
- *Moncocytes:* 4–6% relative value (200–600 absolute value). Monocytosis may be due to either chronic infection, chronic inflammatory disorders, such as Crohn's disease, or carcinoma. However, a transient monocytosis can be seen with the resolution of an infection. A monocytosis may also be seen in the myelodysplastic conditions.

Coagulation

In circulating blood, a series of factors are present that provide the means for clot formation as appropriate when damage to a vessel occurs. Prior to many renal procedures, such as kidney biopsy, it is standard practice to ascertain that the patient has normal clotting function to avoid the risk of haemorrhage. Those with uraemia are more prone to bleeding as urea affects the clotting cascade.

Included in this group of tests are platelets (normally, $150–400 \times 10^9 \, L^{-1}$ are present in the FBC). Platelets adhere to each other and initiate the clotting cascade when damaged endothelium is encountered. Platelet deficiency (thrombocytopenia) is a common cause of prolonged bleeding.

Other coagulation studies likely to be encountered in renal investigations include the bleeding time (normal < 10 min); partial thromboplastin time (PTT); activated partial thromboplastin time (APTT); fibrinogen, and international normalised ratio (INR). Most methods in current use require a very precise amount of blood in coagulation tests; the blood sample should exactly reach the marked line. Blood for coagulation studies during or immediately post-haemodialysis or from heparinised lines (e.g. temporary or permanent dialysis catheters) should not be taken from a central line, as the result will be falsified. It is recommended to use a vein instead.

ERYTHROPOIETIN THERAPY

Anaemia is a major complication of CKD and a contributory factor to cardiovascular disease in patients needing dialysis. The major cause is the lack of production of the hormone erythropoietin (EPO), which is produced by the kidney. Correction of renal anaemia has been shown to improve both cardiac function and the quality of life of dialysis patients (Macdougall 2000). The desired rate of increase in haemoglobin is $1\,g\,dL^{-1}$ month^{-1} until the target haemoglobin is reached. Anaemia treatments are discussed further in Ch. 5. Before starting treatment for anaemia, some basic investigations must be completed in order to correct any deficiencies that may prevent an adequate response to this very expensive therapy.

Symptoms of anaemia

These are: lethargy, dyspnoea and pallor.

Before starting EPO therapy it is important to exclude or treat (if possible) underlying causes such as:

- iron deficiency
- blood loss
- infection or inflammatory disease
- hyperparathyroidism
- aluminium toxicity
- vitamin B12 and folate deficiency
- haemolysis
- haemoglobinopathies.

Haemoglobin

Haemoglobin should be checked to ensure that anaemia is not present. Haemoglobin varies with age, gender and ethnicity. The level at which it is considered that EPO should justifiably be given varies from one centre to another, but a haemoglobin of less than $8\,g\,dL^{-1}$ or haematocrit below 25% is commonly given as a guideline. The recommendation from the European Best Practice Guidelines (2004) is for haemoglobin to be $> 11\,g\,dL^{-1}$ within 3 months of commencing therapy ($1\,g\,dL^{-1}\,month^{-1}$). Normocytic erythrocytes are typical in the patient with renal anaemia. However, in the case of iron-deficiency anaemia, normocytic and hypochromic red blood cells will be seen.

Haematocrit

Haematocrit is the percentage of red blood cells in the whole blood volume, which will be low in the patient with renal anaemia, running in parallel with the low level of haemoglobin. When the patient responds to the effect of EPO, a rise in haematocrit will be seen in conjunction with a rise in haemoglobin and red blood cells.

Other tests

Having ascertained that the patient has renal anaemia, the next step is to carry out certain investigations to check that there is no condition present which may prevent or reduce the effect of EPO. These tests should be repeated if diminished or non-response to EPO occurs at a later date.

Haematinics

In order to maintain the haem component of the healthy red blood cell, an adequate amount of available and stored iron must be present. There are several tests that can be carried out to determine this very important factor – the main cause of non-response to EPO has been found to be low available iron.

Iron-deficiency anaemia is either absolute or functional.

Ferritin

The normal range in health is 15–300 ng mL^{-1}, but an individual with renal failure needs a minimum of 100 ng mL^{-1}. Ferritin is the main stored iron form found in all tissues, but especially in the liver, spleen and bone marrow. Ferritin found in the serum relates to the amount of stored iron, but is not necessarily an accurate assessment of available iron.

Unless ferritin levels are at least 100 µg/L before EPO therapy is started, the response will be short-lived. Ferritin levels should be kept in excess of this by infusing intravenous iron to allow adequate erythropoiesis, as oral iron supplementation is inadequate.

Transferrin

Iron is transported by the specific plasma protein transferrin (or siderophilin). A useful test of available iron for red cell production is the transferrin saturation rate. Transferrin saturation indicates how much iron is circulating in the plasma relative to total iron-binding capacity.

Folic acid

Folic acid is a water-soluble vitamin in the B-complex group that is absorbed from the duodenum and jejunum. Folic acid works along with vitamin B12 and vitamin C to help the body digest and utilise proteins, and to synthesize new proteins when they are needed. It is necessary for the production of red blood cells and for the synthesis of DNA. Folic acid also helps with tissue growth and cell function. Low levels can cause macrocytic anaemia. Stores of this vitamin last only a few months.

Vitamin B12

Vitamin B12 (normal range 150–1000 ng L^{-1}) is a water-soluble vitamin that is part of the vitamin B complex. It is absorbed in the ileum. The uptake is dependent on the production of acid and intrinsic factor in the stomach, adequate oral intake and production of transcobalamin (transport protein). Vitamin B12, like the other B vitamins, is important for metabolism, and helps in the formation of red blood cells and in the maintenance of the central nervous system. Although the body stores can last several years without oral intake, low levels (e.g. in pernicious anaemia) can cause a macrocytic anaemia.

C-reactive protein

C-reactive protein (CRP) is a globulin that is synthesised by the liver and is present in small amounts in a normal individual. An elevated CRP is indicative of infection, inflammation or malignancy. The most important role of CRP is its interaction with the complement system, which is one of the body's immunologic defence mechanisms. It is normally present in the plasma at a concentration of less than $5\,mg\,L^{-1}$.

C-reactive protein increases in virtually all conditions associated with tissue damage and may double its concentration every 6 h. CRP is better than erythrocyte sedimentation rate for monitoring fast changes, as it does not depend on fibrinogen or immunoglobulin levels, and is not affected by red blood cell numbers and shape.

Haptoglobins

Haptoglobin is an acute phase protein, rising in concentration during acute inflammation. Classically, a low haptoglobin concentration is indicative of intravascular haemolysis. It may also occur in extravascular haemolysis, where some free haemoglobin leaks from the phagocytic cells of the spleen, chronic liver disease, metastatic malignancy and sepsis.

Bilirubin (3–17 µmol L⁻¹)

Bilirubin is a bile pigment produced by the breakdown of haem and reduction of biliverdin. Unconjugated bilirubin is insoluble in plasma unless bound to protein, mainly albumin. Salicylates, sulphonamides, non-esterified fatty acids and reduced pH levels result in decreased protein-binding of unconjugated bilirubin. Normally, 95% of the circulating bilirubin is unconjugated.

The bilirubin–albumin complex is dissociated by receptors on hepatocytes. The albumin remains in the plasma. The bilirubin is taken into the hepatocyte and conjugated by the enzyme bilirubin UDP-glucuronyl transferase to form bilirubin diglucuronide. It is this water-soluble glucuronate derivative which is excreted into the biliary system. In the gut, principally the colon, bilirubin glucoronides are degraded by bacteria and converted into a mixture of compounds, known as urobilinogen or stercobilinogen; these are water soluble. Most of the urobilinogen is excreted in the faeces where it is oxidised to urobilin, which is brown. Some is reabsorbed into the liver where it is re-excreted. When the amount of urobilinogen is increased, some passes into the systemic circulation and is excreted in the urine.

Complete biliary obstruction is indicated by:

- the absence of urinary urobilinogen
- the presence of urinary bilirubin.

Jaundice or icterus describes the yellow staining of the tissues due to an excess of bilirubin – unconjugated or conjugated. Jaundice becomes clinically detectable at levels $> 40\,\mu mol\,L^{-1}$.

Coombs' test The Coombs' test is used in the investigation of haemolytic anaemia. A positive Coombs' test is found in cases of autoimmune haemolysis due to the presence of immunoglobulin G (IgG), complement or both, on the surface of the patient's red cells. A positive result may be found in a haemolytic transfusion reaction or autoimmune haemolysis, including drug-induced haemolysis.

Occult blood A faecal occult blood test (FOBT) is a non-invasive test that detects the presence of hidden (occult) blood in the stool. Such blood may arise from anywhere along the digestive tract. Hidden blood in stool is often the first, and in many cases the only, warning sign that a person has colorectal disease, including colon cancer. A positive test result requires further investigation of the gastrointestinal tract, usually with a colonoscopy in the first instance.

Serum iron Serum iron (standard reference range varies between laboratories) in those with CKD is of no great significance (except in iron overload) but is necessary for calculating transferrin saturation rate.

Reticulocytes Reticulocytes (normal range: men 0.5–1.5%; women 0.5–2.5%) are immature red blood cells that have been newly released from the bone marrow and can be recognised as such for about 48 h before reaching a mature state. Patients with renal anaemia have a depressed reticulocyte count before EPO therapy and a rise should be seen when stimulation of erythrocyte production occurs as a response to EPO. If no response occurs, further investigation should be considered.

The percentage of hypochromic red blood cells will assess how much iron is being incorporated into the red blood cell. This level should be < 10%; greater levels indicate iron-deficiency anaemia.

Aluminium The normal range is less than $20 \mu g \, L^{-1}$. In dialysis patients who have been prescribed aluminium hydroxide as a phosphate binder, or who have used dialysate containing aluminium or water with high aluminium levels, a high serum aluminium level may be found. Aluminium has been implicated in osteomalacic bone disease, dialysis dementia and, importantly, in EPO therapy, which is unresponsive due to hypoplasia of the bone marrow (Rao et al 1993). Owing to the current acceptance that aluminium ingestion should be kept to a minimum, especially for patients with kidney disease, measures have been taken to provide purer water and dialysate. Aluminium hydroxide has mainly been discontinued as a phosphate binder in favour of calcium carbonate. However, serum aluminium levels should still be checked. Venous samples (10 mL) are collected in a plain plastic tube, as samples can become contaminated by the aluminium content of glass.

Parathyroid hormone Normal values of para-thyroid hormone vary according to the local assay method being used.

Parathyroid hormone is a hormone produced in the parathyroid gland and it is concerned with the regulation of extracellular calcium.

This test is useful in establishing whether hypercalcaemia is due to an overactive parathyroid. Increased parathyroid hormone is found in chronic kidney disease, vitamin D deficiency and osteomalacia. Hyperparathyroidism has been implicated in reduced response to EPO therapy, possibly due to inducing bone marrow fibrosis or suppressing the erythroid cell growth (Rao et al 1993).

Blood for parathyroid hormone analysis should be delivered immediately to the laboratory for analysis or, if this is impossible, kept on ice for a maximum of 30 min.

Reasons for low or non-response to EPO therapy other than haematinic may be underlying infection or inflammation, occult malignancy, inadequate dialysis, immunosuppressive drugs and chronic blood loss (e.g. haemorrhoids, menorrhagia, gastrointestinal bleeding). These possibilities should be investigated.

URINE INVESTIGATIONS

Urinalysis plays an important part in the assessment of renal disease, as renal damage may allow increased concentrations of various chemicals through to the urine, together with other signs of disease such as haematuria or proteinuria. The quantity of urine passed during the day together with its specific gravity also gives an indication of renal function. Table 6.3 lists the normal volumes of urine passed per day.

Urine is composed of about 95% water and 5% solids, mainly urea and sodium chloride. It is slightly acidic (pH 6.0) and has a specific gravity of 1.010–1.030 (specific gravity of water = 1.000).

URINALYSIS

Measurement of specific gravity can be unreliable in the presence of water and electrolyte imbalance, low-protein diets, chronic liver disease and pregnancy.

APPEARANCE

Urine can vary in colour from pale straw to dark amber for the reasons given below.

- Pale urine is dilute because of:
  - heavy fluid intake

Table 6.3 Normal volumes of urine

Healthy adult	1–1.5 L day^{-1}
Newborn baby	50–300 mL day^{-1}
Infant	350–550 mL day^{-1}
Child	500–1000 mL day^{-1}
Adolescent	700–1400 mL day^{-1}

– polyuria due to renal disease where the tubules fail to reabsorb water
– diabetes-insipidus or diabetes mellitus.
- Dark urine may indicate:
  – concentration due to fluid depletion
  – presence of bile.
- Haematuria can vary in appearance from 'smoky' to 'tea' to red, either bright or dark.
- Coloured urine can be caused by beetroot in the diet and other vegetable food dyes, porphyria and some drugs (e.g. orange-coloured urine is caused by rifampicin).
- Frothy urine indicates heavy proteinuria.
- Smoky urine may indicate the presence of bleeding from the kidney.
- Deposits or turbid urine, which occurs when the urine sample is left to stand, may be crystals of phosphate, oxalate or urates, or due to pus in the presence of infection.

DIPSTICK TESTS

Dipstick tests can be carried out in the clinic or ward situation as well as in the laboratory. Dipsticks are available that accurately show the presence of a variety of substances that may occur in the urine (e.g. protein, glucose, ketones, blood) as well as giving the pH of the urine sample. The stick should be briefly dipped into a fresh sample of urine and read after 1 min or according to the manufacturer's instructions. The results are then compared with those supplied on the instruction sheet.

Caution: these kits are very reliable providing that the container is always kept dry and capped between use, the strips are only briefly dipped into the urine sample and the expiry date is not exceeded.

OSMOLALITY

Osmolality (normal range 500–800 mosmol kg^{-1}) measurement indicates the kidney's ability in concentration and dilution and is considered more reliable than measuring the specific gravity. Collection methods vary from one centre to another (Malarkey & McMorrow 2000).

GLUCOSE

The presence of glucose may indicate diabetes mellitus, proximal tubular dysfunction, Fanconi's syndrome, glomerulonephritis or nephrotic syndrome.

PROTEINURIA

No more than a trace of protein should be found in the normal collection (i.e. less than 25 mg 24 h^{-1}, mainly albumin). However, proteinuria may be present up to 150 mg in 24 h before a dipstick test shows a positive reading. (The procedure for collecting the 24-h sample is the same as is detailed for creatinine clearance, page 125.) The urine should be kept refrigerated during the collection period to minimise bacterial growth.

Persistent proteinuria is a common sign of many forms of renal disease. In nephrotic syndrome, proteinuria may be as high as 4–30 g 24 h^{-1}.

BENCE JONES PROTEIN

This test consists of a sample of urine from the first specimen of the day. In the laboratory the urine is heated; if this protein is present, it will precipitate on heating and dissolve at 100°C; on cooling, the protein will precipitate again. This test is now performed by electrophoresis and immunoelectrophoresis. It is most commonly (70–80% of positive results) found in multiple myeloma due to the proliferation of paraprotein-producing bone marrow. It is also occasionally seen in amyloidosis, cryoglobulinaemia and hyperparathyroidism.

MICROALBUMINURIA

The first sign of kidney damage due to diabetes is very small amounts of protein in the urine (microalbuminuria), this then proceeds to larger quantities (proteinuria) and, possibly, low serum albumin, oedema, deranged blood chemistry and hypertension.

Microalbuminuria is defined as persistent small amounts of albumin not determined by the usual dipstick test and is of importance as a predictor of renal involvement in patients with diabetes mellitus. Whereas a normal sample of urine may contain albumin 2.5–25 mg 24 h^{-1}, microalbuminuria is in the range 30–300 mg 24 h^{-1} and macroalbuminuria is generally > 300 mg 24 h^{-1}.

Annual laboratory testing for microalbuminuria (by early morning urine sample), is of importance in the care of those with diabetic nephropathy, although the cost-effectiveness of screening all those with diabetes for microalbuminuria has been questioned.

MYOGLOBIN LEVELS

Myoglobinuria may occur due to conditions such as rhabdomyolysis, where there is a breakdown of muscle tissue, causing the release of myoglobin into the blood stream. This may occur due to trauma or crush injury to an area, seizures, immobility or severe exercise. The kidneys filter the blood and excrete the myoglobin in the urine. Myoglobin is nephrotoxic and large amounts of this protein can cause the occlusion of the renal tubules, leading to acute tubular necrosis and acute renal failure. This can be diagnosed by a sample of urine – usually the first sample of the day.

URINE MICROSCOPY AND CULTURE

Microscopy will reveal information from the sediment found in urine – casts, crystals, blood cells and bacteria. The site of origin of casts can often be determined, indicating the type and extent of damage to the kidney. It is normal to find red blood cells in urine at approximately $0.8\text{--}2 \times 10^6\,L^{-1}$ and these normally originate from the renal pelvis, ureter or bladder, and are uniform in shape and size. Leukocytes are also present at approximately $2 \times 10^6\,L^{-1}$ but the presence of eosinophils can be indicative of an allergic interstitial nephritis.

Casts

Different types of casts can be found in the urine and these indicate underlying conditions. Hyaline casts, known as Tamm–Horsfall proteins, originate from the renal tubules. They may be present due to the use of diuretics, fever and exercise; however, they also present in renal disease. Granular or cellular casts may be seen in renal parenchymal disease. Red cell casts indicate bleeding and white cell casts indicate pyelonephritis.

If microorganisms are found to be present in the urine specimen – usually determined by the Gram staining method – the laboratory will provide information as to which antibiotic is most appropriate. It is important that the urine sample is collected before a broad-spectrum antibiotic is taken, as this may be given in the interim period before specific sensitivity is ascertained.

A positive microscopy sample shows at least $10\,000$ organisms mL^{-1}; below this figure is not considered significant. However, with very dilute urine, a false-negative result may occur despite infection being present.

KIDNEY FUNCTION TESTS

In chronic kidney disease a regular assessment of kidney function can be useful in monitoring renal decline and in predicting the time when renal replacement therapy is likely to be needed. Glomerular filtration rate tends to decrease in a linear fashion over time in progressive renal disease and so, by extrapolation, predictions can be made as to when end-stage renal failure may occur.

Knowledge of the amount of nephron damage is useful in assisting in making the choice of suitable drug regime. When there is more than 30% of nephron loss, certain drugs should be avoided or used with caution because of the slow excretion of the drug or its metabolites. Glomerular filtration rate declines with age at approximately $10\,mL\,min^{-1}\,decade^{-1}$, starting at the fourth decade.

An *increased* glomerular filtration rate occurs as a result of:

- increased protein intake
- diurnal variation
- pregnancy.

A *decreased* glomerular filtration rate occurs as a result of:

- exercise
- age
- low-protein diet
- liver disease.

Many research studies and clinical trials of pharmaceuticals depend on regular glomerular filtration rate calculations to monitor the effect of treatments with regard to renal function. The kidney function investigations discussed here include creatinine clearance, the [51]chromium ethylenediaminetetra-acetic acid glomerular filtration rate (^{51}Cr EDTA GFR) and estimated glomerular filtration rate.

EGFR (ESTIMATED GLOMERULAR FILTRATION RATE)

The eGFR (calculated from serum creatinine results) provides the best overall assessment of the level of kidney function. However, creatinine clearance estimation (using 24-urine collection) can be helpful in the following situations:

- estimation of GFR in individuals with exceptional dietary intake (vegetarian diet, creatine supplements) or muscle mass (amputation, malnutrition, muscle wasting)
- assessment of diet and nutritional status.

The eGFR can be calculated in adults using the following equations, which take into account the serum creatinine concentration and some or all of the following variables: age, gender, race and body size.

The Cockcroft–Gault equation:

$$(140 - age) \times weight\ /\ 72 \times creatinine\ (\times 0.85\ if\ female)$$

The modification of diet in renal disease (MDRD) (known as the four-variable MDRD):

$$186 \times [serum\ creatinine\ (\mu mol\,L^{-1}) \times 0.011312]^{-1.154}$$
$$\times age^{-0.203}\ (\times 1.212\ if\ black)\ (\times 0.742\ if\ female)$$

For adults, the preferred equation is the MDRD, which uses creatinine, age, sex and ethnicity in its calculation. The Cockcroft–Gault, which uses creatinine, age, sex and weight, may be better at extremes of weight (Lamb et al 2005).

The results and interpretation of eGFR calculations are discussed in Ch. 5.

MEASUREMENT OF PROTEIN EXCRETION

Twenty-four-hour protein estimations are no longer recommended. The total daily protein excretion (in mg) can be estimated simply by multiplying the total protein–creatinine ratio (TPCR) (from a spot urine sample, preferably early morning, measured in $mg\,mmol^{-1}$) by a factor of 10.

For example, if urine protein is $750\,mg\,L^{-1}$ and urine creatinine is $7.5\,mmol\,L^{-1}$, then

$$Total\ protein\text{-}creatinine\ ratio\ (TPCR) = 750/7.5 = 100\,mg\,mmol^{-1}$$

Therefore

$$Daily\ protein\ excretion = 100 \times 10 = 1000\,mg\ (i.e.\ 1\,g)$$

CREATININE CLEARANCE

Note: this test is not recommended for estimating renal function but it is outlined here as some clinicians may still be requesting 24-hour urine samples.

The principle of clearance is that an estimation of a known substance in the plasma is compared with the amount in the urine. This substance must only be excreted in the urine. The calculation by which the clearance of the substance occurs can be measured is thus:

$$\frac{\text{Urine concentration of substance } (U) \times \text{Volume of urine in 24 h } (V)}{\text{Plasma concentration of substance } (P)}$$

Because creatinine is believed to be manufactured at a fairly constant rate by the muscle mass, is circulating in the blood stream and is filtered by the glomeruli (although a very small amount is excreted by the tubules), this is the usual substance measured. When used as in the above example, this is known as creatinine clearance.

About 50% of nephrons will have lost their function before an appreciable alteration occurs in the result of the creatinine clearance test. The normal value of creatinine clearance should be between 70 and 125 mL min^{-1}; the function lessens with age. A creatinine clearance result of less than 10 mL min^{-1} is an indication to start renal replacement therapy.

Procedure

A 24-h urine collection is made, which will provide the urinary creatinine content (U) and volume (V). A blood sample should be taken to indicate the plasma creatinine (P).

Patient information for 24–h urine collection

Patients should be given an explanation of the reason for the test and what is expected of them. One (or more) 2-L collection bottles containing no additives or preservatives should be given to the patient. While male patients can usually void straight into the bottle, female patients should be provided with a suitable receptacle in which they can catch the urine. The patient must be instructed to discard the first urine of the day (on day 1) into the lavatory and then collect all urine passed for the next 24 h into the bottle provided. On the following morning (day 2), the first sample should be collected and then the collection is complete. The completed urine collection should be labelled with the date and time of start and completion of the collection as well as the usual details, such as name, identity number and date of birth.

The urine collection and the blood sample should be delivered together to the laboratory with the request form, which should specify creatinine clearance test. The above formula is then applied and this will calculate the creatinine clearance.

^{51}CHROMIUM EDTA GFR

A more accurate method of assessing renal function than the creatinine clearance test is the ^{51}Cr EDTA GFR. As with the creatinine clearance test, the normal range is a clearance of 70–125 mL min^{-1}.

The patient should be informed of the reason for this test, the fact that a small dose of a radioisotope will be injected, and the necessity of a series of blood samples over a 4-h period, and consent should be sought.

The radiolabelled substance is given by intravenous injection. The patient's weight and height must also be recorded to enable the result to be normalised for the individual patient's body surface area.

Over the 4h following the injection, the usual procedure is for four blood samples to be drawn from the opposite arm to the injection of the radioisotope. (This is to avoid contamination from any activity still lingering around the injection site, which will falsify the result.)

Whilst the ^{51}Cr EDTA GFR is considered to be very accurate, only personnel who have completed a radiation protection course in accordance with the ionising radiation (medical exposure) regulations (Department of Health 2000) are permitted to administer radiolabelled substances.

RENAL BIOPSY

Patients who are referred to the nephrology outpatient clinic with proteinuria, haematuria or renal impairment with no obvious cause require a renal biopsy in order that the nephrologist can make a diagnosis and commence appropriate treatment. Patients referred in acute renal failure may also require a renal biopsy to provide a diagnosis. Whilst in experienced hands renal biopsy is a fairly safe procedure, there are risks which should be taken into consideration. Risks of renal biopsy, which are greater in the acute renal failure patient, are perirenal haematoma, prolonged and severe bleeding necessitating blood transfusion and possible surgery, irreparable damage to the kidney requiring a nephrectomy (1 in 1500), and, rarely, death (Baker et al 2000).

Renal biopsy is contraindicated in the following:

- small kidneys
- a single kidney
- gross obesity
- uncontrolled hypertension
- non-adherent patient
- obvious diagnosis
- severe anaemia
- uncontrolled coagulopathy.

PATIENT PREPARATION

Information regarding the benefits and risks attached to this procedure should be given to the patient, who should be allowed the opportunity to ask questions and time to consider the implications before consenting to the biopsy. Child patients under 16 years need written parental consent.

Patients are usually admitted to the ward on the day planned for biopsy, and a further explanation of the exact procedure and what is expected of the patient should be given prior to signature of a consent form. Children are fasted for 4 h before the biopsy, as they will be sedated with a preparation such as midazolam following a mild premedication. In order to gain full compliance, whilst still in the ward, it is helpful to ask the patient to practise deep breathing and breath-holding. Unless the patient can cooperate with breath-holding on demand, the procedure should not be attempted, as the danger of malplacement of the sharp biopsy needle causing laceration or haemorrhage becomes a possibility.

Blood samples should be taken for bleeding times, FBC, plasma viscosity, INR, group and save, and full biochemical and immunology profile. Biopsies should not proceed if any bleeding disorder is present (platelets $< 100 \times 10^9 \, L^{-1}$, INR > 1.2, bleeding time > 10 min), or if the blood pressure exceeds $160/95$ mmHg, as the highly vascular kidney can haemorrhage even when clotting times are within normal limits.

PROCEDURE

Patients will be asked to empty their bladder before the procedure. Percutaneous renal biopsy is usually done in a ward treatment or side room, or X-ray department, under local anaesthetic. The patient lies in a prone position, with a pillow under the upper abdomen to isolate the kidney, perhaps supported with sandbags to prevent movement. The kidney (usually left) is identified by ultrasound as to position and depth, and the skin is marked as to where the needle should be inserted. After cleaning the ultrasound gel from the skin, using a full aseptic technique, the area is cleaned, the area infiltrated with lidocaine (lignocaine) as a local anaesthetic and a spinal needle is inserted into the lumbar muscle layer until the needle is noted to swing with the patient's respirations. The patient should be asked to hold the breath whilst the needle is advanced 5 mm at a time, leaving the needle to swing free when the patient breathes in and out. When the needle has located the kidney, more local anaesthetic should be injected.

The spinal needle is then withdrawn, a small incision is made at the needle exit site and a Tru-cut renal biopsy needle is inserted along the pathway made by the spinal needle in the same manner, making advances as the patient holds the breath. When the kidney is again located, the biopsy is taken with the patient holding a breath. The biopsy needle is withdrawn and the specimen obtained is immediately placed on a slide and viewed under a dissecting microscope to ascertain that cortex which has been obtained is large enough (about 5 mm length) to divide into three samples. If not enough cortex has been obtained, the biopsy needle will have to be inserted again until a suitable strip of cortex containing sufficient glomeruli has been identified. Samples are sent to the laboratory for histology (in a 10% formalin pot), for immunofluorescence (in sterile normal saline) and electron microscopy (in specific glutaraldehyde fixative, kept cold). These samples should be delivered immediately (within minutes, not hours) to the laboratory, which must have had advance warning of the biopsy.

Finally, after the needle has been withdrawn, a pressure dressing is applied and the patient is asked to remain flat in bed. The patient will need much encouragement and reassurance during the renal biopsy procedure, as it can be painful, despite local anaesthetic. A friendly hand to hold and quiet encouragement to cooperate with breathing requirements from the attending nurse can be very reassuring.

PATIENT CARE FOLLOWING RENAL BIOPSY

It is usual practice to keep patients in the ward on bed-rest for 24h following this procedure. Haemorrhage is the main complication following renal biopsy; the wound site should be frequently checked for surface bleeding, and blood pressure and pulse observations should be carried out until stable, for example, on the time scale of every 15 min for 2h, then every 30 min for 2h, and then hourly for 4h. The signs and symptoms giving an indication of internal bleeding are a rise or fall in blood pressure, and dull aching pain in the abdomen, back or shoulder. The patient should be warned that some degree of haematuria will occur initially, but only persisting or heavy haematuria is of significance. Small urine samples from each void should be retained in transparent specimen containers for observation of diminishing haematuria and dipstick testing. It is becoming common practice for suitable patients to be admitted to day-case units for this procedure. These patients must be carefully chosen and must fully understand instructions for aftercare at home. The patient should be advised not to do any strenuous activity for 2 weeks following renal biopsy.

RENAL BIOPSY IN THE TRANSPLANTED PATIENT

Closed percutaneous biopsies of the transplanted kidney are undertaken to support evidence of rejection (see Ch. 12). The procedure is similar to the biopsy of the native kidney but more straightforward, owing to the superficial position of the transplanted kidney. The patient will be placed in a supine position with a pillow beneath the transplant side to move the intra-abdominal contents away from the site. The amount of tissue required in a transplant biopsy will be less than in a native kidney biopsy as fewer tests will be performed. The patient should remain resting in bed for 4–6 h and may be discharged home the same day, though it is important to ensure the patient has passed urine and a dipstick test has been performed to check for blood.

RADIOGRAPHIC INVESTIGATIONS

Investigations using various radiographic methods are often employed to assist diagnosis and to assess progression of renal disease and its attendant side-effects. The most common techniques are discussed here.

Patients should have received adequate explanations before entering the department in order to allay any fears they may have on finding themselves in a department full of strange machinery, hazard warnings and unfamiliar staff. If they are aware of the reasons for the investigation and what will be expected of them, the likelihood of an accurate result of the examination will be enhanced. The patient will be asked to sign a consent form for some invasive tests and early information will be of help for understanding the procedure.

All investigations involving X-rays must be performed according to the safety regulations in using a potentially hazardous substance, and these techniques must not be used unless the risk to the patient is outweighed by the benefit. Some departments follow the practice that women with reproductive capacity should only be subjected to X-rays and other procedures using ionising radiation during the 10 days following the commencement of the last menstrual period to avoid possible damage of a vulnerable fetus – the so-called '10-day rule'. More recently, guidelines have indicated that minimal exposure to a possible fetus must be ensured with the use of shields, as developing fetal organs are at higher risk of radiation.

PLAIN ABDOMINAL X-RAY

Plain abdominal X-rays incorporating the kidneys, ureters and bladder (KUB) indicate the size, shape, position, and the presence or absence of one or both kidneys, and may be taken before other more complicated radiological procedures in order to provide an overall background picture. Most calculi may be seen as they are usually composed of radiopaque material. KUB X-rays are usually taken from the anterior aspect. A combination of KUB and ultrasound often forms the basic routine screening in those with renal failure.

SKELETAL X-RAYS

Skeletal X-rays may be taken in the dialysis patient. This is to detect renal osteodystrophy, which may become apparent in association with impaired glomerular filtration, and associated disturbed metabolism of calcium and phosphate. The bones most likely to show the characteristic abnormalities are the phalanges, skull, pelvis and vertebrae. Pain and deformity will ultimately develop unless imbalances of calcium and phosphate can be corrected and inadequate metabolism of vitamin D can be halted.

INTRAVENOUS UROGRAM (IVU)

This procedure is also known as the intravenous pyelogram (IVP). This examination indicates the size and position of the kidneys, and the anatomy of the calyces and pelvis. The ureters are also outlined by the progression of the dye containing urine to the bladder and the subsequent use of sequential X-rays, enabling any deformities in these organs to be demonstrated.

Patient preparation

The patient should be told that the investigation will take about an hour to complete – longer if there is renal impairment.

It should be ascertained that the patient is not allergic to iodine or shellfish, and caution should be observed with asthmatics and others who have allergic conditions, as the contrast medium is iodine-based. Therefore, it is standard procedure that injections of adrenaline (epinephrine) 0.5–1 mg (0.5–1 mL of 1:1000 solution = 1 mg mL^{-1}) intramuscular, antihistamine (e.g. chlorphenamine (chlorpheniramine) 10–20 mg intravenous) and hydrocortisone should be immediately available to treat anaphylaxis, should it occur.

Laxatives should be given to the constipated patient prior to this examination to clear the bowel so that there is no interruption to the view of the urinary system. Adult patients should fast for 3 h, but limited fluid is usually allowed until 1 h before the IVU. After an explanation of the procedure with adequate time to ask questions, the patient may be asked to sign a consent form. Emptying the bladder beforehand is important, or the contrast will become overdilute on reaching a full bladder and a poor picture will result.

Following this test, patients should be encouraged to drink fluids, as they may become dehydrated if fluids were restricted prior to the examination. Nurses should be aware that there is a possibility of acute renal failure following this investigation, so urinary output should be monitored.

The IVU gives little useful information in advanced chronic kidney disease and consequently is not the investigation of choice if more than 50% of nephron loss is suspected. If impaired renal function is known and an IVU is indicated, a greater dose than usual of the radiopaque contrast medium may need to be given. This in itself is nephrotoxic and may exacerbate renal failure, at least temporarily.

RETROGRADE PYELOGRAM

In this examination, radio-opaque dye is injected directly into the upper urinary tract via a catheter inserted through a cystoscope into the ureter. A series of X-rays are performed on one or both kidneys. This test is useful in outlining stones, calyceal defects, and masses in the ureter or renal pelvis and in defining deformities such as hydronephrosis or hydroureter. This investigation is sometimes performed after an IVU or ultrasound (US) has demonstrated a hydronephrosis, and more clarification is needed for a diagnosis. After the procedure, the urine should be observed for haematuria, and patients should be watched for signs and symptoms of infection. They should be encouraged to drink copiously to help avoid infection (antibiotics may be given as a prophylaxis).

COMPUTED AXIAL TOMOGRAPHY (CAT)
OR COMPUTED TOMOGRAPHY (CT) SCAN

This investigation is reserved for the patient who needs staging of a renal mass or a diagnosis when other methods of detection have failed to provide a clear picture. CT is an X-ray technique that uses a computer to reconstruct cross-sectional images of 1-cm slices of the organ targeted. The dose of radiation is about the same as that for an IVU. A clear bowel is necessary so a suitable laxative may be given 2 days before the scan. A light diet should be taken for 2 days before the scan and nothing on the day of examination apart from clear fluids. Patients must be able to follow instructions such as when to hold the breath, to be able to lie motionless and not to talk.

NUCLEAR MAGNETIC RESONANCE OR MAGNETIC RESONANCE IMAGING (MRI)

This form of scanning involves application of a strong external magnetic field along with a radio-frequency signal that produces a current in a receiving coil proportional to the density of protons in the body organ being scanned. This signal is processed by computer to create a tomographic slice of the organ similar to a CT scan. In renal medicine, a clear picture of tumour invasion into blood vessels can be demonstrated as well as differentiation of tissue character.

The advantage of MRI over CT imaging is that no ionising radiation or contrast media is used, and many planes can be visualised. However, this method is three times as expensive as CT imaging.

It is vitally important that the patient is not wearing any magnetic metal object, and it must be ascertained that no internal metal objects are present, such as aneurysm clips, screws, pacemakers or shrapnel. Therefore, an X-ray may be taken before the procedure to ensure that no hidden metal objects are within the body.

ULTRASONOGRAPHY

Ultrasound (US) investigations have replaced some X-ray procedures (especially the IVU) to a large degree and, because this procedure does not carry the hazards associated with radiation, this method can be used in women without consideration of the possibility of pregnancy. This is a non-invasive procedure where a transducer (sonar probe) is moved in close contact with the skin over the area of investigation and it can be repeated frequently if necessary, unlike X-ray. US is especially useful in examinations of the abdominal and pelvic organs. It is widely used to determine the size and shape of the kidney, its presence and position, and the composition of cysts or neoplasms, if present, and also in the diagnosis of polycystic kidney disease. However, it is less useful in providing information about the ureters. US is also used to guide the operator in procedures such as renal biopsy.

Patients who are to have renal US scans are usually asked to fast for 6–8h (in order to keep pockets of air in the gut to a minimum) except for drinks of clear fluids.

Ultrasound in renal transplantation

Real-time US scanning is an ideal method of examining the transplanted kidney, as it is a simple and non-invasive technique and provides immediate feedback (Emelianov et al 2000). The most important and common cause of early transplant dysfunction is acute rejection, which occurs in 10–20% of all patients. This is accompanied by inflammation, which leads to swelling of the kidney and an increase in pressure inside the organ.

US is employed to diagnose the increase in size using diameters relating to the local renal anatomy (Nicholson et al 1990a). This procedure should be used daily and two size increases on consecutive days would be strongly indicative of acute rejection. However, dysfunction attributed to other causes must be excluded. Infection may be associated with an increase in the kidney size, but this is easily diagnosed by routine testing of midstream specimens of urine.

Renal vein thrombosis is a serious complication and will cause a rapid increase in size, possibly resulting in a tear of the kidney substance. If this condition is quickly diagnosed with US, rapid surgical intervention is possible and the graft may be rescued. Renal artery thrombosis may be diagnosed ultrasonically by the observation of lack of vessel pulsation. For greater accuracy, duplex scanning using a combination of imaging and frequency waveform analysis is available.

Early complications following transplantation include urine leaks, usually from the site of the ureteric anastomosis. These are seen ultrasonically as a fluid collection around the graft site. Later complications are obstructive lesions, which are often insidious in onset and lead to deteriorating renal function. Routine scanning of outpatients is a simple and easy method of detecting dilatation and stenoses of the urinary tract, which are then treated surgically.

Needle core biopsy of the transplanted kidney remains the best method of detecting rejection and determining the degree of interstitial fibrosis and acute inflammation. Using US guidance of the biopsy needle, a good core of the renal cortex may be safely obtained, carefully avoiding the structures of the renal medulla and damage to the graft. The disadvantage of biopsies is they cannot be performed frequently owing to the preparation, screening and cost involved (Emelianov et al 2000).

Ultrasound is therefore a valuable tool in the detection and diagnosis of renal allograft dysfunction, allowing intervention and early treatment of problems.

RENOGRAMS

Renograms calculate percentages of renal function and indicate the position of obstruction. This investigation can be used in place of IVU if the patient is allergic to iodine contrast medium, and it is also used in transplanted patients. In renal artery stenosis, a renogram may be performed and then repeated, incorporating an injection of captopril to outline any response induced. This test is carried out by injecting a small amount of radiostope and taking a rapid series of imaging. The isotope commonly used is ^{99m}Tc-MAG$_3$ as it is filtered by the glomeruli and eliminated by tubular secreation.

Renal scanning

There are two types of radioisotope scan that can be performed to provide quantitative data on the function of the kidneys.

Firstly, the isotope, ^{99m}technetium-labelled diethylenetriaminepentaacetic acid (^{99m}Tc DTPA), is rapidly excreted by the kidney and shows the blood flow through the kidneys, identifies obstructions, e.g. renal artery stenosis, and provides valuable information about the function and excretion capacity of the kidney. A diuretic may also be given intravenously and the patient should be well hydrated. The procedure takes about 1 h.

The other isotope is ^{99m}technetium-labelled dimercaptosuccinic acid (^{99m}Tc DMSA), which is retained by the cells in the proximal tubules and parenchyma, and enables the identification of areas of cortical scarring, contusions and solid lesions. This will provide quantification of relative renal function between kidneys and within a kidney.

MAG 3

MAG 3 is the isotope ^{99m}technetium-labelled benzoylcaptoacetyltriglycerine, which is a dynamic imaging scan that is rapidly excreted by the kidney via glomerular filtration, or a combination of filtration and tubular secretion. The test enables visualisation of the aorta and renal perfusion. Quantification of renal blood flow can be calculated, and it identifies the overall kidney function and presence of obstruction, thrombus, emboli and stenosis. When patients undergo radioisotopic scans, they should empty their bladder immediately before scanning. Patients should be advised that they are radioactive for 24 h and nursing staff should ensure universal precautions when managing waste disposal.

Renal angiogram

This is performed through a catheter inserted via the femoral vein and fed to the renal artery. Contrast dye is radiopaque; this is injected and a series of X-rays performed. It identifies tumours, trauma and stenosis of vessels. Caution should be taken with patients who have some degree of renal insufficiency as the dye is nephrotoxic. If patients are able, then they should drink plenty of fluids to flush through the contrast. Patient should be fasting for 6–8 h and must be checked for any allergies to iodine and shellfish prior to the procedure.

The most common complication of a femoral angiogram is haemorrhage and haematoma.

After the procedure, observations of the puncture site and haemodynamic status should be performed every 15 min for 1 h, then half-hourly for 2 h for any signs of bleeding. It is also important to check the pedal pulses for any neurological or circulatory changes. The above observations may change depending on the hospital; usually, the patient is required to lie flat for the first 2 h and remain resting in bed for 24 h.

SUMMARY

The investigations that have been discussed above are by no means exhaustive. Since those with renal disease usually have multifactorial disease processes, many other specific investigations may be indicated, especially cardiovascular tests, such as electrocardiography and echocardiography. The gastrointestinal tract in the renal patient is frequently investigated for bleeding problems using techniques involving endoscopy (e.g. gastroscopy and colonoscoscopy).

Such is the commercial pressure to exploit the latest technology, it is inevitable that new methods and procedures will enter the renal field in the near future, condemning some present-day tests to redundancy. However, it is hoped that if nurses understand something of the current techniques used in renal investigations, they will be able to inform and reassure their patients reliably.

ACKNOWLEDGEMENT

With grateful thanks to Jane Hattersley who was the original author of this chapter

References

Baker LRI, Hurst MJ, Rudge CJ et al. Practical procedures in nephrology. London: Arnold, 2000.

Department of Health. Guidance for clinical health care workers, protection against infection with blood-borne viruses – recommendations of the expert advisory group on AIDS and the advisory group on hepatitis. London: HMSO, 1998.

Department of Health. The ionising radiation (medical exposure) regulations, London: HMSO, 2000.

Department of Health. The National Service Framework for Renal Services. Part Two: Chronic Kidney Disease, Acute Renal Failure and End of Life Care. COI: London, 2005.

Emelianov SY, Lubinski MA, Skovoroda AR et al. Reconstructive ultrasound elasticity imagin for renal transplant diagnosis: kidney ex-vivo results. Ultrasonic Imaging 2000; 22: 178–194.

European Best Practice Guidelines for the management of renal anaemia in patients with chronic renal failure. Nephrol Dialysis Transplant 2004; 19(Suppl): 1–47.

Greenhalgh Report. The interface between junior doctors and nurses. Macclesfield, UK: Greenhalgh, 1994.

Lamb E, Tomson C, Roderick P. Estimating kidney function in adults using formulae. Ann Clin Biochem 2005; 42: 321–345.

Macdougall IC. Hematological problems and their management in hemodialysis and peritoneal dialysis patient. In: Lameire N, Mehta R, eds. Complications of dialysis. New York: Marcel Dekker, 2000: 303–325.

Malarkey L, McMorrow ME. Nurse's manual of laboratory tests and diagnostic procedures, 2nd edn. Philadelphia: WB Saunders, 2000.

Nicholson ML, Attard AR, Bell A et al. Renal transplant biopsy using real time ultrasound guidance. Br J Urol 1990b; 65: 564–565.

Rao SD, Shih M-S, Mohini R. Effect of serum parathyroid hormone and bone marrow fibrosis on the response to erythropoietin in uraemia. N Engl J Med 1993; 328: 171–175.

The Management of Health, Safety and Welfare Issues for NHS Staff. London: The NHS Confederation (Employers) Company Ltd, 2005.

United Kingdom Central Council for Nursing, Midwifery and Health Visiting. Perceptions of the scope of professional practice. London: UK CC, 1992.

Further reading

McMurray S, Johnson G, Davis S, McDougall K. Diabetes care and management significantly improve patient outcomes in the dialysis unit. Am J Kidney Dis 2002: 40: 566–575.

Wallach J. Handbook of interpretation of diagnostic tests. Philadelphia: Lippincott-Raven, 1998.

Miles A, Friedman E et al. In: Lameire N, Mehta R, eds. Complications of dialysis. New York: Marcel Dekker Inc., 2000.

Chapter 7

Haemodialysis

Paul Challinor

INTRODUCTION

Haemodialysis is an area of renal nursing that has developed, and continues to develop, at a very fast rate. Expert practitioners in this field are constantly striving to promote excellence in the application of nursing care and are implementing evidence-based practice.

The principles of haemodialysis are dependent upon a number of simple phenomena, namely diffusion, osmosis, ultrafiltration and hydrostatic pressure. The term haemodialysis itself is derived from the roots of two words: 'haemo' meaning blood, and 'dialysis' meaning filtration or cleansing. The process of haemodialysis is the filtration of substances from the blood via a semipermeable membrane (the dialyser), which are then carried away by dialysis fluid. The process primarily employs diffusion for solute removal, and osmosis and ultrafiltration for fluid removal. However, the role of osmosis is limited in haemodialysis.

PRINCIPLES OF HAEMODIALYSIS

'Haemodialysis' is a term used to describe the removal of solutes and water from the blood across a semipermeable membrane (dialyser). Techniques have become increasingly sophisticated, resulting in a variety of highly efficient methods of clearing waste products and excess fluid that would normally be removed by the healthy kidney.

The process of dialysis depends on two major physiological concepts that involve solute removal–diffusion (sometimes referred to as coduction) and filtration (convection). Fluid is removed by the process of ultrafiltration. It is essential to have a clear understanding of how these physiological principles relate to dialysis to appreciate fully both the benefits and limitations of this form of renal replacement therapy (RRT).

DIFFUSION

Diffusion is the term used to describe the movement of molecules from an area of high concentration (of solutes) to a region of low concentration (of solutes) until they are equal. For diffusion to take place, a concentration gradient is essential, and the rate of diffusion is greatest when the concentration gradient is highest. In RRT a physiological solution (dialysate) passes on the opposite side of the semipermeable membrane to the blood. The dialysate contains essential solutes in similar concentrations to normal serum. The dialysate, however, does not contain waste products such as urea and creatinine and so these substances will pass across the membrane from the region of high concentration (the patient's uraemic blood) to the region of low concentration (the dialysate).

The rate of diffusion is dependent upon the difference in concentration of the solute between the dialysate and the blood – the concentration gradient. The higher the concentration difference, the faster the rate of movement.

Diffusion is also proportional to the temperature of the solution (increased temperature increases random molecular movements), and inversely proportional to the viscosity and size of the molecules (small molecules diffuse more quickly).

CONVECTION

Convection involves the transfer of solutes along with the movement of fluid. As fluid is removed during dialysis, solutes are 'dragged' across the dialysis membrane. Convection is the main principle involved in solute movement in haemofiltration, but it also plays a part in haemodialysis. Convection, unlike diffusion, is dependent upon fluid movement across the dialyser (Fig. 7.1). The combination of diffusion and convection results in a total solute removal called mass transfer.

ULTRAFILTRATION AND HYDROSTATIC PRESSURE

As blood is pumped through a dialyser, a positive pressure will be exerted on the membrane. The pressure in the space on the opposite side of the membrane will be lower, whether or not the space is filled with dialysate. As a result, fluid and small solutes will move from the area of greater pressure to the area of lower pressure (Fig. 7.2).

ULTRAFILTRATION AND CONVECTION

As a result of hydrostatic pressure, fluid will move across the semipermeable membrane, and this process is called ultrafiltration. The rate of ultrafiltration depends on the permeability of the membrane and the

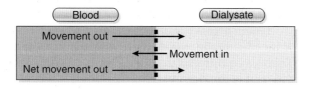

Figure 7.1
Diagram showing the net movement of solutes across the dialyser membrane during dialysis.

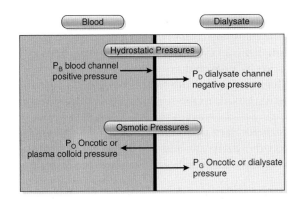

Figure 7.2
Transmembrane pressures. Overall pressure difference over the dialyser membrane = $(P_B + P_D) - (P_O + P_G)$. However, as the osmotic pressures are small in relation to the hydrostatic pressures the transmembrane pressure $(TMP) = (P_B + P_D)$.

hydrostatic pressure exerted upon it. The sum of the positive pressure in the blood compartment and the negative pressure in the dialysate compartment equals the transmembrane pressure (TMP).

The removal of fluid by ultrafiltration also results in the removal of solute, or those molecules dissolved in the water; this process is known as convection or solvent drag. Again, the higher the permeability of the membrane, the higher the removed volume of fluid and contained solute will be.

During conventional haemodialysis treatment, fluid will be removed by ultrafiltration, but this is usually a small amount (2–3 L) and will not provide significant removal of waste products by convection. Haemodialysis has traditionally been the standard form of extracorporeal treatment: haemofiltration and haemodiafiltration are becoming more common therapies in the treatment of patients requiring ongoing renal replacement therapy. Some centres, however, now routinely use intermittent haemodiafiltration in place of conventional haemodialysis. For the purpose of this chapter (due to space constraints), the reference is to standard haemodialysis unless otherwise stated.

MOLECULAR WEIGHT AND SOLUTE MOVEMENT

As well as diffusion and convection, there are a number of other influences on the 'clearance' or removal of a solute across the dialyser membrane. The smaller the molecular size of the solute, the easier it will pass across the membrane. Urea, creatinine and electrolytes will dialyse easily. However, toxins with a larger molecular size, such as β2-microglobubin (β2M) will be cleared in smaller volumes. Movement across the dialyser is also dependent upon the permeability of the membrane, called the coefficient of ultrafiltration (KuF; see the 'Dialysis equipment' section later in this chapter). High-flux dialysers will enable greater clearance of middle-sized molecules, such as β2M, in comparison to low-flux dialysers.

FLOW THROUGH THE DIALYSER

Haemodialysis depends on diffusion for the efficient clearance of waste products. The patient's blood is pumped through the circuit (via blood tubing) on one side of the membrane, whilst a physiological dialysis fluid (dialysate) is passed through the circuit (via dialysate tubing) on the opposite side of the membrane. The faster the blood flows through the dialyser, the greater the amount of blood is 'processed' in a given time. Efficiency of dialysis is also, therefore, dependent upon optimising the blood flow through the dialyser.

To optimise the concentration gradient, the blood and the dialysate flow in opposite directions (countercurrent flow). This maintains an optimum concentration gradient throughout the dialyser.

Dialysate flows through the dialyser at a rate of $500\,mL\,min^{-1}$. Lower flow rates are associated with lower clearances. Some units increase the dialysate flow above the standard $500\,mL$. However, there is conflicting evidence on whether this significantly improves clearance rates.

ACCESS FOR HAEMODIALYSIS

The success of haemodialysis therapy depends almost entirely on the adequacy of the blood flow through the dialyser. Optimal clearance of waste products depends on dialysate flow rate, membrane permeability, membrane surface area, duration of dialysis and, most significantly, blood flow rate. Dysfunctional access will, therefore, adversely affect dialysis adequacy, and consequently increase patient mortality and morbidity (Butterley & Schwab 2001).

The nurse has a responsibility to ensure that the prescribed blood flow is achieved whenever possible. Poor access should be addressed as a priority.

Various types of access can be used for haemodialysis, which fall broadly into two categories:

1. arteriovenous fistulae (AVF) and arteriovenous grafts, and
2. percutaneous access, including jugular, subclavian and femoral lines, which can be either temporary or permanent.

For those with established renal failure, the AVF is preferred, as there is evidence of long-term patency, improved flow rates and fewer complications than other methods (National Kidney Foundation Kidney Disease Quality Outcomes Initiative) (NKF-K/DOQI 2001). The National Services Framework for Renal Services Part 1 (Department of Health 2004) has set down a standard that patients should have vascular access created in a timely manner prior to renal replacement therapy being required. However, the creation and maintenance of long-term access still remains one of the most challenging aspects of caring for those with renal failure, particularly patients with vascular disease, older people and those with diabetes mellitus (Ernandez 2005, Konner 2004).

THE ARTERIOVENOUS FISTULA

The AVF is created during a surgical procedure to anastomose an artery and a vein (Fig. 7.3). Most commonly the radial artery and the cephalic vein are used in the patient's non-dominant forearm. Other sites include the upper arm – the brachial artery and cephalic vein or brachial artery and basilic vein.

As a result of the anastomosis, blood from the artery is forced into the vein, where it flows in a retrograde direction. The increased blood flow and pressure cause the vein to thicken and dilate. Once established, blood flow through the fistula of up to $800–1000\,\text{mL}\,\text{min}^{-1}$ can be achieved.

Ideally, the patient should have the fistula created at least 3–4 months before the need for dialysis arises. This will ensure that the operation is performed when the patient is well, and will allow the fistula time to mature, preventing the need for insertion of temporary access and the associated risk of infection. Many renal centres have a policy that medical and nursing staff should avoid phlebotomy or cannulation into the forearms of patients with suspected renal disease. This precaution will help to prevent damage to vessels that may subsequently be required for fistula formation. Repeated use of subclavian central venous catheters prior to fistula formation can also cause swollen arms and dilated chest veins following fistulae formation, so should be avoided (Butterly 2001).

FORMATION OF THE ARTERIOVENOUS FISTULA

Preoperative care

Patients should be given every opportunity to participate in their plan of care and all aspects of treatment should be discussed with them.

Figure 7.3
Arteriovenous fistula.

Before anastomosis

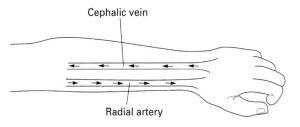

After anastomosis

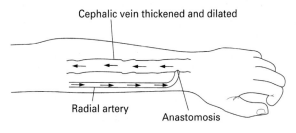

As part of the patient's predialysis preparation and education, a full explanation of the surgical procedure and aftercare should be given to the patient. The patient may wish to visit and speak with someone who has a well-established functioning fistula to find out what it looks and feels like.

Information should include explanation that the fistula will be cannulated each dialysis, often using a different site (see the explanation of the rope ladder puncture later). Also it is helpful if the needles that will routinely be used are available for the patient to see and examine. Patients should be well hydrated before surgery, and above their target weight if recently dialysed. This reduces the chance of postoperative hypotension, which would adversely affect the blood flow through the fistula, increasing the chance of thrombosis.

Postoperative care

In addition to routine postoperative care, the nurse should ensure that the following specific post-operative care is carried out.

- The limb should be kept warm and well supported to help peripheral circulation.
- Blood pressure should be monitored closely and maintained at a minimum of 100 mmHg systolic. If the blood pressure falls below this, peripheral blood flow may be affected, with an increased risk of fistula thrombosis. It may be advisable to avoid antihypertensive therapy in the postoperative period.
- The wound site should be examined regularly for signs of excess bleeding or swelling.
- The blood flow through the fistula should be checked regularly by completing the following observations.
  - Placing a stethoscope lightly over the incision, a 'whooshing' sound should be heard. This is called a bruit. The bruit should be loudest near the incision and gradually becomes softer as the stethoscope is moved further up the vessel.
  - When a hand is placed lightly over the incision site, a buzzing sensation should be felt. This is called the thrill.
- The bruit and thrill should be checked regularly (half-hourly at first) and the patients should be taught how to perform these observations as soon as they are able.
- Before discharge the patient should be informed how to care for the fistula and advised to avoid using the fistula arm for carrying heavy loads and to avoid tight or restrictive clothing on the arm. Hand exercises (such as clenching and releasing pressure on a squash ball or small bandage) may promote fistula maturation. Additionally, the patient must be advised to inform non-renal doctors and nurses that the arm should never be used for phlebotomy, cannulation or for recording blood pressure, as all of these may result in permanent damage to the fistula.
- Patients should be advised to contact the hospital immediately if they notice bleeding, swelling, or absence of bruit or thrill.

CANNULATION OF THE ARTERIOVENOUS FISTULAE

In the first instance, the fistula should be allowed 2–3 months to mature before cannulation is attempted, to allow healing of the anastomosis and some development of the vessels. After this time, the fistula can be safely cannulated but the procedure should only be undertaken by experienced practitioners.

New fistulae may be prone to extravasation and clotting, which can be painful and distressing. Therefore, all attempts should be made to minimise trauma during the initial dialysis treatments when the fistula is still new and maturing.

If the patient is anxious, a local anaesthetic may be offered. Common forms of local anaesthetic include lignocaine or topical creams. Topical creams are a sensible choice; the injection of lignocaine can sting and defeat the object of pain-free cannulation. However, the topical cream needs to be applied at least 30 min before cannulation.

Prior to each cannulation, a thorough physical examination of the fistula should be undertaken to check that there is no evidence of oedema, infection or bruising. and that blood flow through the fistula is evident through the presence of the bruit and thrill.

The unit policy for strict asepsis and cleansing of the arm should be adhered to. Universal precautions should be employed, including wearing gloves, aprons and a face visor, as blood may splash into the face and eyes during cannulation. A tourniquet may be used prior to cannulation to help engorgement of the vessel but in well-established larger fistulae this is often unnecessary.

CANNULATION PROTOCOLS

Many units are now evaluating the use of planned protocols to insert fistula needles, with the aim of reducing complications and extending the longevity of the fistula. The effect of repeated puncture on fistulae can adversely affect elasticity of the surrounding tissue (Kronung 1984). During each cannulation a small area of vessel tissue is displaced. When the needle is removed, this area is filled with a thrombus. Scar tissue is then formed, resulting in increased tissue and subsequent elongation of the vessel wall. Over time, this results in a loss of elasticity of the vessel, and dilation results in aneurysm formation and adjacent stenosis.

Kronung (1984) described three methods of cannulation and the effects of each (Fig. 7.4).

1. *Rope ladder puncture.* This describes the systematic use of the entire length of the vessel. Each needle is inserted at approximately 2 cm above the last site and back again, resulting in a uniform use of the vessel. This has demonstrated less aneurysm formation as the punctures per area are reduced. However, care must be taken to ensure that an area puncture technique is *not* undertaken in the belief that the nurse is following the rope ladder technique.
2. *Area puncture.* This describes the development and use of one or two areas of the fistula that are regularly used. It may result in increased

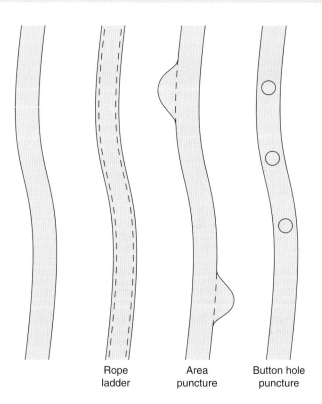

Figure 7.4
Needle protocols (Kronung
1984).

Rope   Area   Button hole
ladder   puncture   puncture

aneurysm formation related to the number of repeated punctures over a small area, causing increased tissue elongation and aneurysm formation.

3. *Button hole puncture*. This describes the repeated puncture of exactly the same site at exactly the same angle into exactly the same hole each dialysis. Over time cylindrical scar tissue develops, guiding the needle into the right place. It is suggested that the button hole technique results in less aneurysm formation and has been shown to have high survival rates (Twardowski 1995).

Whilst the adoption of protocols may be beneficial and ensure high standards of uniform practice, it is acknowledged that additional evaluation is necessary to provide evidence for the long-term effects of any of these protocols on the longevity of fistulae. The use of an access scoring system and staff cannulation programme to decrease access complications and increase staff competence can be beneficial in prolonging the life of the vascular access (Hayes 1998). Both these initiatives are important in ensuring good standards of nephrology nursing practice.

NEEDLE SETS

The achievable blood flow for many patients isoften underestimated. The careful selection of needles will ensure that optimum flows are obtained. Smaller needles (e.g. 16- and 17-gauge) produce high resistance as the blood pump is increased. This results in a 'sucking' effect of the needles and machine arterial alarms. Larger needles (14-g and 15-g) produce lower resistance and, therefore, avoid negative pressure as the blood pump speed is increased.

Needles should be inserted aseptically at 45° to the skin following appropriate skin preparation. The entire needle shaft should be inserted and the butterfly wing secured with tape. On insertion, a syringe should be attached to the end of the needle tubing and blood withdrawn. Any resistance to withdrawal may indicate that the needle position needs adjusting. Often the needle hole is occluded against the side of the vessel wall. This can be corrected by placing a small piece of sterile gauze under the butterfly; this will lift the needle externally and lower the needle tip internally. If flow still cannot be obtained, the presence of a clot may be suspected or there may be complete misplacement of the needle. In this event, the needle should be removed. Arterial and venous needles need to be placed at least 5 cm apart to avoid recirculation.

If the needle punctures the wall of the vessel, extravasation will occur, resulting in a painful visible swelling around the site. The needle should be removed and firm pressure applied for about 10 min before further insertion is attempted. On no account should the nurse push and pull the needle blindly, hoping that the needle will finally find the vessel. This will result in much pain and discomfort for the patient, and will bruise and damage the surrounding tissue, which may in turn cause permanent damage to the fistula.

It is also important that nurses, no matter how experienced, recognise their limitations in relation to cannulation. If a cannulation attempt has failed after more than two or three attempts, assistance should be sought from a colleague, as the increased anxiety of the nurse and patient may negatively influence further attempts at successfully siting the needle.

COMPLICATIONS OF ARTERIOVENOUS FISTULAE

Thrombosis

Thrombosis may occur in the immediate postoperative period or at a later date, sometimes following a hypotensive episode on dialysis. Surgical treatment (thrombectomy) may be indicated but salvage is often unsuccessful. Percutaneous angiopathy using a balloon catheter may be more successful (Rocek & Peregrin 2001). However, if reported promptly, permanent damage may be avoided by the use of thrombolytic agents.

Stenosis

Stenosis of the fistula can occur anywhere along its track. However, irrespective of where it occurs, there is an increased chance of the fistula failing. Stenosis at the anastamosis site will reduce blood flow into the fistula. A stenosis higher up above the needle site will increase pressure within the fistula, reduce blood flow out and increase the percentage of recirculation, all of which could adversely affect the adequacy of dialysis (Bouchouareb et al 1998).

This can be caused by the repeated area puncture (Fig. 7.4). The skin eventually becomes much thinner as the aneurysms dilate. Cannulation in the aneurysm should be avoided. Aneurysms are also associated with the development of stenosis of the vein above the needling site.

Aneurysm

The patient may complain of pain, oedema, coldness or 'pins and needles' as blood is 'stolen' from the hand as a result of the fistula (lower resistance in the arteriovenous anastomosis). Surgical correction to restore blood supply to the hand is usually required, with subsequent loss to the fistula.

Steal syndrome

Infections of established arteriovenous fistulae are uncommon, and are mainly localised to the immediate area, not progressing to bacteraemia. Treatment with antibiotic therapy is usually successful.

Infection

ARTERIOVENOUS GRAFTS

If the peripheral blood vessels are unsuitable for fistula formation, the surgeon may decide to create a graft (Fig. 7.5). Most grafts are created using synthetic materials, such as polytetrafluoroethylene (PTFE). Grafts may be cannulated soon after insertion, preferably after 14 days.

The graft may be configured in a straight line or in a loop. Grafts are less compliant than fistulae, resulting in higher pressure through the vessels. Patients should be taught how to care for the graft in the same way as a fistula.

The nurse should perform the same predialysis physical examination prior to cannulation. Thorough skin preparation is vital and sterile gloves must be used for cannulation of grafts, as there is high infection risk.

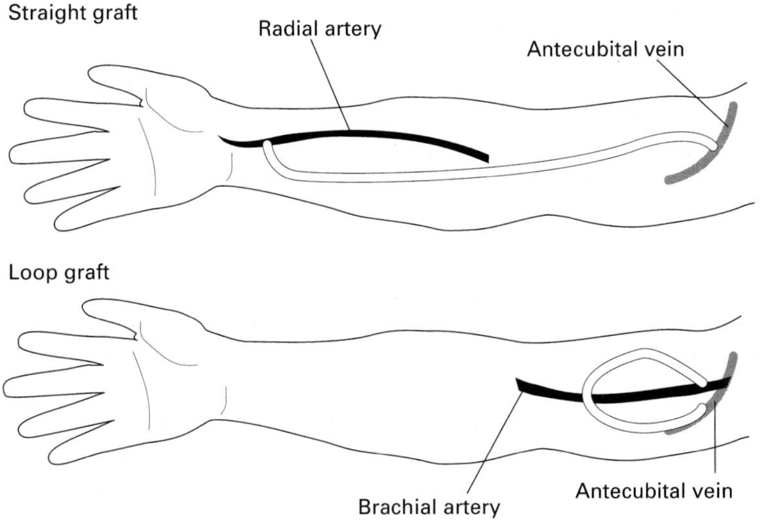

Figure 7.5
Arteriovenous graft configuration.

The arterial needle should be inserted at the arterial end of the graft at least 5 cm from the anastomosis site. The venous needle should be inserted in the venous end with the same considerations. For loop grafts, it is important to identify the arterial and venous sides of the graft, as incorrect needle placement will result in recirculation. Needles may be rotated through 90° following insertion (bevel of needle downwards) to reduce the risk of graft damage.

MONITORING ACCESS PATENCY

Adequacy of dialysis is directly related to the total blood volume that is processed during the dialysis treatment. As such it is important that the access used should be capable of delivering the optimum blood flow. However, stenosis occurring in the anastamosis area will reduce the volume of blood passing through the fistula; while a stenosis above the needling site will likewise decrease blood flow and increase the chance of recirculation. Regular monitoring of the blood flow will provide valuable information and trends on blood flow through the fistula and the percentage of recirculation.

A blood flow through the fistula or graft of less than $600 \, \text{mL min}^{-1}$ is an indicator of access failure (NKF-K/DOQI 2001). Early identification of stenosis associated with radiological or surgical intervention can improve longevity of the access (Besarab 2001, Butterly 1994). Other ways of monitoring access patency are reviewing any changes or trends in the venous and arterial pressures recorded on the dialysis machine. An increase in venous pressure over a period of weeks or months may indicate that a stenosis may be developing above the needle site (Berkoben & Schwab 1995).

VASCULAR ACCESS STANDARD

The Kidney Alliance (2001) has stated that the renal service in the UK should aim to have the percentage of new haemodialysis patients with natural AVF approach the European average of 66%. If this is to be achieved, then there will be increasing pressure on nurses to care for AVF proactively and to ensure that only well-trained competent nurses carry out cannulation. Detailed ways in which the multiprofessional team can work together to achieve this aim are beyond the scope of this book, but Berkoben & Schwab (1995) provide a good review of how to prolong vascular access patency.

PERCUTANEOUS ACCESS

Percutaneous access is the term used to describe the insertion of a cannula or catheter into a major vein (Fig. 7.6). Catheters may be inserted as a temporary measure, as in acute renal failure, or for temporary use whilst a fistula matures. Potential sites include the subclavian, femoral and internal jugular veins. The use of the subclavian vein

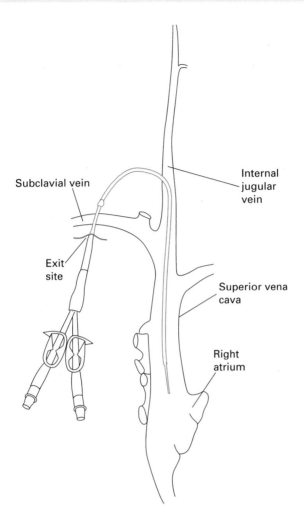

Figure 7.6
Permanent tunnelled
percutaneous catheter.

Subclavial vein

Internal
jugular
vein

Exit
site

Superior vena
cava

Right
atrium

is not recommended in patients with established renal failure, as this may adversely affect the success of the creation of an AVF due to central venous stenosis (Uldall 1996). Femoral catheters should only be used in those who are immobile and should be changed every 1–3 days.

More commonly, percutaneous catheters are being inserted as permanent access for patients whose fistulae have either failed or whose vessels are inadequate to attempt AVF creation in the first place. The permanent catheters are cuffed and inserted through the creation of a subcutaneous tunnel, as this ensures optimal placement of the catheter and helps reduce the rate of infection.

Catheters are invariably double-lumen, but single-lumen catheters are occasionally used. Catheters may be inserted under general or local anaesthetic and nursing care pre- and postoperatively will be the same as for any surgical procedure. Postinsertion it is essential that the correct placement of the catheter is checked by X-ray prior to dialysis, as insertion complications may include pneumothorax and puncture of the adjacent vessels.

The nurse's responsibility includes the maintenance of catheter patency, patient education, prevention of infection and early intervention when infection occurs. Nurses caring for percutaneous access must demonstrate meticulous care, as defined by a strict unit policy. This policy should include the need for strict asepsis during any catheter intervention. The exit site should be examined before each dialysis and observed for signs of infection, such as soreness, redness or the presence of exudate. Exit sites should be covered with a dressing that will maintain an optimum environment conducive to healing (not too wet and not too dry) and one that will repel *Staphylococcus aureus* (Wittich 2001). Chlorhexidine aqueous solution or povidone-iodine can be used to clean the exit site and then a non-occlusive dressing is applied (Pellowe 2001). It is important to note manufacturers' guidelines on the use of cleansing agents. Chlorhexidine alcohol solutions can degrade the material that forms the central line. The catheter hubs and portals are common site of infection, and should be cleaned prior to connection and disconnection from dialysis (Pellowe 2001).

PATENCY

To maintain patency between dialysis treatments it is common to instil a bolus of heparin (usually $5000\,iu\,mL^{-1}$) equal to the volume of each catheter lumen. It is important that the exact volume of each respective lumen is ascertained to prevent giving a systemic dose of heparin to the patient. However, other locks, such as citrate or a mixture of heparin and gentamycin, have been found to be equally effective (Betjes & van Agteren 2004, Easom 2000, McIntyre 2004). The use of antimicrobial lock has the advantage of reducing catheter-related infections, but is more expensive to use than heparin.

Before the next dialysis treatment, the anticoagulant lock must be removed by aspirating the catheter with a syringe and then flushing with 0.9% normal saline before connecting the dialysis lines. Nevertheless, clotting is a common complication, either preventing use of the catheter, or reducing flow rates adversely affecting adequacy of the dialysis. Several attempts may be needed to aspi-rate a clot in the catheter if resistance is felt. It is vital that any clot is removed and no attempt is made to flush a catheter that cannot be aspirated from either lumen. In permanent catheters, the administration of urokinase should dissolve the clot, if all other methods have failed, and should be left for at least 30 min before or between dialysis sessions.

In dual-lumen catheters, it is important to use the arterial and venous lumens appropriately. Occasionally, flow from the arterial lumen is partially occluded owing to poor positioning of the arterial holes against the side of the vessel wall. The lines may have to be reversed to achieve an acceptable blood flow. Reversal of the lines will result in increased recirculation (Twardowski 1993).

HAEMODIALYSIS EQUIPMENT

THE DIALYSER

The dialyser is the functional unit of the extracorporeal circuit just as the nephron is the functional unit of the kidney, and some patients and nurses refer to the dialyser as the 'kidney'.

Manufacturers have made significant advances in the development of membranes, which provide highly efficient clearance of waste products and which are biocompatible for the patient. There are two types of dialyser design: the hollow fibre (Fig. 7.7), and the parallel plate. The hollow fibre dialyser is the most commonly used variety in the UK today.

The hollow fibre dialyser is made up of thousands of hollow fibres or capillaries about the thickness of a human hair. The fibres are secured at each end of the cylindrically shaped dialyser in a polyurethane potting compound. Blood passes through the centre of each fibre like a straw, whilst the dialysate passes on the outside of the fibres in the opposite direction.

The plate dialyser consists of sheets of membranes arranged in layers. Blood passes through the space between one set of layers whilst the dialysate passes through the adjacent layers in the opposite direction. Plates have more compliance (stretch) than hollow fibre dialysers and, therefore, have higher priming volumes.

THE MEMBRANE

The choice of membrane type is becoming increasingly important as part of the patient's individual dialysis prescription. In addition to selecting the membrane that provides the desired clearance and fluid removal,

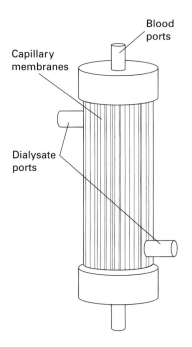

Figure 7.7
Hollow fibre dialyser.

the nurse should also consider the issue of biocompatibility related to the patient's needs.

A large and increasing variety of membrane types are available, but these fall broadly into the following three categories.

1. Cellulose membrane (e.g. Cuprophan): low flux.
2. Modified cellulose membranes (e.g. cellulose acetate, cellulosynthetic, such as Hemophan, cellulose triacetate): mid or high flux.
3. Synthetic membranes (e.g. polysulfone, polyacrylinitrile (PAN), poly methylmetacrylate (PMMA), polycarbonate (Gambrane) and polyamide): mid or high flux.

The efficiency with which a membrane clears water and solutes is described as its flux properties. Thin membranes with large pores are very permeable to water and large molecules, and are called high-flux membranes, as they have the ability to clear solutes with a molecular weight of up to 30 kDa. Low-flux membranes are less permeable to water and solutes, but will provide adequate clearance of solutes up to a molecular weight 10 kDa. The membrane's permeability to water is described as its ultrafiltration coefficient (KUf), and is measured in $mLh^{-1}mmHg^{-1}$ (the number of millilitres per hour of fluid that is removed for every one unit of pressure across the membrane). The efficiency of solute clearance is measured by the mass transfer urea coefficient or KoA, indicating the effectiveness of the membrane for allowing solute to pass across its surface.

High-flux membranes have a high KUf (> 10) and moderate-water-permeability membranes have a KUf of between 5 and $10 mLh^{-1}mmHg^{-1}$. Details of the properties of each dialyser can be found on the dialyser specification sheet, which is provided with each box of dialysers.

Solute removal by modified cellulose and synthetic membranes is similar, although β2-microglobulin clearance is greater with synthetic membranes, and this may translate into fewer amyloid dialysis deposits (Jaradat & Moe 2001, Levy & Morgan 2001).

BIOCOMPATIBILITY

It is ironic that the very process of haemodialysis, whilst providing an effective treatment for established re nal failure, can result in significant side-effects due to the interaction of the blood with the various components that make up dialysis equipment. The process of dialysis requires the repeated exposure of the patient's blood to foreign substances, including the dialyser membrane, blood lines, dialysate, chemicals, drugs and water. Biocompatibility can be defined as the use of a material that elicits the least amount of inflammatory response during dialysis.

At its simplest, the exposure of blood to the artificial surfaces of the dialysis circuit results in coagulation within the dialyser and dialysis line. Although all membranes illicit an increased incidence of thrombogenesis and fibrinolysis, cellulosic membranes create a more marked increase than synthetic membranes (De Sanctis 1996). However, dialysis may also initiate subtle, but long-term effects on immunological responses that include activation of the complement system, and release of cytokines involved in the inflammatory process and anaphylactic reactions.

Recent moves to ensure that the products used during dialysis (the dialyser and dialysis lines) are sterilised now though gamma-irradiation has reduced one serious issue of bioincompatibility, namely the incidence of 'first use syndrome' associated with sterilisation using ethylene oxide (see 'Dialyser reactions').

Dialysis-related amyloidosis leading to conditions such as carpal tunnel syndrome is associated with elevated $\beta2$-microglobulin levels. This was initially thought to be related to exposure of cellulose membranes; however, subsequent studies have found no significant evidence that bioincompatible membranes have a marked increase on the production of $\beta2M$ (Shaldon & Koch 1995). Interestingly, biocompatible high-flux dialyser membranes have been shown to increase the clearance of $\beta2M$, slowing the development of amyloidosis (Copley & Lindberg 2001, Jaradat & Moe 2001). More focus is now on the use of high-flux dialysis and haemodiafiltration as the treatment of choice for renal replacement therapy (Winchester et al 2003).

Other more subtle effects of biocompatibility should not be ignored. Parker et al (1996) suggest that bioincompatible membranes adversely affect the nutritional parameters of patients in comparison to those dialysed with biocompatible membranes.

Poor water quality can also induce inflammatory reactions. Bacterial and endotoxin contamination resulting from biofilm development has been implicated in increased morbidity of haemodialysis patients (Hoenich & Levin 2003, Lonnemann 2004). Standards aim to define safe levels of chemical and bacteria contaminants, outlining regular monitoring to identify potential quality problems (Association for the Advancement for Medical Instrumentation (AMMI) 2004). Regular testing of water used for dialysate should show a total viable bacterial count of less than $100\,cfu\,mL^{-1}$ and an endotoxin level less than $0.25\,IU\,mL^{-1}$. The importance of water quality cannot be emphasized enough in units using high-flux or haemodiafiltration. The larger pores in the dialysis membrane increase the risk of exposure to bacteria or endotoxin.

WATER TREATMENT

Undertaking simple mathematics, a patient dialysing for 4h, 3 times a week, is exposed during treatment to approximately 6240 L of water a year. Because of this level of exposure, the water used during dialysis should be well controlled and regularly monitored for impurities and contamination. Raw water coming into the dialysis unit from the mains supply contains many contaminants that pose a potential risk to the patient. The clinical effects on dialysis patients caused by various contaminants can be seen in Table 7.1.

Table 7.1
Dialysis contaminants and
symptoms

Symptom	Related contaminants
Anaemia	Aluminium, choramine, nitrate, lead, copper, zinc
Bone disease	Aluminium, fluoride
Hypertension	Calcium, magnesium, sodium
Hypotension	Bacteria, endotoxin, nitrate
Acidosis	Low pH, sulphate
Muscle weakness	Calcium, magnesium
Nausea/vomiting	Bacteria, endotoxin, chloramine, low pH, nitrate, sulphate, calcium, magnesium, copper, zinc
Neurolical disturbance	Aluminium, lead, calcium, magnesium

Figure 7.8
Typical water treatment
plant.

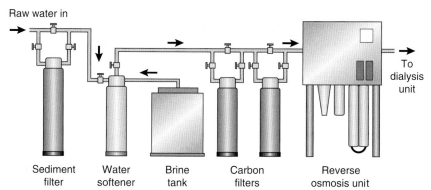

Raw water in

Sediment filter   Water softener   Brine tank   Carbon filters   Reverse osmosis unit

To dialysis unit

In order to avoid these symptoms, raw water is treated to reduce the concentration of contaminants to safe levels. The most common standard of contaminant concentration used is defined by the AMMI (2004). A simplified schematic drawing of a typical water treatment plant can be seen above in Fig 7.8.

Water first passes through a sediment filter to remove particulate matter, before passing through the water softener removing calcium and magnesium via ion exchange. The water softener is charged (usually on a daily basis) with salt from the brine tank.

Chlorine added to the mains water supply to reduce the bacterial count can induce anaemia and nausea/vomiting in the dialysis patient (Ward 1996). The carbon filters remove the chlorine and chloramines (free chlorine) from the incoming water, before passing through the reverse osmosis (RO) unit. The RO uses a semipermeable membrane to filter water and works by rejecting 90–95% of univalent and divalent ions in addition to microbiological contaminants that may still be in the water.

Standards for water quality have existed for many years, but in many countries in Europe there is no legal obligation to comply with the European Pharmacopoeia and testing is not mandatory. Water should be regularly analysed to measure endotoxin levels and numbers of organisms to ensure that they do not exceed the standard for the dialysis unit. There is evidence, however, that many European dialysis facilities do not routinely check the quality of their water (Lindley et al 2001).

PREPARATION OF THE DIALYSER

Priming and rinsing of the extracorporeal circuit is a crucial process in the preparation of the dialysis treatment. Manufacturers provide guidelines and recommendations for priming volume and rinsing time; however, there are two important aspects to consider.

1. The removal of air. Air must be removed from the blood lines and from all surfaces of the dialyser membranes. Pockets of air retained in the dialyser will result in less efficient dialysis and will promote clotting in the dialyser.
2. The removal of any chemicals or sterilising agents used during the dialyser manufacturing process. Of most concern is ethylene oxide (ETO), a gas which is a highly effective sterilant against all micro-organisms. It may, however, have toxic effects and cause hypersensitivity reactions in some patients (see 'Dialyser reactions'). Alternative sterilising methods are now routinely used, including heat sterilisation and gamma-radiation. Typically a minimum of 1 L of saline is required to remove residual ETO.

DIALYSATE COMPOSITION

Dialysate is the term used to describe the fluid that is pumped through the dialyser on the opposite side of the semipermeable membrane to the patient's blood. The function of dialysis fluid is to correct the chemical composition of uraemic blood to normal physiological levels, the removal of excess uraemic wastes and electrolytes. In addition, it is also responsible for the movement of buffering agents from the dialysate into the blood to restore the acid–base balance of uraemic patients.

Dialysate is produced by mixing a concentrated electrolyte solution (concentrate) with a buffer (bicarbonate) and purified water. Dialysate composition can be tailored to individual patient requirements (particularly potassium and calcium levels, and sodium levels, if sodium profiling is being used to minimise hypotension) but on the whole the solution

Table 7.2	Usual composition of haemodialysis dialysate
Solute	Concentration
Sodium (mmol L^{-1})	135–143
Potassium (mmol L^{-1})	0–4
Chloride (mmol L^{-1})	100–111
Calcium (mmol L^{-1})	1.25–1.75
Magnesium (mmol L^{-1})	0.75–1.5
Bicarbonate (mmol L^{-1})	30–35
Glucose (g 100 mL^{-1})	0–0.25

will be physiological, i.e. it will resemble normal serum biochemistry with specific deviations (Table 7.2).

Sodium

Physiological sodium   This is the most common sodium dialysate concentration (usually 135–140 mmol L^{-1}) and is normally adequate to remove enough sodium and water during the dialysis procedure. The use of physiological sodium means there is no large concentration gradient between plasma and dialysate; thereforethere is little or no net diffusion of sodium.Fluid movement is therefore not dependent upon variations in the sodium concentration, but upon ultrafiltration. Sodium, if any, is removed by convection. Dialysing with a sodium concentration of 140 mmol L^{-1} results in a reduced incidence of dialysis-related hypotensive episodes when compared with a lower sodium dialysate (Gerrish & Little 2003).

High sodium

Improvements in dialysis machine technology now allow the nurse to alter the sodium concentration during dialysis. Patients who cannot tolerate fluid removal during dialysis (suffering hypotensive episodes, cramping and other cardiac-related events), may benefit from part of the dialysis being conducted using a higher sodium dialysate – sodium profiling. Sodium diffuses into the blood from the dialysate, increasing the sodium concentration of the plasma. This osmotic imbalance helps to mobilise the intracellular fluid reserves, increasing the fluid shift from the intracellular fluid compartment to the intravascular compartment. Ultrafiltration is facilitated and the blood pressure remains stable (Dheenan & Henrich 2001, Gerrish & Little 2003, Song et al 2004). Care must be taken to ensure that the dialysate sodium is reduced during dialysis to physiologic levels otherwise the patient will finish dialysis with a positive sodium load, leading to experiences of thirst, resulting in an increased fluid intake and risk of hypertension (Stiller et al 2001).

Low sodium

In hypernatraemic patients, a low sodium dialysate may be considered an option. Low sodium dialysate leads to the transport of sodium from blood to the dialysis fluid. This creates an osmotic imbalance between the extracellular and intracellular fluid compartments, leading to greater fluid shifts and intracellular swelling, resulting in a form of dialysis disequilibrium. The lower the sodium dialysate level, the more efficient the dialysis and the more pronounced the effect of sodium clearance. Care needs to be taken when using low sodium dialysate owing to the resultant extracellular volume depletion and hypotension.

Potassium

Many renal patients present for dialysis with raised potassium levels, which are associated with morbidity and death among dialysis patients (Ahmed & Weisberg 2001). Most dialysis concentrates use a hypotonic concentration of potassium of 2 mmol L^{-1}. This is usually enough to reduce serum potassium levels of patients with hyperkalaemia. However, nopotassium dialysate can be used for severely hyperkalaemic patients, but should be used with care. Potassium-free concentrates should be used only at the start of dialysis, and then changed to concentrate of $2\,mmol\,L^{-1}$. If this is not done, then the patient may become severely hypokalaemic with attendant cardiac arrhythmias. Extra potassium can be added to concentrates if the patient is hypokalaemic. Patients who routinely present with lower potassium levels or those who are dialysing for the first time should dialyse against a solution containing $3.0\,mmol\,L^{-1}$, reducing the risk of disequilibrium.

Calcium

Normal calcium dialysate levels are usually in the range of 1.25–$1.75\,mmol\,L^{-1}$, slightly below physiological levels. The use of higher concentrations causes a positive calcium balance, with the long-term risk of development of metatastic calcifications. Lower concentrations induce release of parathyroid hormone, exacerbating the risk of secondary hyperparathyroidism. The increased use of calcium carbonate as a phosphate binder instead of aluminium derivatives has led to the need to reduce calcium levels in dialysis fluid. Despite the use of lower calcium dialysate, care needs to be exercised to ensure the patient does not develop a negative calcium balance leading to increased secondary hyperparathyroidism (Fernandez et al 1995). This emphasises the complex nature of calcium and phosphate management in patients needing dialysis.

BUFFERS (ACETATE AND BICARBONATE)

Haemodialysis patients tend towards a moderate to severe acidosis owing to their inability to excrete excess hydrogen ions. The aim of the buffer in dialysis is to normalise the patient's acid–base balance as far as possible. Bicarbonate is the body's major buffer and is the preferred choice to use in the dialysate.

The use of acetate is largely historical and there is no feasible argument for its use as a first choice. In the early days of dialysis, bicarbonate was the buffer used but this caused many operational problems, largely due to dialysate preparation. In the 1960s, acetate was used as an alternative to bicarbonate, so acetate dialysis became the norm, and was convenient and cheap to use. Acetate is an organic ion that generates bicarbonate when metabolised. Metabolism in the body takes place in the muscle cells and the mitochondria of the liver. However, as dialysis techniques have become increasingly efficient, the disadvantages of acetate have become apparent. Symptomatic hypotension, nausea and vomiting, and dialysis fatigue were shown to increase with acetate dialysis, and to decrease or disappear with bicarbonate dialysis. A patient's ability to metabolise acetate is considered critical. It is essential that patients are able to metabolise acetate at a rate equal to the rate at which they lose bicarbonate. Patients who are at risk of poor metabolism include those with reduced muscle mass and those with liver failure (Ledebo 1990).

Unlike acetate, bicarbonate has no direct pharmacological effect on the cardiovascular system. A better preservation of plasma volume during bicarbonate dialysis has been shown, especially during the first part of dialysis. The better tissue oxygenation in combination with normal pCO_2 values during bicarbonate dialysis are thought to contribute to increased sympathetic tone and vasoconstriction. Bicarbonate dialysis has been shown significantly to reduce the incidence of hypotensive episodes, nausea and vomiting during dialysis (Oettinger & Oliver 1989). Because of its biocompatibility in comparison to acetate, bicarbonate is now used as the buffer of choice.

ANTICOAGULATION

Heparin is the most common form of anticoagulant used, mainly because of its relative cost and short half-life. Heparin regimes are given either via intermittent or continuous infusion. Both require a loading dose, usually between 25 and 50 units kg^{-1} body weight, with further bolus doses given during the dialysis, if on intermittent regimen, or continuously via syringe pump. The amount given depends upon the needs of the patient and should be individually assessed using activated clotting times (ACT). Continuous infusion is the preferred regimen, as bolus heparinisation is associated with over- or under-anticoagulation (Ward 1995). Once a patient has been established on the appropriate regimen, it should be checked monthly, or if there is a change in the patient's condition.

Regular anticoagulation (as defined by Box 7.1) is given to maintenance haemodialysis patients who have no or little risk of bleeding.

Box 7.1 Anticoagulation guidelines

Baseline
ACT range 165–212 s
Patients pre-heparinisation. It is useful to measure the patient's baseline when establishing the heparin regime. Most patients will fall into this range unless clotting abnormalities are present.

Tight reduced control
ACT range 206–265 s
Clotting time: 120% of baseline
Suggested start regime: no loading dose; maintenance rate 500 unit h^{-1}
Adjust as required
Moderate bleeding risk:

- pericarditis
- recent surgery
- thrombocytopenia
- any active bleeding
- new/acute patients
- haematological disorders

For any high bleeding risk, consider heparin-free

Normal control
ACT range 250–320 s
Clotting time: 150–200% of baseline
Suggested start regime: 1000 units loading dose; maintenance rate 500 units h^{-1}
Adjust as necessary
Low bleeding risk
Suitable for all chronic haemodialysis patients
Consider lower end of range for diabetics

Extra control (to be used with caution)
ACT range 330–424 s
Clotting time: 200% of upper baseline
Suggested start regime: increase loading dose; maintenance rate 1000 units h^{-1}
Adjust as necessary
Chronic haemodialysis patients who continue to clot despite being in normal range
Consider other factors before using this range, i.e. blood flow, ultrafiltration rate, haemoglobin

Patients with acute renal failure, or patients having dialysis for the first time should be dialysed against a moderate regimen. Individuals at risk of bleeding (i.e. postoperative, post-transplant, bleeding diathesis, pericarditis) should be carefully dialysed with minimal or no heparin, if at all possible, to reduce the risk of bleeding complications.

In patients being dialysed via a fistula or graft, the heparin infusion should be switched off 30 min before the end of the dialysis session to prevent the risk of bleeding from the access site postdialysis. Prolonged pressure on the fistula postdialysis, waiting for a clot to form after removal of the needles, could damage the fistula. Patients dialysed via a subclavian or femoral line should not have the heparin discontinued until the end of dialysis.

Regional heparinisation

Patients at high risk of bleeding can be dialysed using regional heparinisation. Here the heparin is given as usual in the arterial dialysis lines (those entering the dialyser), but before the blood re-enters the body, protamine sulphate is infused continuously to counteract the effects of heparin. This is a very tedious approach and has since been superseded by low-molecular heparin.

Low-molecular weight heparin

Low-molecular-weight heparin (LMWH) is created by chemical degradation of crude heparin. It inhibits factors X and XII, but has little effect on thrombin and factors IX and XI, thereby increasing clotting time *in vivo* but having a minimal *in-vitro* effect. There are no direct bedside tests that can ascertain clotting times, so LMWH is given on the basis of body weight. Owing to the reduced systemic anticoagulant effect, LMWH is increasingly being used on patients with acute renal failure (ARF) or with an increased risk of bleeding. Bolus doses of LMWH can be as efficient in preventing clot formation within the filter as continuous infusion heparin (Kerr et al 1994).

Heparin-free dialysis

Prostacyclin has been used as an anticoagulant in ARF for both intermittent dialysis and haemofiltration. Some reports have suggested that prostacyclin is inferior to heparin in its effectiveness, but in the case of patients with a high risk of haemorrhage, prostacyclin is more effective at maintaining the integrity of the haemofiltration system than heparin (Davenport et al 1994).

Assessing effectiveness of anticoagulation

All patients should have regular assessment to determine their anticoagulation needs. Many of the assessments are quick and easy to conduct. Following the dialysis session, when the dialyser has been flushed there should be no clots visible and the patient should not be at risk of increased bleeding times. During dialysis, visual checks of the filter can indicate undercoagulation. If the colour of the blood within the filter becomes darker or dark streaks appear, then clotting of the filter has occurred. Changes in venous pressure and an increase in transmembrane pressure could also indicate the presence of clots forming in the filter or bubble trap. Prolonged bleeding from the needling site postdialysis is an indication that the patient may have been over-heparinised during dialysis.

An objective form of assessment that can be conducted at the bedside is through activated clotting times (ACTs). In new patients, a baseline should be established before dialysis to compare results during the procedure and heparin given accordingly. ACTs are a simple, effective and timely method of assessing clotting times of haemodialysis patients. A sample is taken prior to any heparin being given to establish a baseline. Depending upon the patient's condition, bleeding risk and anticoagulation requirements, the clotting times vary. Patients with a clotting risk (e.g. postsurgery) would require their clotting times to be maintained between 1.2 and 1.5 times their baseline. Other low-risk haemodialysis patients would be maintained at 1.5–2.0 times their baseline.

PRESCRIBING THE DIALYSIS DOSE

For many years patients were given dialysis treatments based entirely on the subjective evaluation of blood biochemistry along with a general assessment of perceived patient well-being. Patients themselves have been held responsible for the success of their treatment in relation to these parameters by being instructed to adhere to restricted diets aimed at maintaining biochemistry within acceptable limits. Limited resources and lack of understanding have compounded this philosophy over time.

More recently, there have been attempts to provide a more objective and scientific method of assessing dialysis adequacy. The aims of nursing care, utilising the dose of dialysis and nutritional parameters, should be to measure dialysis adequacy as well as encouraging patients to eat well.

UREA KINETIC MODELLING

Many years ago, the direct relationship between dialysis dose and long-term patient survival was demonstrated (Lowrie et al 1981). Today, the positive correlation between good dialysis adequacy and dialysis outcome also exists (Charra 2000). It is therefore essential that dialysis prescription be aimed at preventing or reducing the mortality and morbidity of patients receiving haemodialysis. High levels of urea clearance are correlated with improved patient outcomes.

One method of determining the dose is by the use of Kt/V. Kt/V is estimated by measuring pre- and postdialysis urea concentrations. K equals the dialyser clearance of urea, t equals the treatment time and V equals the amount of urea distributed in the body water. To complete the equation, it is necessary to know the clearance of urea through the dialyser. This is estimated by the pre- and postdialysis urea ratio. To ensure an accurate assessment of V, the nutritional status of the patient must be optimised, ensuring that the patient has an adequate protein intake. The patient's weight, height and gender are included in the calculation to estimate the percentage of body weight that is water (usually 55% in women and 65% in men).

For accurate assessment of K, it is essential to calculate the pre- and postdialysis urea ratio. The dialyser data sheet may be cautiously used to estimate the dialyser clearance but it is wise to assume a 10–20% reduction on the manufacturers' *in-vitro* values. An approximate example is given but more precise information is essential (i.e. the patient's height, etc.) for accurate calculation.

For example, a woman weighs 60 kg, therefore, an approximate estimation of $V = 33$ L.

$$K = 150 \, \text{mL} \, \text{min}^{-1}, \, t = 4 \, \text{h} \, (240 \, \text{min}), \, K \times t = 36 \, \text{L}$$

$$(150 \times 240 = 36\,000 \, \text{ml}), \text{divided by}$$

$$V = 36/33 = 1.09$$

Therefore, $Kt/V = 1.09$

Another, and possibly the simplest, method of assessing dialysis adequacy is through calculating the urea reduction ratio (URR). This is expressed as a percentage reduction:

$$\text{URR} = 100 \times (1 - Ct/Co)$$

where Ct = postdialysis urea and Co = predialysis urea.

These parameters can now provide an acceptable standard for dialysis dose. The Renal Association (Renal Association 2002) recommends the following: URR of 65% or a Kt/V of greater than 1.2 in patients dialysing three times per week. However, it should be noted that these recommendations are individual targets that each patient should reach or exceed, and if a patient is found to be receiving less than this amount, steps should be taken to increase the blood flow, the dialyser size or the duration of dialysis.

The Kidney Alliance (2001) states that haemodialysis adequacy should be assessed regularly and the above targets should be achieved in more than 90% of patients. Haemodialysis should be provided three times per week for > 90% of patients.

The mathematical concepts of urea kinetic modelling (UKM) can be complicated, but there are many computer software packages available to complete the calculations and to advise on corrective measures to achieve the desired Kt/V. However, it is important to be aware that there is no internationally agreed method for measuring Kt/V in everyday practice (Renal Association 2002). Some of these computer packages also measure protein catabolic rate (PCR), and this has been shown to be an increasingly important variable in patient morbidity and mortality, as it estimates daily protein intake (see Ch. 9).

What is vital is a clear understanding of the need for highly accurate sampling of pre- and postdialysis blood specimens, and the comprehensive dietary support of the patient. Postdialysis blood samples should be collected either by the slow-flow method, the simplified stop-flow method, or the stop-dialysate-flow method (Renal Association 2002). Whichever process is used, it is important that consistency is applied throughout the unit and across all samples collected.

Another significant role of the nurse is to ensure the delivery of the prescribed dialysis, and to understand the effect of deviations in treatment on the dialysis dose and the subsequent effect this may have on the patient's well-being.

- *Prescribed dialysis dose versus delivered dialysis dose:* the dialysis prescription may be affected by a number of events that will effectively reduce the dialysis dose.
- *Errors of time (t):* the patient starts dialysis late; the machine is in bypass due to concentrate running out; there is another machine fault or isolated ultrafiltration; the patient comes off dialysis early.
- *Errors of clearance (K):* reduction in blood flow; incorrect dialyser used; recirculation.
- *Errors of volume (V):* residual renal function increases or decreases; excessive or inadequate protein intake; incorrect sampling.

High-flux/high-efficiency dialysis by *Kt/V* measurement and high-flux membrane dialysis treatment time can be shortened using rapid blood and dialysate flow rates. The benefits for the patient of less time on dialysis may be outweighed by the potential complications such as increased hypotensive episodes.

PREPARATION FOR HAEMODIALYSIS

The period of time from diagnosis to commencement of RRT may be sudden, but often there is a period of time from a few months to several years when patients will have time to adjust their lifestyle and prepare for whichever form of dialysis is appropriate. The need for predialysis care, including psychological support as well as clinical monitoring of the progression of the renal failure, cannot be overemphasised.

For those requiring long-term haemodialysis, there are a number of options to be considered in relation to the location of the haemodialysis treatment.

IN-CENTRE HAEMODIALYSIS

Regional dialysis centres may provide both an acute and chronic haemodialysis service. In-centre haemodialysis may be offered, but the service may be overstretched in terms of available dialysis space. For this reason, the options of home haemodialysis or satellite haemodialysis should be explored for those who choose haemodialysis.

HOME HAEMODIALYSIS

The patient who expresses a desire to take the home haemodialysis treatment option should receive support and encouragement from the multidisciplinary team. The patient, once established and familiar with the dialysis regime, may want to learn the technique quickly in order to be self-supporting at home at the earliest possible time. With support and cooperation, a training programme can be completed in 6 weeks, if the patient is well and has no other complications, such as poor access, but most training programmes aim to get the patient home within 12 weeks.

To optimise training and learning opportunities, the patient can be encouraged to come to the unit on non-dialysis days to practise lining and priming the machine. Partners should be encouraged to attend as often as they can, but will need to negotiate a minimum amount of time with the nurse to learn emergency procedures. It should be emphasised to the patient and partner that the overall management of the treatment (setting up, monitoring and discontinuing the treatment) is primarily the responsibility of the patient. The partner is there to provide support and help, not to accept complete responsibility for the procedure.

There was evidence that home haemodialysis was declining in popularity in the UK (Ansell & Feest 2000); however, with the proposed increase in provision of haemodialysis (Department of Health 2004, Mowatt 2002, National Institute for Clinical Excellence (NICE) 2002), it has been recognised that there is a role for home haemodialysis in delivery of quality treatment to patients. This is supported by reports highlighting the benefits of home haemodialysis for selected individuals (NICE 2002).

SATELLITE HAEMODIALYSIS

The availability of satellite dialysis is increasing within the UK. Satellite centres provide an ideal setting for patients on maintenance haemodialysis. The centres are community-based, closer to the patient's home, making them more convenient and accessible. These important considerations for siting renal units are acknowledged by the Department of Health (2004).

Satellite centres are essentially nurse-managed and led. A nephrologist will oversee patient dialysis prescription and consultation, but day-to-day dialysis management is the responsibility of the nurse.

ASSESSMENT OF THE PATIENT

Before dialysis, the nurse must carry out a comprehensive predialysis assessment (Fig. 7.9). This includes discussing any concerns the patient may have in general or about the last dialysis session, reading the notes of the previous dialysis session and asking about any intradialytic problems. Measurement of blood pressure, fluid allowance and clinical assessment all contribute to the correct dry-weight assessment.

WEIGHT

Regular assessment of dry weight is essential to enable the nurse and patient to determine the amount of fluid removal required during dialysis.

Figure 7.9
Simple schematic drawing of a
typical water treatment plant.

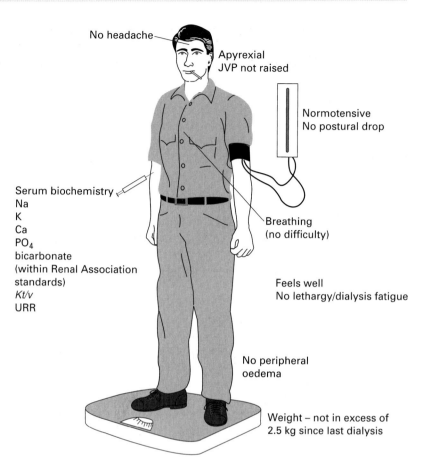

No headache

Apyrexial
JVP not raised

Normotensive
No postural drop

Serum biochemistry
Na
K
Ca
PO$_4$
bicarbonate
(within Renal Association
standards)
Kt/v
URR

Breathing
(no difficulty)

Feels well
No lethargy/dialysis fatigue

No peripheral
oedema

Weight – not in excess of
2.5 kg since last dialysis

The term 'dry weight' refers to the weight at which there is no clinical evidence of oedema, shortness of breath, increased jugular venous pressure or hypo/hypertension.

The initial determination of dry weight should involve the expertise of the nurse, doctor and dietitian. However, on a day-to-day basis this remains the responsibility of the nurse and many nurses are now trained in the routine clinical skills of fluid assessment.

The aim of dialysis is to remove the excess volume of fluid to ensure that the patient comes off dialysis at the dry weight. To calculate this, the following formula is used:

Actual weight	68.5 kg
Target weight	66 kg
Weight gain	2.5 kg

Add any additional fluid intake during treatment
Washback of saline (300 mL)
Two drinks (300 ml)
Total fluid to be removed   (2.5 + 0.3 + 0.3) = 3.1 L

Blood volume monitoring (BVM) is a relatively new addition to the armoury in assessing dry weight. The system relies on measuring a relative reduction in blood volume while continuously monitoring the patient's haematocrit during treatment. The aim is to reduce the blood volume by 10–15% through the treatment. A higher reduction of > 15% that is also associated with hypotension and/or cramps indicates that the patient has been dialysed to below their dry weight. A lower blood volume reduction of < 10% indicates that fluid is still retained and the dry weight may need to be reduced. BVM should still be used in conjunction with the global subjective assessment of dry weight.

BLOOD PRESSURE

Systolic hypertension with or without diastolic hypertension is a major problem in haemodialysis (HD) patients, and is associated with increased mortality (Agarwal 2003). Recommended predialysis blood pressures should be < 140/90 mmHg, and 130/80 mmHg postdialysis (Renal Association 2002).

Blood pressure should be recorded predialysis to provide a baseline from which to measure any significant changes during treatment. If a patient is overloaded prior to dialysis, blood pressure may be raised due to an increased circulating volume. A number of authors suggest that treatment of hypertension should first consider fluid and sodium control prior to the introduction of hypertensive medication. In the author's experience, correct assessment of dry weight has led to a reduction in reliance on antihypertensive medication in a number of patients.

Patients taking antihypertensive medication who become hypotensive on dialysis may find it necessary to omit the dose before or nearest to the next dialysis session, allowing greater cardiovascular compensatory systems to act during fluid removal on dialysis.

TEMPERATURE AND PULSE

The patient's temperature should be routinely recorded pre- and postdialysis for patients with central lines, and if clinically required for fistulas and grafts. Pyrexia prior to dialysis should be investigated immediately. Pulse should be recorded on all patients.

SERUM BIOCHEMISTRY AND HAEMATOLOGY

Blood tests are routinely carried out monthly but more frequent tests may be ordered as necessary. Target predialysis values recommended by the Renal Association (2002) are:

- Kt/V: > 1.2 (three times a week dialysis)
- URR: > 65%
- albumin: > 35 g L^{-1} (using a Bromocresol Green assay); > 30 g L^{-1} (using a Bromocresol Purple assay)
- potassium: 3.5–6.5 mmol L^{-1}

- phosphate: $< 1.8\,mmol\,L^{-1}$
- calcium: between 2.2 and 2.6 $mmol\,L^{-1}$ (adjusted for albumin concentration)
- haemoglobin: $> 10\,g\,dL^{-1}$, although there is evidence that $> 11\,g\,dL^{-1}$ should be aimed for.

Anaemia management is an increasingly important issue for those caring for patients with renal disease, and many renal units are now employing specialist anaemia coordinators.

INFECTION CONTROL

In 1972, The Rosenheim Report set standards for infection control in relation to hepatitis B in renal units. Now patients and staff within renal units must acknowledge daily the risks associated, not just with hepatitis B, but with other blood-borne viruses (BBV), such as hepatitis C and human immunodeficiency virus (HIV). Recent guidelines (Department of Health 2002) provide clear guidelines on prevention of cross-infection within the renal unit, providing details on disinfection of equipment, routine protective testing of patients and staff, and immunisation protocols.

The guidelines suggest that carriers of hepatitis B should be dialysed separately on dedicated machinery, and carriers of hepatitis C should be dialysed in separate or single shifts, on dedicated machines but not necessarily isolated in separate rooms.

The practicalities of providing isolation for every patient with BBV will need to be explored, along with the desired philosophy of care towards patients with BBV. Whilst the identification of patients with hepatitis is, on the whole, accepted, the screening of patients for HIV is controversial. Nurses must ensure that they advocate for patients and are satisfied that the rationale for testing is in the patient's interests and is only carried out with informed consent.

Facilities and policies for the containment of methicillin-resistant *Staphylococcus aureus* (MRSA) in renal units must be available and should be drawn up with the local infection control team. Patients colonised with MRSA must be isolated from other patients (Renal Association 2002). Universal precautions should be used as standard practice in the haemodialysis unit for the protection of the patients and the staff. Universal precautions require that body fluids of all patients are treated as potentially infectious and therefore protocols for hand-washing, protective clothing, eyewear and disinfection of machinery should be strictly adhered to prior to nursing interventions with all patients. When universal precautions are used effectively, the isolation of patients should be unnecessary unless it is to protect the immunocompromised patient from opportunistic infections.

Postdialysis clinical observations of blood pressure and weight are completed to check that the patient has lost the desired weight and is not hypo/hypertensive. It is important that patients are advised to wait until blood pressure is normalised, particularly if they are travelling home alone.

HAEMODIALYSIS COMPLICATIONS

Continuous and progressive development of equipment and expertise has ensured that haemodialysis is a safe procedure and, if prescribed and monitored correctly, serious complications should be rare. The treatment should only be carried out under the supervision of an expert practitioner. The aim of nursing care should be to prevent the occurrence of complications through comprehensive assessment and planning.

HYPOTENSION

Hypotension is a very common complication associated with haemodialysis, estimated to occur in around 15–25% of dialysis treatments (Maggiore 2002, Orofino et al 1990), and is probably a reflection of the large amount of fluid that is removed during the procedure as the patient nears their target weight.

Sympomatic hypotension associated with relative hypovolaemia usually occurs towards the end of the dialysis session. Maintaining blood pressure is dependent upon the replacement the fluid removed from the blood volume by fluid from the surrounding tissues. If fluid removal exceeds this intercompartmental shift, then the venous return will be reduced, resulting in a decreased cardiac output and hypotension.

To prevent hypotension, fluid removal should be controlled throughout the session. To achieve this, an ultrafiltration (UF) control should be used. Without this, fluctuation in fluid removal can occur owing to changes in pressure across the dialyser membrane. If a large amount of fluid needs to be removed, owing to an excessive intradialytic weight gain or a previously short dialysis, then consideration should be made to prolonging the treatment time to remove the fluid without resorting to an aggressive ultrafiltration rate. Large amounts of fluid can be removed by stopping dialysis and putting the machine into sequential ultrafiltration mode. Because relatively few electrolytes are removed in UF, only fluid, the patient is able to tolerate greater fluid removal. It is advisable to dialyse the patient for a short time (1 h) to remove potassium, before placing the machine into UF. This prevents haemoconcentration of potassium as fluid is removed, reducing the risk of cardiac arrhythmias. Once enough fluid has been removed, the session can then be returned to dialysis with a reduced TMP (see 'Principles of haemodialysis').

If the patient is dialysed below their dry weight, hypotension results. The symptoms persist after dialysis and are associated with cramps and a 'washed-out feeling'. Dry weights should be reviewed on a regular basis, using global subjective assessment in conjunction with blood volume monitoring, especially if symptoms persist after dialysis.

Reducing the temperature of the dialysate has been found to reduce the incidence of dialysis-related hypotension. Many dialysis patients have a subnormal temperature (Fine & Penner 1996) and, with the standard dialysate temperature at approximately 36.8–37°C, the result is a warming effect on the patient, causing peripheral vasodilation. Reducing the dialysate temperature to 36–36.5°C or lower, reduces this effect.

Lower temperature dialysis has been related to a significant reduction in hypotensive episodes on dialysis (Gjessing et al 1976, Maggiore et al 2002). Some dialysis machines incorporate a biofeedback system that reduces the dialysis temperature as the blood pressure falls, providing further patient protection.

In patients who cannot tolerate fluid removal, possibly due to cardio-vascular stability, may benefit from sodium and ultrafiltration profiling (Gerrish & Little 2003). Profiles that result in an overall neutral sodium balance at the end of dialysis have been associated with postdialysis weights close to dry weight targets (Song et al 2004, Stiller et al 2001).

Dialysis-related hypotension can also be induced by eating whilst on dialysis and is associated with a decrease in the systemic vascular resistance (Shibagaki & Takaichi 1998). It may be appropriate to suggest to patients that they do not eat large amounts of food whilst dialysing.

NAUSEA AND VOMITING

Nausea and vomiting occurs in approximately 10% of dialyses. The causes are multifactorial. Although in the majority of cases it is probably due to hypotension, it may also be associated with disequilibrium, and eating whilst on dialysis.

The prime point of caring for patients who may be suffering from nausea and vomiting during dialysis is to treat the cause. If the symptoms persist, then antiemetics may be necessary.

The most obvious preventative measure is to avoid hypotensive episodes. Reducing the blood flow rate at the beginning of dialysis occasionally helps, but may mean increasing the overall time of dialysis to ensure an adequate dialysis.

CRAMP

The pathogenesis behind the incidence of cramps associated with dialysis is generally unknown, but appears to be linked with a number of predisposing factors: hypotension, an incorrect dry weight, too low a sodium dialysate and/or large ultrafiltration volumes. Cramps usually occur late on in dialysis, when the net amount of fluid removed is at its greatest.

When cramp occurs on dialysis it can be a very painful and distressing condition for the patient. They are unable to move very much to alleviate the discomfort because they are still attached to the machine. A bolus infusion of normal saline or hypertonic saline may be beneficial, but care should be taken not to infuse too much fluid. A bolus of 50–100 mL of 50% glucose can bring relief within 5 min. The resulting period hyperglycaemia is short. However, this treatment is rarely used in the UK. Massaging the affected area helps to bring relief to the affected site, but also the physical contact helps to calm the patient.

Reducing the dialysate temperature has also been found to be beneficial in reducing the incidence of cramp during dialysis (Marcen 1988). If cramps persist, then altering the dialysate sodium to a higher concentration may prevent any further incidences. The use of variable-sodium dialysis has been found to reduce the problem of dialysis-induced cramps.

The link between the removal of large fluid volumes and cramp suggests that preventing too rapid fluid removal may result in a lower incidence of cramp. Educating the patient to prevent large interdialytic fluid gains should be a priority. Increasing the dialysate sodium concentration may be an option; however, this may increase postdialysis thirst and consequent interdialytic weight gain. Administration of quinine sulphate prior to dialysis decreases the incidence of cramps on dialysis. The use of quinine sulphate has been found to be useful as a prophylactic measure. However, because cramp is a subjective symptom, the effectiveness of quinine may be open to question (Mandal et al 1995).

DISEQUILIBRIUM

Dialysis relies upon the diffusion of solute across the semipermeable membrane of the dialyser. At the same time, diffusion will be taking place across the semipermeable membranes between all body compartments from the intracellular, interstitial and intravascular compartments. The rate of diffusion should be equal to maintain equilibrium. If diffusion in the dialyser is highly efficient, the result will be disequilibrium in the body compartments. Rapid urea removal will result in the plasma in the intravascular compartment being hypotonic to the fluid in the cells. This will result in osmotic shifts of fluid from a region of low concentration to a region of high concentration. This is particularly significant in the cerebrospinal fluid and brain cells. Additionally, rapid changes in the pH of the cerebrospinal fluid may predispose to disequilibrium (Bregman et al 2006).

Symptoms of disequilibrium can be mild or severe. Mild symptoms may include headache, dizziness, nausea and vomiting, or disorientation. Severe symptoms include fits, coma and potentially death.

Patients who are acutely ill, who have a very high urea predialysis or who are dialysed for the first time, are considered most at risk of disequilibrium. For those considered at risk, the nurse undertakes the following dialysis prescription to ensure that the blood urea level is only reduced by a maximum of 30%:

- blood flow rates should not exceed 150–200 mL min^{-1}
- dialysers with low surface area should be used
- treatment time is limited to approximately 2 h.

This type of prescription may need to be performed daily until the patient is considered stable and risk of disequilibrium is reduced. If disequilibrium is suspected, the dialysis should be discontinued; infusion of hypertonic solutions such as mannitol may help to correct the fluid shifts.

ELECTROLYTE IMBALANCE

Haemodialysis is a relatively aggressive treatment. Plasma electrolyte balances are subject to large alterations during dialysis, and these changes now occur over shorter periods of time with the trend towards shorter dialysis times. Because of these factors, selection of the appropriate dialysate concentrate takes on greater importance. Inappropriate selection can at least lead to mild but distressing complications, through to potentially life-threatening situations at worst.

Hyponatraemia

This is associated with using a dialysate containing a hypotonic concentration of sodium. Because of the osmotic imbalance between plasma and dialysate, sodium is removed from the plasma during dialysis leading to hypotension, nausea, vomiting cramps, headaches and, in extreme cases, symptoms associated with disequilibrium syndrome. If a patient complains of any of these symptoms, the dialysate and conductivity should be checked, and dialysis reinitiated with an appropriate concentrate solution.

Hypernatraemia

This results when a hypertonic sodium concentrate is used, purposely or accidentally, or the dialysis machine is programmed incorrectly during sodium profiling. It may also be due to inaccurate proportioning systems (Blagg 1992) or inappropriate monitoring of the conductivity. Patients complain of headache, nausea and thirst. Dialysis should be discontinued and recommenced using the correct dialysate.

Hypercalcaemia

This complication is usually associated with water treatment system failure, and primarily occurs in 'hard water areas' (hence the term 'hard water syndrome'). This emphasises the need for regular checks of the water quality, although it can also occur if a hypocalcaemic patient is dialysed against a high calcium dialysate. Symptoms include nausea and vomiting, agitation, muscle twitching and hypertension, which appear about an hour after starting dialysis. Again dialysis should be stopped and recommenced with the correct dialysate or when the water softener is repaired. Because of the risk in hard water areas, the water should be checked daily before dialysis is started for the day.

Hypokalaemia

Hypokalaemia in patients undergoing maintenance haemodialysis is often associated with gastrointestinal loss through vomiting or diarrhoea (Kaplan 1994). The use of a concentrate with no potassium can also be the cause. Hypokalaemia is also common in normokalaemic patients in acute renal failure. Care should be taken to avoid hypokalaemia because of the risk of cardiac arrhythmias, especially in a patient on digoxin (Morrison et al 1980, cited by Kaplan 1994). Dialysis against a dialysate concentrate with a higher potassium concentrate should be considered, though this is not advisable for the whole dialysis, altering to a lower concentration towards the end of the treatment.

Potassium levels at the end of dialysis should be reviewed with care; there is a considerable potassium rebound 1–2 h postdialysis.

Hyperkalaemia

Hyperkalaemia is usually associated with non-adherence to dietary advice. Although it is not associated with the dialysis treatment, it does affect decisions regarding time of dialysis, concentrate and filter to be used. Haemolysis during dialysis may the most likely cause of acute hyperkalaemia, initiated by transfusion incompatibility, overheated dialysate or chloramine breakthrough (Ward 1996).

DIALYSER REACTIONS (MEMBRANE REACTION/ FIRST–USE SYNDROME)

Allergic responses may occur as the patient's blood is exposed to foreign materials. Some examples include the dialyser membrane, the chemical sterilising agents, such as ETO, and bacteria or endotoxin (Hoenich & Van Holder 1993). However, the incidence of dialyser reactions has dropped considerably in recent years with the increase in gamma-irradiation use for sterilising dialysis products.

Allergic reactions can be type A or type B. Type A is a severe anaphylactic reaction, usually occurring within the first 5 min of dialysis. Symptoms can begin with an itchy rash and become severe, including dyspnoea and a burning sensation throughout the body. There may be laryngeal oedema and possibly cardiac arrest.

Treatment necessitates the immediate discontinuation of dialysis; the blood should not be returned to the patient. Maintenance of the airway is paramount and the administration of oxygen is required. The administration of adrenaline (epinephrine), chlorphenamine (chlorpheniramine) and hydrocortisone may be necessary. Patients who have suffered this type of reaction should be dialysed against membranes that have been gamma-irradiated or steam-sterilised. Extra rinsing of the dialysis circuit may also be advised.

Type B reactions are less severe and include chest pain, and may occur up to 1 h after dialysis is commenced. The cause is unknown but it is suggested that the use of synthetic membranes is beneficial (Bregman et al 2006).

HAEMOLYSIS

Haemolysis is the damage to or rupture of red blood cells. As most of the body's potassium is contained within the cells, massive haemolysis can quickly lead to hyperkalaemia and cardiac arrest. Haemolysis may be caused by dialysing against dialysate that is too hot, or dialysing against water or hypotonic dialysate.

Modern blood pumps have low shearing stresses and should not cause haemolysis but, if wrongly adjusted, the rollers of the blood pump may cause damage to cells. The high venous pressure resulting from occluded or obstructed (kinked) venous access or blood lines may also damage red blood cells. The patient will complain of chest pain and dyspnoea, and may be in a state of collapse. If haemolysis is suspected, the dialysis should immediately be discontinued and the blood should not be returned to the patient. Another machine should be prepared as a standby, as emergency dialysis may be needed to treat hyperkalaemia.

AIR EMBOLISM

Modern monitoring equipment with integral ultrasonic air detectors provides some assurance to patients and nurses for the prevention of air embolism. However, the equipment is only as good as its user, and strict adherence to alarm and safety checks prior to initiating each treatment is essential.

Extreme care should be taken during the priming procedure and when connecting the patient to the extracorporeal circuit. The air detector should be activated during the priming procedure, and any problems with false alarms resolved prior to the patient commencing dialysis. An air detector that persistently or intermittently alarms with no obvious cause should not be accepted as troublesome or oversensitive. The machine should not be used, and should be sent to the technicians for service.

In the event of a patient receiving an air embolus, the nurse must stop dialysis and lay the patient on the left side with the head lower than the rest of the body. This will force air in the circulation into the ventricle to act as a bubble trap. Immediate medical assistance must be sought and emergency resuscitative measures commenced. Outcome may be related to the volume of air infused.

CLOTTING OF THE BLOOD LINES AND DIALYSER

Clotting of the circuit will occur if anticoagulation is inadequate, if blood flow is inadequate or not continuous and if there is air in the circuit. A change in the pressure of the circuit will occur as a result of clotting. If the dialyser has clotted, there will be a decrease in the venous pressure and possibly a rise in the arterial pressure. Clotting of the venous chamber will result in a raised venous pressure. If clotting occurs, the treatment should be discontinued without returning the blood to the patient. The cause should be investigated (i.e. anticoagulation regime, access or dialyser preparation).

Table 7.3 summarises the complications of haemodialysis.

SPECIAL CARE ON HAEMODIALYSIS

An increasing number of those requiring haemodialysis have very special nursing needs and, although a detailed analysis of the care required is beyond the scope of this book, an outline of the care required and some useful further reading now follows.

DIABETES MELLITUS

Diabetes is the leading cause of established renal failure in western countries (Zimmet et al 2001), and many UK renal replacement

Table 7.3 Complications of haemodialysis (summary)

Complication	Cause	Prevention	Treatment

Hypotension	Dry weight too low
	Excess UF rate
	Antihypertensive drugs
	Eating on dialysis
		Accurate and regular
		  assessment of dry weight
		Correct UF calculation
		Suggest taking antihypertensive
		  postdialysis
		No eating on dialysis
			Lay patient flat
			Reduce UF rate
			0.9% NaCl bolus 100 mL if no
			  response to the above
			Recalculate UF rate

Cramp	Excessive UF rate	Correct UF calculations Re-educate patient regarding fluid gains Quinine sulphate prior to dialysis	0.9% NaCl or hypertonic solution Heat pad/massage
Disequilibrium	Dialysis is too efficient	Small surface area dialyser Reduce blood flow < 150 mL min^{-1} Reduce time 2 h Consider daily dialysis until biochemistry satisfactory	Discontinue dialysis Mannitol i.v.

Arrhythmias	Underlying hypertension
	Coronary artery disease
	Excess potassium shifts
	Digoxin
		Identify cause
		Consider dialysis against
		  dialysate of 3 mmol L^{-1}
		  potassium or greater
			Monitor

Membrane reaction	Complement activation
	  on exposure to
	  membrane and/or ETO
		Use gamma-irradiated
		  membranes
		Correct rinsing of disposables
		  during preparation
			Stop dialysis
			Do not return blood to patient
			Treat as anaphylaxis
			Adrenaline/hydrocortisone/piriton i.v.

Air embolus	Air entry into the patient's
	  circulation via dialysis
	  circuit
		Ensure all lines are secure
		Ensure correct and safe
		  use of air detector
		Regular observation of circuit
			Stop treatment
			Lay patient on left side
			Give 100% oxygen

Haemolysis	Damage to red blood cells
	  through pump or
	  kinked lines
	Dialysate temperature
	  too high
		Low shearing pumps
		Ensure venous pressure is
		  not high
		Check dialysate temperature
		  during dialysis
			Give oxygen
			Test for hyperkalaemia from damaged
			  red cells
			Dialysis

Clotting of blood
  lines
	Inadequate
	  anticoagulation
	Incorrect priming
	  procedure
		Review anticoagulation
		  regime
		Review priming procedure
			Stop treatment
			Discard circuit and line to continue
			  dialysis
			
			Review anticoagulation needs

Blood leak	A tear or rupture in the
	  dialyser membrane
		Careful handling of
		  the dialyser
		Keep pressures within
		  safe limits
			Stop dialysis
			Discard circuit, do not return blood
			  to the patient

ETO, ethylene oxide; HD, haemodialysis; i.v., intravenous; UF, ultrafiltration.

programs have in excess of 30% of the dialysis population having diabetes as the primary cause of renal failure. Many renal programmes in the UK have up to 25% of their dialysis population with diabetes as their underlying renal disease.

The following points should be considered when caring for those with diabetes on dialysis.

- Care of those with diabetes and renal failure should be through joint renal–diabetes management (Renal Association 2002), e.g. joint clinics.
- Those with diabetes should continue to attend specialist diabetes centres or specialist practice nurse clinics for annual review, to monitor complications of retinopathy, neuropathy and cardiac disease.
- Glucose monitoring should be individualised according to patient requirements – tight glycaemic control is preferable to avoid further complications of diabetes. Insulin requirements may either be reduced (dialysis reverses insulin resistance) or increased (dialysis may reverse anorexia and may increase dietary intake). Dialysate should contain glucose to avoid hypoglycaemia.
- Tight blood pressure control is recommended (< 135/75 mmHg), although it is recognised that hypotension on dialysis may be common. Sodium profiling may be helpful.
- Good nutrition is important, as patients may suffer gastroparesis, and subsequent nausea and vomiting.
- Dialysis nurses should carry out foot examination at least once per month, as foot lesions are the most commonly mismanaged problem (de Francisco 1999). Patient teaching on foot care is vital.

de Francisco (1999) has written a useful review article on diabetes and renal failure, which is recommended for further reading. Patients with diabetes have a decreased survival rate associated with increased interdialytic weight gain, so the importance of good patient education in this group is warranted (Kimmel et al 2000). The poor survival rate for older people with diabetes on dialysis has been highlighted by Khan et al (2000), and the importance of reducing or preventing the cardiovascular complications that cause high mortality rates is described.

OLDER PEOPLE

Nearly 50% of those requiring renal replacement are aged 65 or more (Ansell & Feest 2000), and it is increasingly recognised that this group requires special nursing care. The occupational therapist can make a valuable contribution to the multiprofessional team in rehabilitating those who are elderly and frail (Williams 2001). The implications of the increasing numbers of older people on dialysis are discussed by

Bevan (2000). The renal health care team may not be fully conversant with the physiological or mental changes that old age makes to the body, and this can have a detrimental impact of the quality of care offered to this group of patients. The conclusion is that, because the renal population is growing older, the renal team needs to be more aware of the changes that occur as people grow older and to deliver care acknowledging these changes.

Another important issue that is often overlooked by the renal care team is that of fatigue, a phenomenon that is poorly understood by healthcare professionals (McCann & Boore 2000). They found that fatigue was significantly associated with the presence of symptoms such as sleep problems, poor physical health status and depression. An individually prescribed exercise programme and exercise (cycling) whilst on dialysis showed an improvement in physical functioning (Painter et al 2000), which may in turn have an effect on health outcome.

SUMMARY

Those requiring haemodialysis should have a named nurse who is responsible for the planning, delivery and evaluation of the highest standards of individual care. Patients should have the opportunity to participate in decision-making related to all aspects of their care and have a right to be cared for by nurses who are competent in all aspects of haemodialysis treatments. Ideally this competence should be assessed in a formal and structured training programme. Finally, the skills needed to provide comprehensive nursing care to patients on haemodialysis cannot be measured solely by a nurse's competence to set up and use a haemodialysis machine, or by the ability to insert a pair of fistula needles first time. The haemodialysis nurse is constantly demanding access to the skills and knowledge that tacitly underlie the rapidly expanding scope of professional practice. There is a professional expectation of all nurses to ensure continuous learning and development in order to keep abreast of new research findings, new technology and the ever-increasing needs and demands of the patient.

The nurse working within the haemodialysis unit is faced on a day-to-day basis with a practical dichotomy. On the one hand, the working environment is highly technical and the delivery of optimal treatment is a cognitive challenge. On the other hand, the nursing focus must acknowledge the very special affective skills required in providing support, counselling and rehabilitative interventions to patients with chronic ill health. Although units will function with nurses whose strength or preference lies in one or other domain, it is the careful combination of the skills, knowledge and attitudes of both aspects that results in the advanced and expert practice of the nurse on the haemodialysis unit.

Case study 7.1

An 85-year-old woman with renal failure secondary to diabetes mellitus was dialysing for 4 h twice a week. Following adequacy studies, the nurses found a *Kt/V* of 0.9 on two consecutive measurements taken 3 months apart. It was likely that the value of *Kt/V* had dropped because of recent blood flow difficulties with her permanent central venous catheter.

As increasing the blood pump speed was not possible, and a large dialyser was already in use, it was proposed that this patient should attend the dialysis unit three times a week to improve her dialysis dose. The patient was very reluctant to do this.

- What benefits of increasing the *Kt/V* could be explained to this patient?
- Is it the quantity or quality of dialysis that is important in this case?
- Who should be involved in making the final decision about dialysis treatment times

References

Agarwal R. Systolic hypertension in hemodialysis patients. Semin Dial 2003; 16(3): 208–213.

Ahmed J, Weisberg LS. Hyperkalemia in dialysis patients. Semin Dial 2001; 14(5): 348–356.

Ansell D, Feest T. Third annual report of the UK Renal Registry. Bristol: UK Renal Registry, 2000.

Association for the Advancement for Medical Instrumentation (AAMI). Dialysate for hemodialysis. AAMI, 2004, Arlington, VA.

Berkoben M, Schwab SJ. Maintenance of permanent haemodialysis vascular access patency, Am Nephrol Nurses Assoc J 1995; 22: 17–24.

Besarab A. Intervention for intra-access stenosis. Semin Dial 2001; 14(5): 401–402.

Betjes MG, van Agteren M. Prevention of dialysis catheter-related sepsis with a citrate-taurolidine-containing lock solution. Nephrol Dial Transplant 2004; 19(6): 1546–1551.

Bevan M. The older person with renal failure. Nurs Stand 2000; 14: 48–52.

Blagg C. Acute complications associated with haemodialysis. In Replacement of Renal Function by Dialysis, 3rd edition (ed. JF Maher), 1992. Dordrecht: Kluwer Academic Publishers.

Bouchouareb D, Saveanu A, Bartoli JM, Olmer M. A new approach to evaluate vascular access in hemodialysis patients. Artif Organs 1998; 22: 591–595.

Bregman H, Daugirdas JT, Ing TS. Complications during haemodialysis. In: Daugirdas JT, Ing TS, eds. Handboook of dialysis, 2nd edn. New York: Little Brown, 2006: 149–168.

Butterly DW, Schwab SJ. Catheter access for hemodialysis: an overview. Semin Dial 2001; 14(6): 411–415.

Butterly DW. A quality improvement program for hemodialysis vascular access. Adv. Ren Replace Ther 1994; 1: 163–166.

Charra B. Improving adequacy improves haemodialysis outcome. EDTNA ERCA J 2000; 26(1): 6–10, 19.

Copley JB, Lindberg JS. Nontransplant therapy for dialysis-related amyloidosis. Semin Dial 2001; 14(2): 94–98.

Davenport A, Will EJ, Davison AM. Comparison of the use of standard heparin and prostacyclin anticoagulation in spontaneous and pump-driven extracorporeal circuits in patients with combined acute renal and hepatic failure. Nephron 1994; 66(4): 431–437.

de Francisco AL. Clinical outcomes for patients with diabetic nephropathy, EDTNA ERCA J, 1999; 25(1): 23–27.

De Sanctis LB, Stefoni S, Cianciolo G et al. Effect of different dialysis membranes on platelet function. A tool for biocompatibility evaluation. Int. J Artif Organs 1996; 19(7): 404–410.

Department of Health. Good practice guidelines for renal dialysis/transplantation units: prevention and control of blood-borne virus infection. London: Department of Health, 2002.

Department of Health. The national service framework for renal services, part 1: dialysis and transplantation. London: Department of Health, 2004.

Dheenan S, Henrich WL. Preventing dialysis hypotension: a comparison of usual protective maneuvers. Kidney Int 2001; 59(3): 1175–1181.

Easom A. Prophylactic antibiotic lock therapy for hemodialysis catheters. Nephrol Nurs J 2000; 27(1): 75.

Ernandez T, Saudan P, Berney T, Merminod T, Bednarkiewicz M, Martin PY. Risk factors for early failure of native arteriovenous fistulas. Nephron Clin. Pract 2005; 101(1): c39–c44.

Fernandez E, Borras M, Pais B, Montoliu J. Low-calcium dialysate stimulates parathormone secretion and its long-term use worsens secondary hyperparathyroidism. J Am Soc Nephrol 1995; 6(1): 132–135.

Fine A, Penner B. The protective effect of cool dialysate is dependent on patients' predialysis temperature. Am J Kidney Dis 1996; 28(2): 262–265.

Gerrish M, Little J. The effect of profiling dialysate sodium and ultrafiltration on patient comfort and cardiovascular stability during haemodialysis. EDTNA ERCA J 2003; 29(2): 61, 65, 70.

Gjessing J, Barsa J, Tomlin PJ. A possible means of rapid cooling in the emergency treatment of malignant hyperpyrexia. Br J Anaesth 1976; 48(5): 469–473.

Hayes J. Prolonging access function and survival, the nurse's role. EDTNA ERCA J 1998; 24(2): 7–10.

Hoenich N, Van Holder R. Allergic reactions associated with haemodialysis: biocompatibility monograph. EDTNA. ERCA J 1993; (Suppl): 3–6.

Hoenich NA, Levin R. The implications of water quality in hemodialysis. Semin Dial 2003; 16(6): 492–497.

Jaradat MI, Moe SM. Effect of hemodialysis membranes on beta 2-microglobulin amyloidosis. Semin Dial 2001; 14(2): 107–112.

Kaplan AA. Maintenance haemodialysis: prescription and management. In Renal Dialysis (JD Briggs, BJR Junor, RSC Rodger, JF Winchester, eds) 1994. London: Chapman & Hall.

Kerr PG, Mattingly S, Lo A, Atkins RC. The adequacy of fragmin as a single bolus dose with reused dialyzers. Artif Organs 1994; 18(6): 416–419.

Kidney Alliance. End-stage renal failure – a framework for planning and service delivery. Kidney Alliance, 2001.

Kimmel PL, Varela MP, Peterson RA et al. Interdialytic weight gain and survival in hemodialysis patients: effects of duration of ESRD and diabetes mellitus. Kidney Int 2000; 57(3): 1141–1151.

Konner K. Vascular access for dialysis in diabetic patients. EDTNA ERCA J 2004; 30(3): 148–150.

Kronung G. Plastic deformation of Cimino fistulae by repeated puncture. Dial Transplant 1984; 13: 635.

Ledebo I. Acetate vs. bicarbonate in everyday dialysis. Lund: Gambro, 1990.

Levy J, Morgan JBE. Oxford handbook of dialysis. London: Oxford University Press, 2001.

Lindley EJ, Lopot F, Harrington M, Elseviers MM. Treating and monitoring water for dialysis in Europe. Nephrol News Issues 2001; 15(2): 27, 30, 33–27, 36.

Lonnemann G. When good water goes bad: how it happens, clinical consequences and possible solutions. Blood Purif 2004; 22: 124–129.

Lowrie EG, Laird NM, Paker TF et al. Effect of the haemodialysis prescription of patient morbidity. Report from the National Co-operative Dialysis Study. N Engl J Med 1981; 305: 1176–1181.

Maggiore Q. Isothermic dialysis for hypotension-prone patients. Semin Dial 2002; 15(3): 187–190.

Maggiore Q, Pizzarelli F, Santoro A et al. The effects of control of thermal balance on vascular stability in hemodialysis patients: results of the European randomized clinical trial. Am J Kidney Dis 2002; 40(2): 280–290.

Mandal AK, Abernathy T, Nelluri SN, Stitzel V. Is quinine effective and safe in leg cramps? J Clin Pharmacol 1995; 35(6): 588–593.

Marcen R, Quereda C, Orofino L, Lamas S, Teruel JL, Matesanz R, Ortuno, J. Hemodialysis with low-temperature dialysate: a long-term experience. Nephron 1988; 49(1): 29–32.

McCann, K, Boore JR. Fatigue in persons with renal failure who require maintenance haemodialysis. J Adv Nurs 2000; 32(5): 1132–1142.

McIntyre CW, Hulme LJ, Taal M, Fluck RJ. Locking of tunneled hemodialysis catheters with gentamicin and heparin. Kidney Int 2004; 66(2): 801–805.

Mowatt G, Vale L, Perez J et al. Systematic review of the effectiveness and cost-effectiveness of home versus hospital or satellite unit haemodialysis for people with end stage renal failure. London: National Institute for Clinical Excellence, 2002.

National Institute for Clinical Excellence (NICE). Guidance on home compared with hospital haemodialysis for patients with end-stage renal failure. London: NICE, 2002.

NKF-K/DOQI. NKF-K/DOQI clinical practice guidelines for vascular access: update 2000. Am J Kidney Dis 2001; 37: s137–s181.

Oettinger CW, Oliver JC. An economical new process for incenter bicarbonate dialysate production: comparison with acetate in a large dialysis population. Artif Organs 1989; 13(5): 432–437.

Orofino L, Marcen R, Quereda C et al. Epidemiology of symptomatic hypotension in hemodialysis: is cool dialysate beneficial for all patients? Am J Nephrol 1990; 10(3): 177–180.

Painter P, Carlson L, Carey S, Paul SM, Myll J. Physical functioning and health-related quality-of-life changes with exercise training in hemodialysis patients. Am J Kidney Dis 2000; 35(3): 482–492.

Parker TF, Wingard RL, Husni L et al. Effect of the membrane biocompatibility on nutritional parameters in chronic haemodialysis. Kidney International 1996; 49(2): 551–556.

Pellowe C, Pratt R, Loveday H, Harper P, Robinson N, Jones SR. Guidelines for preventing infections associated with the insertion and maintenance of central venous catheters. J Hosp Infect 2001; 47(Suppl 1): S47–S67.

Renal Association. Treatment of adult patients with renal failure. Recommended standards and audit measures, 3rd ed. London: Royal College of Physicians, 2002.

Rocek M, Peregrin J. Percutaneous interventions for vascular dialysis access. EDTNA ERCA J 2001; 27(2): 83, 91.

Shaldon S, Koch KM. Biocompatibility in hemodialysis: clinical relevance in 1995. Artif.Organs 1995; 19(5): 395–397.

Shibagaki Y, Takaichi K. Significant reduction of the large-vessel blood volume by food intake during hemodialysis. Clin Nephrol 1998; 49(1): 49–54.

Song JH, Park GH, Lee SY et al. Effect of sodium balance and the combination of ultrafiltration profile during sodium profiling hemodialysis on the maintenance of the quality of dialysis and sodium and fluid balances. J Am Soc Nephrol (www.jasn.org/cgi/content/abstract/ASN.2004070581v1), 2004.

Stiller S, Bonnie-Schorn E, Grassmann A, Uhlenbusch-Korwer I, Mann H. A critical review of sodium profiling for hemodialysis. Semin Dial 2001; 14(5): 337–347.

Twardowski ZJ. Constant site (buttonhole) method of needle insertion for hemodialysis. Dial Transplant 1995; 24(10): 559.

Twardowski ZJ, Van Stone JC, Jones MRE et al. Blood recirculation in intravenous catheters for haemodialysis. J Am Soc Nephrol 1993; 3: 218–221.

Uldall R. Vascular access for continuous renal replacement therapy. Semin Dial 1996; 9: 93–97.

Ward DM. Chloramine removal from water used in hemodialysis. Adv Ren Replacement Ther 1996; 3(4): 337–347.

Ward RA. Heparinization for routine hemodialysis. Adv Renal Replacement Ther 1995; 2(4): 362–370.

Williams M. Rehabilitating the frail and elderly on renal replacement therapy. EDTNA ERCA J 2001; 27(2):64–5, 74.

Winchester JF, Salsberg JA, Levin NW. Beta-2 microglobulin in ESRD: An in-depth review. Adv Renal Replacement Ther 2003; 10(4): 279–309.

Wittich E. Maintaining an optimum haemocatheter exit site. EDTNA ERCA J 2001; 27(2): 81–82.

Zimmet P, Alberti KG, Shaw J. Global and societal implications of the diabetes epidemic. Nature 2001; 414: 782–787.

Chapter 8

Peritoneal dialysis

Janet Wild

LEARNING OUTCOMES FOR THIS CHAPTER	■ To recognise the importance of individualised care for those on peritoneal dialysis (PD)
	■ To review the anatomy and physiology of the peritoneum
	■ To identify best practice for the care of the PD catheter and exit site, and the best use of each PD therapy option
	■ To understand the criteria for good patient selection for PD
	■ To review all factors required to dialyse a patient with PD adequately
	■ To review the complications of PD
	■ To understand the importance of good ongoing education for those on PD

INTRODUCTION

Peritoneal dialysis (PD) as a treatment for established renal failure (ERF) is a relatively simple and very effective technique. As such, it has been successfully developed as the preferred first option of home dialysis.

From its introduction in the late 1970s, PD has been refined and developed into a flexible and adaptable therapy that is the treatment of choice for many patients. It has been found to be most effective if performed as a continuous treatment, either by the patient during the day (continuous ambulatory peritoneal dialysis or CAPD), or by a machine, whilst the patient sleeps (automated peritoneal dialysis or APD). Owing to its continuous nature, patients who are treated by this therapy tend to have a more stable biochemical and fluid profile. Its flexible nature makes it suitable for almost all patients with ERF.

This chapter discusses the importance of having an individualised treatment for each patient, which is structured around both clinical and lifestyle needs. The chapter starts with an overview of the anatomy and physiology of the peritoneum and practical aspects of the therapy, and different therapy options on PD; complications and patient education and training are also discussed. It should be noted here that the role of the nurse working within the field of PD has changed markedly over the last decade (Bender & Swartz 1999, Jacobs et al 1997, Kelman 1995, Renal Competency Framework 2005). As the therapy is performed by the patients themselves, in the community, the main focus is on providing patients with not only an individualised treatment, but also adequate psychological and nursing care, which are essential elements for the successful treatment of those needing PD and their families.

PHYSIOLOGY OF PERITONEAL DIALYSIS

The peritoneal membrane, so called because it covers the abdominal cavity and is derived from the Greek word *peritonaion*, meaning to stretch around, has a surface area of up to 2 m². The peritoneal cavity is the potential space between the parietal membrane (which lines the abdominal cavity) and the visceral membrane (the inner layer that closely covers the organs and includes the mesenteries). Under normal circumstances this cavity contains between 50 and 100 mL of fluid, which acts as a lubricant (Fig. 8.1).

During PD, physiological solution or dialysis fluid is instilled into the peritoneal cavity. Uraemic toxins and solutes move across the membrane by the process of diffusion, from the bloodstream into the dialysis fluid, or vice versa, depending on the concentration gradient. The composition of the dialysis fluid is near to that of normal extracellular fluid.

Fluid removal takes place by osmosis. The dialysis fluid is made hypertonic to plasma by the addition of osmotic agent, usually glucose. Other osmotic solutions are discussed later in this chapter.

The membrane is made up of three layers (Fig. 8.2).

- *The mesothelium:* underneath this lies the connective tissue. The luminal side of the mesothelium is covered with numerous microvilli, which are believed to increase the surface area of the peritoneum to up to 40 m² in a healthy individual. During PD the density of these microvilli appears to be reduced (Williams et al 2003).
- *The peritoneal interstitium:* this is composed of fibres and bundles of collagen.
- *The capillary endothelium:* this forms a complex branching system.

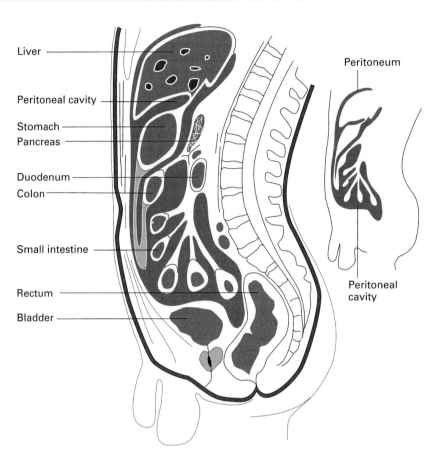

Figure 8.1
Location of the peritoneal cavity.

Liver

Peritoneum

Peritoneal cavity

Stomach

Pancreas

Duodenum

Colon

Small intestine

Rectum

Bladder

Peritoneal cavity

BLOOD SUPPLY

The visceral peritoneum is supplied by the superior mesenteric artery. The parietal peritoneum is supplied by the intercostal, epigastric and lumbar arteries. Venous return from the visceral peritoneum is to the portal circulation, whereas that from the parietal peritoneum goes into the caval circulation. This is important because it means that any drugs administered via the peritoneum will be transported to the liver, the normal route.

LYMPHATIC DRAINAGE

Lymphatic drainage from the peritoneal cavity returns excess fluid and proteins into the systemic circulation. Its other function is to remove foreign bodies from the peritoneal cavity. Lymphatic drainage is a one-way system, the flow rate of which may be affected by respiratory rate, intra-peritoneal hydrostatic pressure, posture or peritonitis.

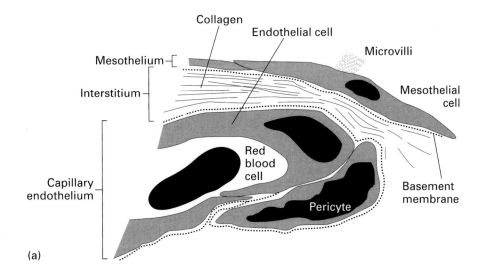

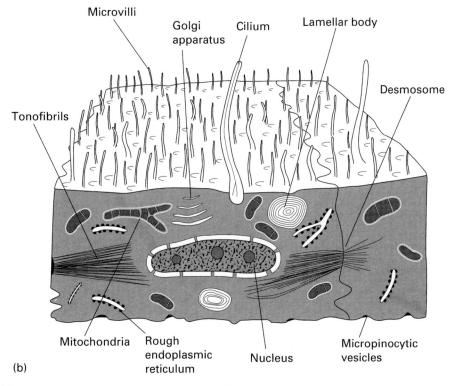

Figure 8.2 (a) The three layers of the peritoneal membrane. (b) Diagrammatic representation of a normal mesothelial cell.

PERITONEAL MEMBRANE TRANSPORT CHARACTERISTICS

The peritoneal membrane is semipermeable and allows the passage of both water and solutes.

During PD three processes are involved in removing fluid and wastes from the bloodstream and balancing electrolytes. These are osmosis, diffusion and convection.

Osmosis

This is the movement of water through a semipermeable membrane from a solution of low concentration into a solution with a higher concentration. The solution into which the water moves in PD contains an osmotic agent, usually glucose (other osmotic agents are discussed later in this chapter). The higher the glucose concentration, the greater the osmotic effect will be, so removing more water from the patient's bloodstream (Fig. 8.3).

Diffusion

This is solute exchange between two solutions, usually separated by a semipermeable membrane. The solutes will travel in either direction across the membrane until equilibrium is achieved. The direction and speed at which the solutes flow depend on the concentration gradient. Solutes will flow from the stronger solution into the weaker solution (Fig. 8.4). Therefore, solutes can pass in either direction across the peritoneal membrane.

Other factors that affect diffusion rate are molecular weight and membrane resistance.

Molecular weight

Diffusion is a spontaneous process whereby solutes move randomly. Lighter, smaller molecules will move quicker than larger, heavier molecules. Urea (which has a molecular weight of 60 Da) diffuses from blood

Figure 8.3
Osmotic ultrafiltration across the peritoneal membrane with a glucose dialysis solution in the peritoneal cavity.

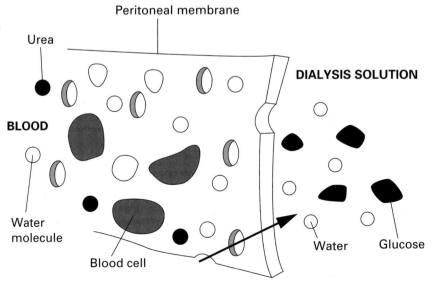

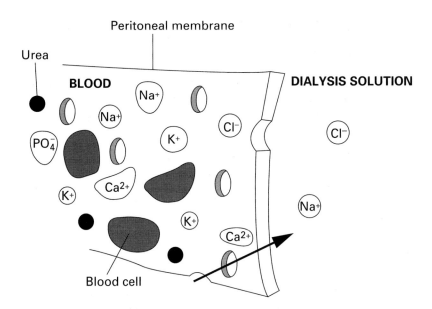

Figure 8.4
The peritoneum acts as a semipermeable membrane, allowing small solutes and water to diffuse through, but retaining large particles such as blood cells.

to dialysate more rapidly than creatinine (molecular weight 113 Da) or vitamin B12 (molecular weight 1352 Da). Unlike haemodialysis, where the membrane pore size is controlled, the peritoneal membrane allows transport of large molecules and even proteins. Protein transport into the dialysate is unfortunate as this is an essential nutrient, particularly in dialysis patients, who may be catabolic.

Membrane resistance

The permeability of the individual's membrane is an important factor controlling diffusion of solutes. Measurement of this is discussed later in this section.

A patient's peritoneal permeability may be changed during illness. Acute episodes of peritonitis appear greatly to increase the membrane permeability to both solutes and water. However, fibrotic thickening of the membrane may lead to a severe reduction in its permeability (Williams et al 2003).

Convection

Owing to the large amount of osmotic ultrafiltration that takes place during PD, convective flow transports or 'drags' water and solutes across the membrane. This occurs at a much faster rate than that which may be accounted for by diffusion alone.

The ability of glucose to exert an effective osmotic pressure depends on its ability to stay in solution in the dialysate. If the peritoneal membrane were perfectly semipermeable (i.e. only permeable to water), the osmotic pressure would be maximised. However, the peritoneum is permeable to solutes as well as water, and so allows the glucose through. The osmotic gradient is, therefore, maximum at the beginning of the exchange. The ultrafiltration will decrease during the dwell time as glucose is absorbed into the bloodstream. It is estimated that the ultrafiltration is maximised at the beginning of the PD fluid exchange when the concentration gradient is highest (Khanna 1999). The total dialysate and ultrafiltrate volume continues to decrease after this point owing to lymphatic absorption.

MEASUREMENT OF PERITONEAL PERMEABILITY

The characteristics, pore size and dimensions of the peritoneal membrane are not printed on the side of a packet as are for haemodialysis. It is therefore important to determine the characteristics of the patient's peritoneal membrane before an appropriate prescription can be written. A number of methods have been described including the SPA test, the PET and Fast PET, and the PDC test.

The peritoneal equilibrium test (PET) is the most commonly used. This test, which was described in 1987 by Twardowski et al, determines solute transport rates over time and the ultrafiltration capacity of the membrane. The results of the test can therefore be used to determine the optimum length of time that PD fluid should be left inside the peritoneal cavity to gain maximum fluid and solute removal. It also alerts the practitioner to any changes in membrane function that could affect patient's dialysis adequacy and outcomes.

Performing a PET

An experienced PD nurse completes the test in the outpatient clinic. Prior to performing the test, the patient's catheter function should be checked so that poor drainage due to mechanical problems with the catheter, such as constipation, is not associated to membrane function. In addition, patients should be uvolemic, and diabetic patients should have serum glucose levels within normal limits. This enables the results of the test to be interpreted accurately.

To enable accurate reproduction of the test according to Twardovski's original work, the following protocol should be followed.

1. The patient attends the clinic with a 2.27% bag, which has dwelled in the peritoneum for between 8 and 12 hours. This is drained out, the volume and dwell time recorded, and a sample taken.
2. The patient's peritoneal cavity is then instilled with another bag of 2.27%. The volume should be the same as the overnight bag but ideally no smaller than 2000 mL.
3. This is drained in over 10 min with the patient in a supine position rolling from side to side to ensure mixing whilst the fluid is infused.
4. Dialysate samples are taken at 0 h, 2 h and 4 h with a serum sample at 2 h.
5. It is essential to record the drain-out time and the drained out volume at 4 h to assess the ultrafiltration capacity of the membrane.
6. Finally, the patient's usual PD solution is instilled before they are sent home.

The samples are then sent for analysis of glucose and creatinine levels as soon as possible.

Calculating results

In order to determine the patient's membrane solute transport characteristics, the level of creatinine that is in the PD fluid at 0, 2 and 4 h is compared to the level of creatinine in the patient's plasma (D/P ratio). This gives a ratio of between 0 and 1. The closer the dialysate to plasma ratio is to 1, the faster solutes equilibrate across the membrane. Glucose absorption, from the PD solution into the patient's serum, is calculated in the same way. The level of glucose in the PD fluid at 0, 2 and 4 h is compared to the level in the patient's serum (D/P ratio). The closer the ratio is to 1, the faster glucose crosses the membrane. Patients who equilibrate solutes fast will therefore have good solute removal during PD; however, as glucose will also be absorbed quicker, the glucose concentration gradient will not be sustained. Thus, fluid removal will be poor.

The results can be plotted to determine transporter status.

Corrected creatinine

Owing to glucose interference with creatinine assays, corrected creatinine values may need to be determined. A corrected creatinine result may be provided by individual laboratories, depending on the type of laboratory test used. Enzymatic tests do not require correction. Analysis of samples must always be carried out on the same analyser to avoid erroneous results. If corrected creatinine is not available, the standard creatinine results should be used throughout (Baxter Healthcare 1992).

Analysis of results

When the patient's transport characteristics have been identified, it is easy to tailor the treatment to suit the membrane. The patient's peritoneal membrane is categorised into one of the four membrane classifications. Each membrane classification has specific characteristics that guide the clinician in tailoring the patient's prescription (see Table 8.1).

RECOMMENDATIONS FOR OPTIMAL USE OF PET RESULTS

Patients who have high transport membranes should have rapid exchanges of fluid, usually achieved by using APD. Patients who transport glucose and solutes more slowly are better suited to receiving CAPD, where the fluid remains in the peritoneal cavity for longer periods. Any prescription modification should be accompanied by an assessment of the patient's lifestyle to ensure that the treatment is achievable within work and social constraints. By performing this test regularly, it is possible to monitor peritoneal membrane function over time and, therefore, diagnose acute membrane injury, inadequate ultrafiltration and poor solute clearance.

A PET should be performed after 4–8 weeks on dialysis (European Best Practice Guidelines for PD 2005). It has been suggested that repeat

Table 8.1 Classification of membrane type

% of patients	Membrane type	4-h D/P creatinine	Characteristics
10	High	0.82–1.03	Very efficient membrane Transports solutes easily Increased glucose absorption May have difficulty achieving ultrafiltration At risk of low albumin
53	High average	0.65–0.81	Efficient membrane Transports solutes well Ultrafiltrates well
31	Low average	0.50–0.64	Less efficient membrane Transports solutes slowly Ultrafilters well
6	Low	0.3 –0.49	Inefficient membrane Transports solutes slowly Ultrafilters well

tests should be routinely performed every 1–2 years or if problems arise, such as an apparent loss of ultrafiltration or if there is a change in therapy, such as transfer from CAPD to APD (Bozfakioglu et al 2002, Renal Association 2002). Changes over time in the test results can then be related to clinical performance and treatment regimens may be altered accordingly.

PERITONEAL DIALYSIS ACCESS AND EXIT-SITE CARE

Although inserting a catheter for peritoneal dialysis is a relatively simple procedure, the implications of this going wrong can be catastrophic for the patient at a most vulnerable time – when they are new to PD. Not only can poor insertion technique lead to a malfunctioning catheter, it can also be responsible for infections and the failure of PD in about 25% of patients (Ash 2003), which can be devastating for a patient who has chosen this therapy. Unsuccessful PD catheter insertion also has cost implications and can adversely affect the management of a renal unit.

There are many facets to successful PD access:

- choosing the right catheter
- good insertion technique
- meticulous preoperative and postoperative care.

However, what is fundamental is effective teamwork from the multidisciplinary team, in particular the medical and nursing staff.

TYPES OF CATHETERS

The perfect PD catheter is one that provides reliable and rapid inflow and outflow from the peritoneal cavity without leaks or infections. Catheters should be designed to stay in pelvic cavity and be easy to insert.

PD catheters generally have the following three portions (Fig. 8.5).

- *The outer segment*, which connects via an adapter to the solution transfer set.
- *The intramural segment*. This has Dacron cuffs, spaced about 8 cm apart. By creating an inflammatory response, fibrous tissue fixes the catheter into position, thereby minimizing leakage of dialysate and preventing bacteria entering the catheter 'tunnel' and intraperitoneal segment.
- *The intraperitoneal part*, which has many small holes up the side, is situated inside the peritoneal cavity for the in and outflow of the solution.

Variations in the design of catheters include the number of cuffs (one vs. two), the design of the intramural segment (permanently bent vs. straight) and the intraperitoneal portion (straight vs. curled). Despite the number of types of catheters available, the most widely used are the straight (Fig. 8.6) and curled (Fig. 8.7) Tenckhoff catheters. They are easily inserted under local or general anaesthetic, and choice of catheter will usually depend on local preference.

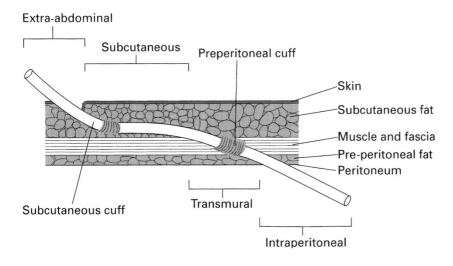

Extra-abdominal

Subcutaneous   Preperitoneal cuff

Skin

Subcutaneous fat

Muscle and fascia

Pre-peritoneal fat

Peritoneum

Subcutaneous cuff

Transmural

Intraperitoneal

Figure 8.5
Functional parts of the peritoneal catheter.

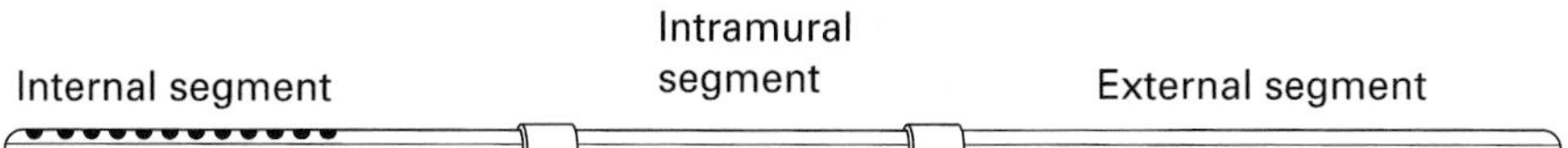

Internal segment

Intramural segment

External segment

Figure 8.6
Straight Tenckhoff catheter.

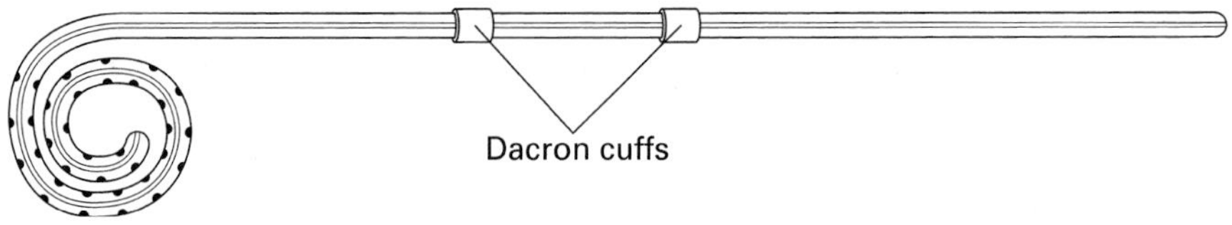

Figure 8.7
Curled Tenckhoff catheter.

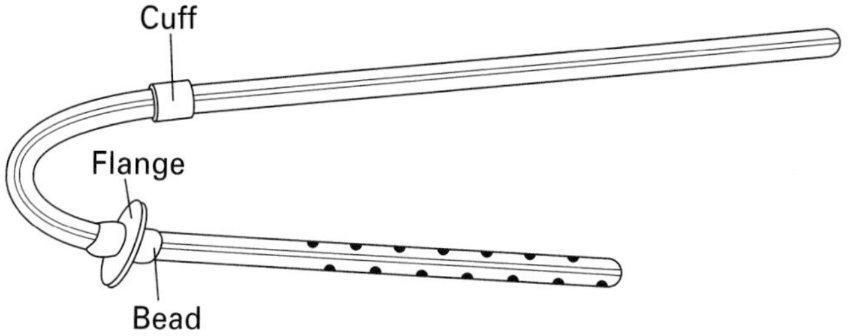

Dacron cuffs

Figure 8.8
Swan-neck catheter.

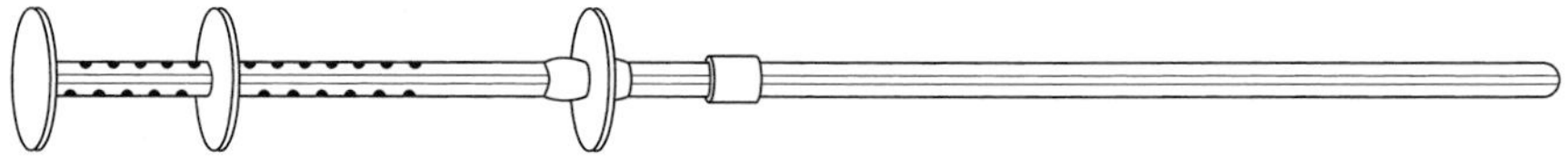

Cuff

Flange

Bead

Figure 8.9
Toronto
Western catheter.

The swan-neck (Fig. 8.8) and Toronto Western (Fig. 8.9) catheters were both developed to aid outflow of the dialysate.

- *Swan-neck:* with two downward-pointing segments, migration of this type of catheter is rare thereby serving to aid outflow. It is also thought to prevent infections at the exit site as this segment of the catheter also points downwards, thus preventing accumulation of sweat and pus.
- *Toronto Western:* this has two discs at the intraperitoneal segment helping to prevent migration. It also has a Dacron flange and bead at the deep cuff, which is sewn in position by a purse-string suture, helping to reduce leaks at the exit site.

Literature shows that there is little difference between risk of infection for the various types of catheters; however, one study showed that there was increased catheter survival in the coiled catheter when compared to the straight (36% vs. 77%, $p = 0.01$; Neilson et al 1995). If properly placed, dual-cuff Tenckhoff catheters have a lower incidence of infection and a longer lifespan than single-cuff catheters (Ash 2003). Overall there seems to be no superior catheter to the standard straight Tenckhoff catheter (Piraino et al 2005 and European Best Practice Guidelines 2005).

PRE-INSERTION PREPARATION OF THE PATIENT

A full preoperative assessment of the patient is essential to identify existing or potential hernias. If present, these can be repaired during the catheter insertion. The catheter exit site should be determined before the catheter is inserted. The preferred site should first be discussed with the patient to help promote participation in, and an understanding of the therapy. The following points should be followed when determining the exit site of the patient's catheter.

- The site should be determined whilst the patient is in a relaxed sitting or standing position.
- It should be either above or below the belt line, whichever the patient prefers.
- Skin folds and abdominal scars should be avoided.
- The catheter exit site should be located where the patient can effectively carry out exit-site care.
- Once the exit site has been determined, it should be marked clearly with a permanent skin marker.

PREOPERATIVE CARE OF THE PATIENT

On the morning of the operation, the patient should bathe or have a shower. If necessary, abdominal hair should be clipped. A major cause of catheter failure, particularly at the start of PD, is constipation. It is therefore recommended that a powerful aperient, such as Picolax, is given the day before catheter insertion. It is also important that the patient has an empty bladder before the insertion procedure takes place. Other usual preoperative practices should also be followed.

Staphylococcus aureus screening

There is evidence (Bernardini et al 1996, Mupirocine Study Group 1996) that patients who have nasal carriage of *Staphylococcus aureus* have an increased risk of exit-site infection and peritonitis, and that the use of mupirocin cream or ointment at the exit site is recommended to reduce the incidence of infection (European Best Practice Guidelines 2005). It is, therefore, advisable to screen all patients for *Staphylococcus aureus* prior to catheter insertion and treat accordingly.

Prophylactic antibiotics

There is evidence that prophylactic antibiotics prevent catheter infections and peritonitis (Gadallah et al 2000, Golper & Tranaeus 1996, Lye et al 1992). In a controlled study using cefuroxime (1.5 g intravenously (i.v.) 1–2 h preoperatively, and 250 mg intraperitoneally (i.p.) perioperatively, the prophylactic group had fewer peritonitis episodes than controls (Wikdahl et al 1997). However, more recently, Gadallah et al (2000) concluded that vancomycin (1 g i.v., single dose) is superior to cephalosporin (1 g i.v., single dose) when preventing early peritonitis. Indeed, all the recently published guidelines recommend that prophylactic antibiotics should be administered at the time of catheter insertion (European Best Practice Guidelines 2005, Piraino et al 2005).

Psychological preparation of the patient

This is of great importance for someone who is new to PD and is discussed in detail in Ch. 3.

INSERTION TECHNIQUES

Peritoneal dialysis is a life-maintaining therapy. Access to the peritoneal cavity, via the PD catheter, is therefore particularly important in ensuring its success (see Fig. 8.10 for the correct position of the catheter in the abdomen). The insertion technique should be treated as a skill acquired by experienced surgeons and physicians, rather like implantation of a pacemaker or similar device. A team approach is essential and nurse involvement is most important. The nurse's role in insertion of PD catheters starts with the preoperative preparation described above, all of which can be carried out by the nurse. In many centres, the PD nurse accompanies the patient to the operating theatre to ensure correct procedures are carried out and that the catheter is functioning well before final wound closure is made.

Figure 8.10
The position of a peritoneal dialysis catheter in the abdomen.

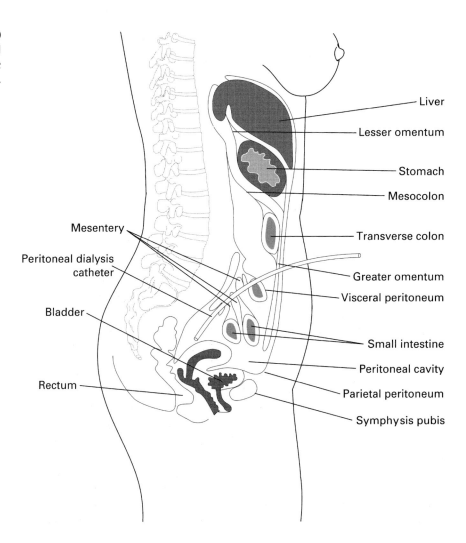

The four most frequently performed methods of catheter insertion include:

1. surgical placement by dissection (Ash & Daugirdas 1994, Ash & Nichols 1994)
2. blind placement using Tenckhoff trocar (Ash & Daugirdas 1994, Gokal et al 1998)
3. blind placement using guidewire (Seldinger technique: Ash & Daugirdas 1994, Ash & Nichols 1994)
4. minitrocar placement using peritoneoscopy (Ash & Daugirdas 1994, Ash & Nichols 1994).

Another implantation technique that has recently been described is the 'buried catheter technique', which involves prolonged subcutaneous implantation of the catheter for up to 6 weeks before being brought to the surface and used. In preliminary studies, this technique seemed to show a reduction in the rate of infection (Park et al 1996). However, prospective trials have not confirmed its success long term (Danielsson et al 2002, Esson et al 2000, Park et al 1998).

Catheters may also be placed surgically, using a laparoscope, or by percutaneous radiological or peritoneoscopic insertion (Gadallah et al 1999), the latter showing longer catheter survival rates, better infection rates and fewer postoperative leaks.

POSTOPERATIVE CARE OF THE PATIENT

The goals of postoperative catheter care are to:

1. minimise any bacterial colonisation of the exit and tunnel during the early healing period
2. prevent trauma to the exit site and traction on the cuffs by immobilisation of the catheter
3. minimise intra-abdominal pressure to prevent leakage.

Ideally, the exit site should remain undisturbed for 7–10 days following insertion of the catheter. The patient may be discharged home during this period. If, during the first 10 days, the dressing becomes soiled, it should be redressed by a nurse. If it merely becomes dislodged, it should simply be replaced with a fresh sterile dressing. During this period, the catheter tubing must be immobilised by securely taping it to the patient's abdomen.

Before discharge from hospital, during this resting of the patient's catheter, clear instructions must be given as to the correct procedures for caring for the catheter at home. It may be appropriate to involve the community district nursing team if no specific community PD nurse is available. In this case, adequate training and support must be provided for the nursing team.

Directly following insertion of the catheter, it may be flushed with 500–1500 mL of PD fluid to check patency. It may then be 'capped off' using a small locking cap on the catheter adapter (this adapter is available in titanium metal or plastic) and left covered until PD commences.

Ideally, PD should not be started until healing of the exit site and tissue ingrowth into the catheter's Dacron cuffs have taken place, usually after 5 days. If dialysis is necessary before this time, and if haemodialysis is inappropriate or unavailable, automated PD would be the preferred method. This is because this treatment will help to minimise the risk of leakage of PD fluid by allowing the patient to be treated using small fill volumes of fluid in a supine position. It is worth noting that patient healing mechanisms may be altered in those patients who are uraemic or who have diabetes mellitus (Flanigan & Gokal 2005).

LONG-TERM CARE OF THE EXIT SITE

As with any wound, care is aimed at keeping the site clear of exudate or debris that could encourage bacterial growth (Prowant & Twardowski 1996). A method of exit-site care that best fits in with the patient's lifestyle is most likely to encourage full participation in the treatment and therefore reduce the risk of complications. A number of studies have been undertaken to attempt to ascertain which particular method of exit-site care is preferred. Various protocols do exist, for example, cleansing with soap and water, or cleaning with povidone–iodine (Piraino et al 2005); however, there is to date no consensus on which method will reduce the incidence of infection.

Whichever solution is chosen, the following points should be considered.

- Harsh solutions should be avoided as they have the potential to cause skin damage, which may predispose to bacterial colonisation.
- Different agents may be preferred in different circumstances. In an immunosuppressed patient the normal skin flora may represent an infection risk; in this case, an antiseptic solution may be preferred.
- Whichever method is used, it is important to ensure that the exit site is carefully dried to avoid skin maceration, which could predispose the site to bacterial colonisation.

There is also some debate as to whether it is necessary to keep the catheter exit-site covered. The use of no dressing and a simple exit-site care routine for a well-healed exit site would appeal to many; however, most centres do use some kind of cover (Prowant & Twardowski 1996).

CATHETER IMMOBILISATION

From the moment the catheter is inserted, it should always be securely anchored to the patient's skin to avoid torque movements at the exit-site. This has been shown to reduce the risk of exit-site infection (Piraino et al 2005), and can be achieved by using tape or a commercially available immobilisation device or tube holder.

SWIMMING AND BATHING

According to a consensus of opinions of leading nephrologists (Gokal et al 1998), PD patients may swim following healing of the catheter, usually

4–8 weeks following insertion. The exit site may be covered with either clear occlusive dressing or a colostomy bag. Diving should be avoided, as this may put tension on the catheter at the exit site. Following swimming, the patient should shower, clean and dry the exit site, and cover it with the usual dressing. Soaking the exit site, for example, in a tub bath, is not recommended (Gokal et al 1998). However, recent published guidelines do not include advice on swimming.

INDICATIONS FOR CATHETER REMOVAL

A PD catheter is designed to be a permanent access device, and its removal should not be routine. However, catheters may have to be removed under the following conditions:

- if they are no longer needed
- in recurrent peritonitis without an identifiable cause
- in peritonitis due to an exit-site and/or tunnel infection
- with an unusual causative organism of peritonitis, e.g. fungus or tuberculosis
- in bowel perforation accompanied by peritonitis
- with persistent and severe pain due either to the catheter impinging on internal organs or during solution inflow
- when there is Dacron cuff erosion and infection.

PERITONEAL DIALYSIS THERAPY OPTIONS

Dialysis should be prescribed according to each individual patient's clinical and lifestyle needs. The dose of PD can be increased or decreased by adjusting any one of the following parameters:

- dialysis fluid fill volume per exchange
- number of dialysis fluid exchanges
- length of dialysis fluid dwell time
- osmotic strength or type of dialysis fluid.

By using the PET each patient's membrane characteristics can be determined, therefore allowing optimisation of the therapy.

There are two general methods of performing peritoneal dialysis, CAPD and APD.

CONTINUOUS AMBULATORY PERITONEAL DIALYSIS

Continuous ambulatory peritoneal dialysis (CAPD) (Fig. 8.11) is carried out during the day-time, manually by patients themselves or sometimes by a carer. Dialysis fluid is infused into the peritoneal cavity and left to dwell for between 3 and 10h. After this time, the dialysate is drained from the cavity, fresh solution is infused and the whole process starts again. Patients usually perform four exchanges of PD fluid each day, fitting them in as appropriately as possible with their normal lifestyle. For example,

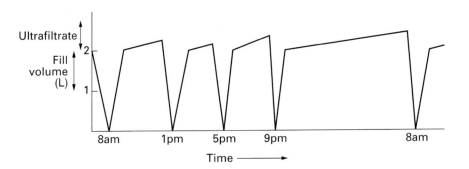

Figure 8.11 Continuous ambulatory peritoneal dialysis.

exchanges may be performed at breakfast, lunch and supper time with the last exchange of the day being carried out at bedtime. Each exchange takes about 20–30 min to complete.

CAPD is most suited to those patients whose membranes transport solutes at an average rate (i.e. low, low-average, and high-average 'transporters'), as it provides the opportunity for longer dwell times. This long dwell period is best achieved during the night time whilst the patient sleeps. Those patients whose membranes transport solutes quickly ('high transporters') may need to use an icodextrin solution for the longest dwell overnight. This will avoid dialysate fluid absorption, which could occur in these patients during long dwell periods.

Patients who require a fifth exchange (for increased dialysis dose) can use a night-time exchange device, which performs one exchange at a predefined time in the middle of the night. Patients connect themselves to the machine before going to bed, and the machine automatically drains out the used fluid and instils fresh fluid whilst the patient sleeps.

AUTOMATED PERITONEAL DIALYSIS

Automated peritoneal dialysis (APD) is carried out by a machine, which performs the dialysis fluid exchanges at night whilst the patient sleeps. An APD machine automatically controls the fill volume, dwell time and length of treatment the patient receives. The dose of dialysis can easily be increased during APD, as it is easy and convenient to alter the parameters of the treatment. Dialysis fluid fill volumes can be more safely increased owing to the reduction in intra-abdominal pressure achieved whilst the patient is supine. This not only decreases the risk of problems associated with high intra-abdominal pressure, such as leaks around the catheter exit site, abdominal hernias and back pain, but it also increases the amount of dialysis the patient can achieve.

The length of the dwell time and the number of exchanges can effectively be altered without disruption to the patient's lifestyle. This is a major advantage to 'high transporters'. Performing frequent exchanges is essential for these patients to achieve adequate dialysis but this can be inconvenient if the patient is on CAPD. APD provides an effective and convenient alternative by enabling rapid exchanges of dialysis fluid whilst the patient sleeps. This increases clearances of solutes whilst maintaining maximum ultrafiltration. As with CAPD, the osmotic strength of the fluid can be altered according to each patient's need.

Automated peritoneal dialysis is particularly suitable for those patients needing to be free during the day-time. Patients who work or who are studying can benefit from this treatment, as the preparation time for the treatment is short and the dialysis takes place whilst they sleep, leaving them free during the day. APD is also suitable for those patients who rely on a carer to perform their dialysis, for example, children, older people or those with disabilities. The carer simply prepares the machine, connects the patient to the machine at bedtime and disconnects them the following morning. APD is therefore an effective therapy option for those patients who require more dialysis and/or freedom during the day-time. However, in order to achieve adequate dialysis, many patients will also need to perform an exchange in the early evening.

Some APD machines have the facility to store information regarding the patient's therapy on a data card that is fitted inside the machine. This data card also stores the patient's individual prescription, enabling the prescription to be altered by a healthcare professional, without the need for the patient's intervention.

There are three different types of APD:

- continuous cycling peritoneal dialysis (CCPD)
- tidal peritoneal dialysis (TPD)
- optimised cycling peritoneal dialysis (OCPD).

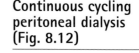

Continuous cycling peritoneal dialysis (Fig. 8.12)

The 'continuous' part of the acronym is derived from the fact that the patient has dialysis fluid in constant contact with the peritoneal membrane. There are typically between five and seven exchanges of fluid with relatively short dwell periods, so maximising the ultrafiltration and clearance capabilities of those patients whose membrane transports solutes quickly. The treatment regime can be programmed to end with a 'fill', giving the patient a 'wet day' (the fluid would be left inside the peritoneal cavity during the day and drained when the patient next starts treatment on the machine at bedtime).

Rarely, the treatment ends following the 'drain', giving the patient a 'dry day'. This may help to prevent absorption of the PD fluid in 'high transporters'. It should be noted, though, that utilising a 'dry day'

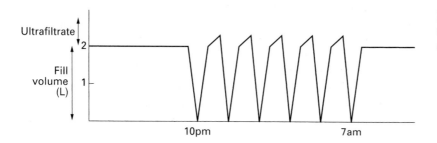

Figure 8.12
Continuous cycling peritoneal dialysis.

will result in severely reduced clearances and possibly underdialysis. Icodextrin solution, designed for long dwells, should preferably be used in these circumstances.

Tidal peritoneal dialysis (Fig. 8.13)

Tidal PD is a form of APD where the dialysis fluid fill volume is not fully drained after each cycle. It is typically used for patients who experience pain at the end of each drain phase. By leaving a small 'sump' volume of about 10% of the dialysis fill volume in the patient's peritoneal cavity at the end of each drain phase, pain is minimised. A full drain takes place at the end of the therapy during the final drain.

Optimised cycling peritoneal dialysis (OCPD) (Fig. 8.14)

This method of APD enables the delivery of more dialysis as the patient's residual renal function declines. During OCPD the patient performs overnight CCPD or TPD as well as adding a day-time exchange of PD fluid. Some APD machines are designed so that the patient can perform both the night and day exchanges using the same disposable equipment and solution bags. The longer dwell of fluid during the day-time will optimise clearance opportunities, and the shorter dwells of the night-time dialysis will help to achieve ultrafiltration goals.

Another form of APD called intermittent peritoneal dialysis (IPD; Fig. 8.15) is rarely carried out in the UK, as it is difficult to achieve adequate dialysis with this technique. Where it is done, it is generally carried out on a hospital ward in sessions of between 12 and 20h, two or three times each week.

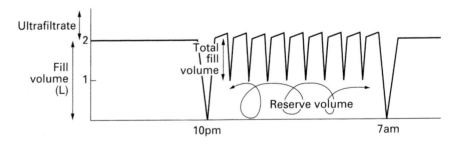

Figure 8.13
Tidal peritoneal dialysis.

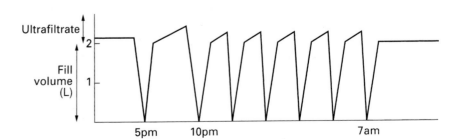

Figure 8.14
Optimised cycling peritoneol dialysis.

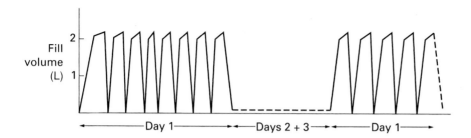

Figure 8.15
Intermittent peritoneal dialysis.

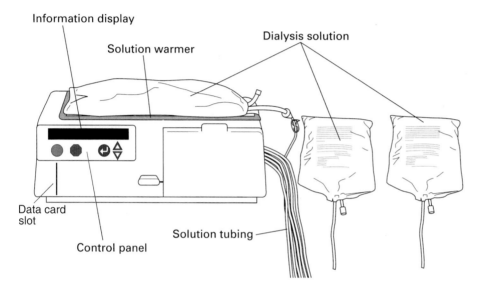

Figure 8.16
Baxter Healthcare Ltd HomeChoice Pro automated peritoneal dialysis machine (with permission).

Whichever method of PD is chosen for the patient at any particular time, it should provide a balance between clinical and lifestyle needs.

Figure 8.16 shows an example of an APD machine.

PATIENT SELECTION

An important consideration when developing a successful PD programme is good patient selection. Treating the most appropriate patients with PD will avoid the patient being subjected to increased risk of morbidity and mortality. In the early years of PD, selection was mainly based on the patient's inability to have haemodialysis, for example, those patients with poor or no vascular access, poor biochemical control on haemodialysis with high predialysis serum levels of creatinine, those patients with severe anaemia (i.e. haemoglobin of $< 5\,g\,dL^{-1}$) with a need for frequent blood transfusions, those patients with poorly controlled hypertension, those with excessive fluid gain between dialysis sessions, and those who had progressive metabolic and neurological complications. Although these criteria do recommend patients for PD, positive selection criteria are now preferred, as PD has proven to be a successful viable alternative to haemodialysis as a treatment for chronic renal disease.

Table 8.2   Patients who are suited to continuous ambulatory peritoneal dialysis (CAPD) or automated peritoneal dialysis (APD)

Suited to CAPD	Suited to either CAPD or APD	Suited to APD
Patients whose membranes transport solutes slowly or at an average speed	Promotion of home dialysis Patients with complicating cardiovascular disease Children with small body size Patients with poor vascular access Patients with diabetes mellitus Patients with severe hypertension Patients with anaemia Patients who wish to travel	Patients who seek day-time freedom to attend work or school Patients at risk of complications associated with raised intra-abdominal pressure Patients who require a carer to perform their dialysis Patients with chronic backache Patients who require enhanced dialysis, i.e. those without residual renal function

Table 8.3   Patients who are unsuitable for continuous ambulatory peritoneal dialysis (CAPD) or automated peritoneal dialysis (APD)

Unsuitable for CAPD	Unsuitable for either CAPD or APD	Unsuitable for APD
Patients with chronic back pain Patients at risk of complications associated with raised intra-abdominal pressure	Patients with documented loss of peritoneal function Patients who are unable to care for themselves and do not have the assistance of a full-time carer	

As there are two different therapy modes within the broad title of PD (i.e. CAPD and APD), the selection criteria for each are seen to be slightly different with many overlaps. Tables 8.2 and 8.3 indicate which patients are more suited to APD and those who are more suited to CAPD.

PERITONEAL DIALYSIS FOR THOSE WITH DIABETES

Diabetic nephropathy is the leading cause of end-stage renal disease worldwide. Although death rates of patients with diabetes on haemodialysis and peritoneal dialysis have decreased substantially, they remain higher than rates in non-diabetics on both modalities. PD offers equal or better survival than haemodialysis for younger diabetic patients during early years of dialysis (Lee et al 2001).

BLOOD GLUCOSE CONTROL

A PD patient using only glucose-based solutions will absorb between 100 and 150 g of glucose per day from the dialysis fluid. This can lead to problems, such as hyperinsulinaemia and premature arteriosclerosis. Alternative solutions offer benefits for those with diabetes. Glucose-free solutions (Icodextrin and amino-acid solutions) provide an excellent solution for diabetics, as the use of these fluids significantly reduces the amount of glucose absorbed by the patient. In addition, the use of more biocompatible solutions, such as bicarbonate/lactate solutions, also reduce the amount of glucose absorbed (Marshall et al 2003).

There are a number of methods of blood sugar control for patients with diabetes on PD. These include subcutaneous or intraperitoneal insulin, oral agents or dietary control. Any combination of these methods can be used. No single method has been shown to be more suitable than another for all patients, as there appear to be no studies that compare the effectiveness of different methods of insulin administration; however, all methods appear to be effective in achieving metabolic control of blood sugar.

INTRAPERITONEAL INSULIN

There are many benefits to adding insulin via the intraperitoneal route. Insulin administered by the i.p. route crosses the peritoneal membrane by passive diffusion, and is predominantly delivered to the liver via the portal circulation before reaching the systemic circulation. Following i.p. administration, the concentration of peripheral free insulin is lower when compared to the peripheral free insulin concentration achieved following subcutaneous dosing. A proposed advantage of i.p. insulin administration is that insulin is delivered to the liver without creating hyperinsulinaemia, a situation thought to be potentially atherogenic.

Absorption of insulin from the peritoneal cavity is concentration dependent. Insulin administered into an empty peritoneal cavity will be absorbed more rapidly and completely than if the insulin is administered in a large volume of dialysis solution. Direct injection of multiple daily doses of insulin into the peritoneum may be impractical for most patients. Therefore, i.p. insulin is usually administered via the routine dialysis fluid exchange. Conversion from a stable subcutaneous insulin dose to i.p. insulin dosing at initiation of PD usually requires a 2.5–3.5-fold increase in the insulin dose. This increase is needed because of the incomplete absorption during the dialysate dwell period, an increased insulin requirement due to the hypertonic dextrose-containing dialysate and possible adsorption (binding) of the insulin to the polyvinyl chloride surface of the dialysis bags. Approximately 10–20% of the administered dose may bind to the surface of the PD bag and tubing. Regular (short-acting) insulin should be used for i.p. dosing.

For patients using CAPD, the total daily insulin dose should be divided among the exchanges according to anticipated calorie intake from food and dialysate dextrose. Additional amounts of insulin may need to be added to exchanges containing more hypertonic dextrose concentrations. The exact amount varies between patients but may be assessed at onset by using a sliding scale of insulin with capillary blood glucose monitoring.

Dose stabilisation may require several days. Insulin requirements often increase during episodes of peritonitis (Bailie et al 2005). At present, there are no published recommendations for i.p. insulin administration when automated peritoneal dialysis is used.

There are a few issues that should be taken into consideration when deciding to use this method of administration: Patients who have dexterity and/or visual problems may experience difficulties injecting insulin into the medication port and the potential exists for contamination of the sterile dialysate solution when adding any medicine i.p. Patients also require frequent blood glucose monitoring when attempting to regulate i.p. insulin initially (Farina 2004).

Insulin should be added to the bag of dialysis fluid before it is connected to the patient. In this way, the bag may be discarded if accidentally contaminated or punctured by the needle. Strict aseptic technique must be followed when adding the insulin, which is usually done through the specially designed medication port. All bags should be inverted several times before the fluid is drained into the patient to ensure thorough mixing of the insulin. There is no evidence to suggest that i.p. insulin administration increases the risk of peritonitis (Williams et al 2000).

SOLUTION FORMULATION

Peritoneal dialysis solution is presented in sterile plastic bags with a protective overpouch in volumes of 1500, 2000, 2500 and 3000 mL. Bags of 5000 mL are available for use with APD machines. The electrolyte concentration of dialysis fluid is similar to that of normal serum, with lactate acting as a bicarbonate-generating agent to combat metabolic acidosis, which is common amongst patients. Electrolyte composition of the dialysis fluid has been changed several times over the years. A major challenge when treating patients with kidney disease has been effective phosphate control. Consequently, dialysis fluid does not contain any phosphate, and patients are given oral phosphate-binding agents to help eliminate dietary phosphate intake from the body. In the past, these phosphate-binding agents were aluminium-based. However, these were implicated in aluminium-related bone disease, which many patients experienced (Armstrong & Cunningham 1994). Aluminium toxicity may also cause microcytic anaemia and encephalopathy, and so its use as a phosphate-binding agent in the present day has been reduced (Hutchison 1992). The alternative ingredient for an effective phosphate binder is calcium given in the form of calcium carbonate or calcium acetate. These binders have their problems too, leading in some patients to raised serum calcium levels, particularly if the patient is also having vitamin D therapy. This led to the manufacture of a dialysis fluid containing physiological levels of ionised calcium and this solution is compared to the original solution in Table 8.4.

	a (mmol L⁻¹)	b (mmol L⁻¹)
Sodium (Na)	132	132
Chloride (Cl)	95	95
Lactate	40	35
Magnesium (Mg)	0.25	0.75
Calcium (Ca)	1.25	1.75

Table 8.4
Comparison of dialysis fluid containing ionised calcium (a) with the original solution (b)

GLUCOSE-BASED SOLUTIONS

Up until the early 1990s, the most commonly prescribed and the most widely available osmotic agent used in PD was glucose. Glucose-based dialysis fluid comes in three strengths (1.36%, 2.27% and 3.86% monohydrate glucose). The strong (hypertonic) solutions provide the greater osmotic strength. Patients should use 1.36% glucose most often whilst their weight is within 0.5 kg of their 'dry' or 'target' weight. Hypertonic solutions should be used when the patient has fluid overload. Most patients ultrafiltrate an extra 200–600 mL by using a 2000-mL medium (2.27%) glucose solution bag and an extra 400–1000 mL by using a 2000-mL strong (3.86%) glucose solution bag. Patients should be taught to record their body weight on a daily basis and choose the appropriate solution strengths for that day.

Ultrafiltration by hypertonic solutions is maintained for approximately 8 h in most patients (Fig. 8.17). After this time, some reabsorption of fluid may occur. In those patients whose membranes transport solutes quickly

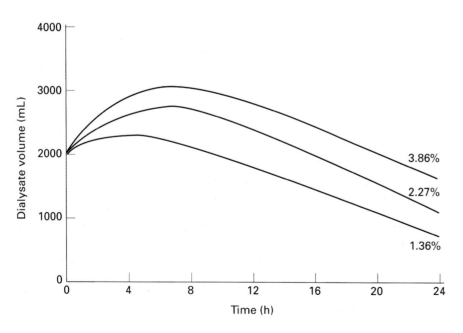

Figure 8.17
Dialysate volume versus time (approximate averages).

(high transporters), reabsorption may occur sooner than 8 h, giving rise to the need to use an Icodextrin fluid exchange for the longer dwell times (i.e. the overnight dwell in CAPD or the day-time dwell in APD; Davies et al 2003).

ICODEXTRIN PERITONAL DIALYSIS SOLUTION

There are problems associated with the use of glucose as an osmotic agent, such as hyperglycaemia and hyperlipidaemia. Patients who have poor ultrafiltration provide the greatest challenge in this area. Worsening fluid balance results in reduced technique and patient survival. Icodextrin solution is known to improve ultrafiltration in the long dwell during PD (Davies et al 2003).

Icodextrin 7.5% is a formulation of a large-molecular-weight glucose polymer, which is a more biocompatible solution as it is approximately iso-osmolar with serum. The use of this larger molecule means that less glucose is available for absorption through the peritoneal membrane. Its long-acting ultrafiltration performance (up to 12 h) is combined with low carbohydrate absorption. Icodextrin reduces the exposure of the peritoneal membrane to glucose for more than 50% of the dialysis time, if used for the long dwell, and improves fluid balance and blood pressure control compared to 2.27% glucose (Woodrow et al 1999).

Johnson et al (2001) demonstrated that using Icodextrin solution as a substitute for one glucose exchange resulted in an average 1 year extension of technique survival in patients on PD who were otherwise about to be transferred to haemodialysis due to refractory fluid overload.

The 2002 Renal Association standards recommend that specialised solutions such as glucose polymers (Icodextrin) are preferable to standard solutions for patients with high small-solute transfer rates, and little or no residual renal function. Similarly, the International Society for Peritoneal Dialysis Ad Hoc Committee on Ultrafiltration Management in PD (Mujias 2000) makes the following recommendation:

> For patients with net ultrafiltration (UF) less than 400 mL/4 h and a high transport profile of small solutes, APD and Icodextrin for the long dwell are the recommended therapeutic approaches. This profile can also be seen during peritonitis and several studies have indicated that UF during an episode of peritonitis can be satisfactorily achieved with Icodextrin.

BICARBONATE/LACTATE–BASED PERITONEAL DIALYSIS SOLUTIONS

Bicarbonate/lactate solutions were developed following extensive research to identify the most suitable alternative formulation to the traditional lactate-buffered solutions. The commercially available solution comes in a double-chambered bag because some of the compounds of the bicarbonate/lactate solution are not stable during the steam sterilisation process. Glucose needs to be in acidic conditions (low pH) in order to prevent caramelisation. Since the bicarbonate/lactate solution is neutral, the glucose has to be separated from the other compounds. The glucose sits in the upper, smaller chamber, together with calcium and magnesium salts, under acidic conditions. The bicarbonate, lactate and sodium salt sit in the lower, larger chamber. The two solutions are mixed just before infusion (usually whilst the patient is draining the used fluid during CAPD or during the set-up of the APD machine).

This solution, with a combination of bicarbonate 25 mmol and lactate 15 mmol as the buffer, is intended for all exchanges. The solution has a physiological buffer system, with a physiological pH of 7.4, and reduced glucose degradation product levels. It allows a significant reduction of inflow pain and/or discomfort in sensitive patients, and has a high potential for improved long-term preservation of the peritoneal membrane (McEnzie et al 1998).

The composition of bicarbonate /lactate-based solution is:

- glucose monohydrate: 1.36%, 2.27% or 3.86%
- sodium chloride: $5.38 \, g \, L^{-1}$
- calcium chloride: $0.184 \, g \, L^{-1}$
- magnesium chloride hexahydrate: $0.051 \, g \, L^{-1}$
- sodium bicarbonate: $2.10 \, g \, L^{-1}$
- sodium lactate: $1.68 \, g \, L^{-1}$.

It has several advantages as a buffer for PD solutions.

- physiological pH and bicarbonate concentration
- reduced pain on infusion
- improved membrane preservation.

Physiological pH and bicarbonate concentration

Bicarbonate is the natural buffer of the body. As a result of the metabolism of ingested foods, our body produces hydrogen ions (protons). This acid must be excreted or neutralised in order to maintain the body's acid–base balance. The kidneys play a key role in maintaining the acid–base balance. Not only do they excrete hydrogen ions, but they also regenerate bicarbonate. In people with renal failure, this function is impaired or lost. Therefore, it is important to replace the lost bicarbonate to maintain the acid–base balance and prevent the occurrence of acidosis. Using bicarbonate in the PD solution is the most natural way of restoring the bicarbonate level in renal patients. Alternative buffers, like lactate, need some conversion (metabolism) before they result in bicarbonate.

The biocompatibility of a PD solution has been defined as the ability of a solution formulation to permit adequate long-term dialysis without a clinically significant undesirable host response (Consensus Conference on Biocompatibility 1994). Di Paolo et al (1995) defined biocompatibility of a PD solution as its capacity to leave the anatomical and functional characteristics of the peritoneum unmodified in time. These objectives will best be met by solutions whose composition is identical to the composition of extracellular fluid in the body, in particular to the composition of blood. Bicarbonate and lactate PD solution has been developed as an alternative buffer component.

Reduced pain on infusion

A clinical study on the treatment of pain on infusion (Mactier et al 1998) compared a bicarbonate/lactate solution and another experimental solution based on 38 mmol L^{-1} of bicarbonate (without lactate). The experimental solution and the bicarbonate/lactate solution both reduced the infusion pain, but the bicarbonate/lactate mix appeared the most effective.

Improved membrane preservation

Results of phase III clinical trials showed that the use of bicarbonate lactate solutions reduced peritoneal membrane inflammation and improved mesothelial cell mass compared to the use of traditional lactate-based PD solutions (Jones 2001).

AMINO-ACID-BASED PERITONEAL DIALYSIS SOLUTION

Intraperitoneal amino-acid (IPAA) solution contains 15 amino acids. Eight are essential amino acids, two are considered essential to patients with kidney disease and five are non-essential. The electrolyte formulation is shown in Table 8.5. The osmotic agent glucose is replaced by 1.1% amino acids, which have the comparative ultrafiltration capability of 1.36% glucose solution. After a 4–6 h dwell, 65–95% of the amino acids are absorbed, the equivalent to about 18 g (from a 2000-mL bag containing 22 g of amino acids) or 0.3 g kg^{-1} day^{-1} in a 70-kg patient. This is approximately 25% of the daily protein requirement for a PD patient.

The IPAA solution is administered in the same way as other PD solutions. It is prescribed for one exchange per day, replacing one of the usual glucose dialysis solution bags or mixed with overnight glucose solutions during APD. If given during the day, it should be given either at a main meal or with a high-calorie snack, as this will ensure that the amino acids are used in the anabolic process to generate protein rather than being expended as an energy source.

The use of 1.1% amino-acid PD solution, when used instead of one glucose exchange, decreases both peritoneal membrane glucose exposure and systemic glucose absorption.

It now seems obvious that patients will benefit from using a combination of all the available solutions formulations, including amino acid, polyglucose, bicarbonate/lactate and glucose.

Table 8.5
Electrolyte formulation of intraperitoneal amino acid solution

Sodium	132 mmol L^{-1}
Chloride	95 mmol L^{-1}
Lactate	40 mmol L^{-1}
Magnesium	0.25 mmol L^{-1}
Calcium	1.25 mmol L^{-1}

ASSESSING PERITONEAL DIALYSIS ADEQUACY

It is well documented that patients survive well on dialysis and this is due to its ability to remove nitrogenous waste products, correct electrolyte and acid–base imbalance, and remove excess fluid. Patients feel unwell if they are inadequately dialysed; they eat less, become malnourished, and are therefore at increased risk of infection. Inadequate fluid removal causes hypervolaemia, which results in hypertension, fluid overload and cardiac complications.

The goals of PD are to prolong life, reverse the symptoms of uraemia, maintain patients in positive nitrogen balance, have an adequate energy intake and have their maximum level of quality of life in a way that is least disruptive to their lifestyle. This can be summarised by saying that well-dialysed patients feel well enough to eat a sufficient diet rich in protein and experience a minimum of complications to their treatment.

There are a number of ways in which dialysis adequacy can be measured and all parameters must be taken into consideration:

- creatinine clearance – a solute-removal test based on body surface area
- Kt/V – a urea index relating urea clearance to the volume of urea distributed in the body (see below)
- protein nutrition
- general well-being.

CREATININE AS A MEASURE OF DIALYSIS ADEQUACY

Creatinine is a metabolic product from the breakdown of muscle. Patients who have a larger muscle mass, therefore, tend to have higher serum creatinine levels. Creatinine, with a molecular weight of 113 Da, will equilibrate more slowly across the peritoneal membrane than urea (molecular weight 60 Da).

A normalised body surface area (BSA) of $1.73 m^2$ is used to enable an assumption of the creatinine generation rate based on a patient's size, provided that the patient is infection free and in nitrogen balance. Creatinine clearance for both the patient's dialysis regime and residual renal function can be calculated by using the worksheet (Fig. 8.18).

UREA AS A MEASURE OF DIALYSIS ADEQUACY

Urea is a metabolic product of the protein we eat. As more protein is eaten, more urea is generated. It therefore follows that, when examining a patient's serum urea levels, it is important to take into consideration recent protein intake. A low serum urea in a patient with ERF may simply be due to a low protein intake, rather than adequate dialysis. A high serum urea on the other hand may indicate increased catabolism, deterioration in residual renal function or inadequate dialysis. Urea is a small molecule (molecular weight 60 Da), which is distributed in body water. It diffuses readily and is therefore easily removed from the blood.

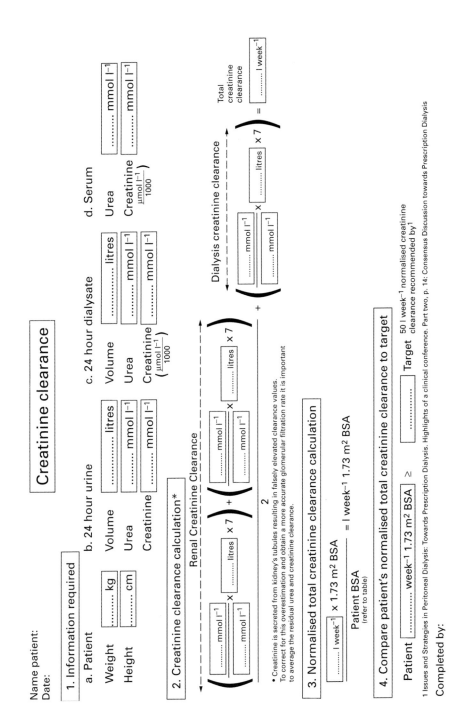

Figure 8.18   Creatinine clearance.

The prescription index, *Kt/V*, was developed by Gotch et al (1983) and Gotch & Sargent (1985) in the National Co-operative Dialysis Study of haemodialysis patients. *Kt/V* is an index of urea removal, which is patient-specific, as it looks at urea removal achieved over time ($K \times t$) and measurement of urea in the body water (*V*) for each patient. Therefore, *K* = clearance, *t* = time, and *V* = volume of body water in which urea is distributed (Figs. 8.19 and 8.20).

The index does not account for dietary protein intake, protein catabolic rate or urea generation rate. It is just as important to measure residual renal *Kt/V* as it is to measure dialysis *Kt/V*. The two should be added together to give a total weekly *Kt/V* value. *Kt/V* for both the patient's dialysis regime and residual renal function can be calculated using the worksheet shown in Figure 8.21.

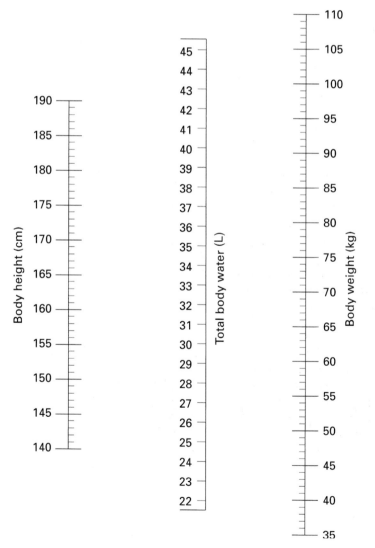

Figure 8.19
Nomogram for the estimation of total body water in females.

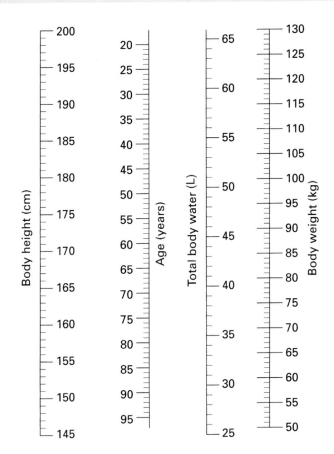

Figure 8.20
Nomogram for the estimation
of total body water in males.

PROTEIN NUTRITION

Malnutrition has been shown to be a major risk factor in survival of PD patients (Dasgupta et al 2002). Various terms have been used to identify a patient's nutritional status; these include serum albumin level, dietary protein intake (DPI), protein catabolic rate (PCR) and subjective global assessment (SGA; Detsky et al 1987). A patient's nutritional status is an important factor in assessing a patient's dialysis adequacy but, as with all measures, it should not be taken in isolation.

Protein intake and PCR are important issues to be considered for those on PD. It is vital that the PD nurse, dietitian and the patient work closely together to avoid the complications associated with malnutrition. SGA is a simple and reliable tool that is increasingly being used in the diagnosis of malnutrition amongst patients with ERF (see Ch. 11 for further details).

GENERAL WELL-BEING

Despite the efficacy of a combination of the above physical parameters for measuring adequacy of dialysis, there can be no doubt that the ultimate gauge of treatment success must increasingly become the overall quality of life of the patient. There is now widespread agreement that

Name patient:
Date:

Kt/V*

1. Information required

a. Patient

- Weight: .... kg
- Height: .... cm

b. 24 hour urine

- Volume: .... litres
- Urea: .... mmol l^{-1}
- Creatinine: .... mmol l^{-1}

c. 24 hour dialysate

- Volume: .... litres
- Urea: .... mmol l^{-1}
- Creatinine $\left(\frac{\mu mol\ l^{-1}}{1000}\right)$: .... mmol l^{-1}

d. Serum

- Urea: .... mmol l^{-1}
- Creatinine $\left(\frac{\mu mol\ l^{-1}}{1000}\right)$: .... mmol l^{-1}

2. Kt/V calculation

a. Residual renal Kt/V

Step 1:

$$\frac{\text{.......... mmol l}^{-1}}{\text{.......... mmol l}^{-1}} \times \frac{\text{.......... litres} \times 1000}{1440\ (\text{min. in 24 h})} = \text{.......... ml min}^{-1}\ \text{(Residual renal clearance)}$$

Step 2:

$$\frac{\text{.......... mmol l}^{-1} \times 1440 \times 7}{\text{.......... kg} \times \begin{matrix} ♂\ 0.6 \\ ♀\ 0.55 \end{matrix} \times 1000} = \text{.............. Weekly residual } Kt/V$$

b. Dialysate Kt/V

$$\frac{\dfrac{\text{.......... mmol l}^{-1}}{\text{.......... mmol l}^{-1}} \times \text{.......... litres} \times 7}{\text{.......... kg} \times \begin{matrix} ♂\ 0.6 \\ ♀\ 0.55 \end{matrix}} = \text{.............. Weekly dialysate } Kt/V$$

3. Total Kt/V

.... Weekly residual Kt/V + ... Weekly dialysate Kt/V = ... Weekly total Kt/V

4. Compare patient's weekly Kt/V with target

Patient .... Weekly total Kt/V ≥ .... Target

* K = Urea clearance (l week^{-1}) - T = Number of days per week the patient dialyses
V = Volume of urea distribution

Figure 8.21 *Kt/V* worksheet.

in assessing the effects of a treatment it is essential to assess both the quality and quantity of life. Healthcare purchasers are increasingly under pressure to demonstrate cost-effective utilisation of the limited resources available to them. Quality-of-life assessment is a key outcome measure in determining this cost effectiveness, but its multidimensional and subjective nature means that it is problematic to measure.

There are a number of tools available for the measurement of quality of life amongst renal patients; however, to date, there is no consensus on which measure is best to use.

Most studies looking into the effectiveness or adequacy of dialysis have concentrated on the impact of small-solute clearance. For peritoneal dialysis, clinical practice guidelines, such as the UK Renal Association, were mainly based on the results of the CANUSA study (Churchill et al 1996). This was one of the largest studies of PD patients and was conducted in 14 centres across the USA and Canada. It investigated the impact of demographic, nutritional and adequacy parameters on morbidity and mortality, and defined adequate PD according to estimates of solute clearance (e.g. urea and creatinine). The CANUSA study showed that estimates of patients' nutritional status and dialysis adequacy had clinically important and statistically significant associations with patients' survival, technique survival and hospitalisation. This study also indicated that increasing creatinine clearance and Kt/V will lead to higher survival rates.

Churchill et al (1996) also stated that total creatinine clearance and Kt/V decreased during the trial period because loss of residual renal function was not compensated for by increasing the dialysis dose. The CANUSA study suggested that patients on CAPD with high membrane permeability had increased mortality, possibly because of poor ultrafiltration and consequent fluid overload. However, it is now understood that the data from the CANUSA study in fact suggested that peritoneal clearance and clearance achieved through the patient's residual renal function are not equivalent (Bargman et al 2001).

In 2001, the ADEMEX (ADEquacy of PD in MEXico) study was published (Paniagua et al 2001). This is the largest interventional study ever conducted in peritoneal dialysis and it examined the effects of increased peritoneal small solute clearances on mortality rates among almost 1000 patients on CAPD. Over the entire 2-year study period, interventions were successful in achieving better clearances in the interventional group compared to the control group with regard to the mean peritoneal weekly creatinine clearance (46.1 vs. 56.9 L week^{-1} 1.73 m^{-2}) and Kt/V (1.62 vs. 2.13). However, the results showed that there was no effect of increased peritoneal clearances on mortality, with death rates being similar in both groups. As in the CANUSA study, the presence of residual renal function did impact favourably on outcome. It is therefore absolutely essential to take a patient's residual renal function into account when assessing adequacy of dialysis.

Preservation of residual renal function (RRF) is an important goal for dialysis and patients treated with peritoneal dialysis have been shown to have a 65% lower risk of RRF loss than those on haemodialysis (Moist et al 2000).

The results of the ADEMEX study highlight the need to think of adequacy of dialysis as being more than just small molecule clearance. A comprehensive approach to improve ultrafiltration management, preserve residual renal function, optimize nutritional status and reduce cardiovascular disease risk factors, in both the predialysis and ERF phases of chronic kidney disease, is important in significantly and positively influencing the clinical outcomes in PD patients.

A further study has now been conducted to demonstrate that PD can be a successful treatment for anuric patients (Brown et al 2003). The European APD Outcome Study (EAPOS) is a 2-year, prospective, multicentre study. A total of 177 patients were enrolled. The APD prescription was adjusted to aim for creatinine clearance (C_{crea}) of 60 L week^{-1} 1.73 m^{-2} and ultrafiltration of 750 mL 24 h^{-1} during the first 6 months. Baseline solute transport status (D/P) was determined by peritoneal equilibration test. At 1 year, 78% and 74% of patients achieved C_{crea} and UF targets, respectively, with 50% of patients using icodextrin. The 2-year patient survival was 78% and technique survival was 62%. This study showed that anuric patients can successfully use APD. Baseline UF, not C_{crea} or membrane permeability, is associated with patient survival.

Targets for adequate dialysis should include targets for both solute clearance and fluid removal (European Best Practice Guidelines for PD 2005). A total weekly creatinine clearance (dialysis + residual renal function) of greater than 50 L week^{-1} 1.73 m^{-2} and/or a weekly dialysis *Kt/V* urea of greater than 1.7, checked 8 weeks after beginning dialysis are recommended as the minimum. Higher targets are desirable especially for high average and high transporters and APD patients (UK Renal Association Clinical Practice Guidelines 2007). The weekly goal for *Kt/V* for haemodialysis patients is 3.0–4.2 a week (1–1.4 per session). The reason that this level is higher than for PD patients is explained by the peak concentration hypothesis proposed by Keshaviah et al (1989) (Fig. 8.22). *Kt/V* for haemodialysis patients has to be increased to equate the peak urea concentrations reached between dialysis sessions.

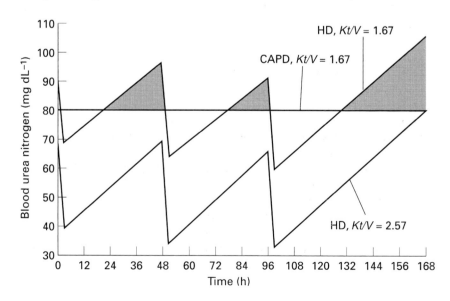

Figure 8.22
Keshaviah's peak concentration hypothesis. HD, haemodialysis; CAPD, continuous ambulatory peritoneal dialysis.

There are a number of computer programmes available on the market that will calculate the patient's *Kt/V*, creatinine clearance and nutritional status. Some of these programmes will also model the patient's treatment, allowing the nurse or physician to look at a wide range of PD therapy options for the optimal regime that meets the adequacy needs of each individual patient. This enables the clinician to eliminate the trial-and-error process of prescribing PD, takes away the need to perform manual calculations, and provides the renal unit with a database of their patients' quality of dialysis.

LONGITUDINAL CHANGES TO THE PERITONEAL MEMBRANE

The peritoneal membrane has proven to be remarkably resilient and there are a number of studies that have shown it to be stable over time (Davies et al 2001, Krediet et al 1996, Selgas et al 1998).

Long term changes, such as thickening of the peritoneal membrane, cause a loss of ultrafiltration (Davies et al 2005). This may be associated with exposure of the membrane to the harmful effects of glucose-based solutions (such as glucose degradation products), peritonitis or uraemic toxicity. In fact, a marked thickening of the membrane is only seen in patients who experience more than two episodes of peritonitis but thickening was shown in patients who used hypertonic glucose solutions (Plum et al 2001).

Davies et al (2001) have demonstrated that, by avoiding the use of hypertonic glucose solutions, functional changes in the peritoneal membrane can be avoided for at least 5 years. It is worth noting also that thickening of the peritoneal membrane has been seen in uraemic patients before the onset of dialysis (Plum et al 2001), suggesting that uraemia itself may cause peritoneal membrane changes.

FLUID MANAGEMENT IN PERITONEAL DIALYSIS

During PD, hyperosmolar dialysis solution removes fluid by the process of osmosis. Water transport across the peritoneal membrane depends upon the concentration of glucose in the dialysis solution and the size of the pores in the peritoneal membrane. At the same time as fluid is being removed from the blood through osmosis, it is continually being reabsorbed through the lymphatic system. In addition, the osmotic gradient is continually reducing owing to dilution of the PD solution (by the ultrafiltrate) and absorption of glucose into the blood. Therefore, there comes a point in time during the PD fluid exchange when fluid removal no longer takes place and fluid is reabsorbed back into the patient. This will occur before solute equilibrium.

Fluid removal and fluid balance can be enhanced in PD patients by increasing the glucose concentration of the dialysate, increasing the volume of fluid used (although a substantial increase in intra-abdominal pressure may reduce UF owing to the increased pressure), optimising the dwell time using APD, restricting sodium intake and by using Icodextrin solution (Konings et al 2003, Plum et al 2001).

SODIUM SIEVING

Most ultrafiltration takes place during the first 30 min of an exchange (Venturoli & Rippe 2005). Owing to the nature of the peritoneal membrane and the fact that the ultra small pores are responsible for transporting water during the initial part of the exchange, no convection or diffusion takes place during this time. This results in a sieving process where no solutes are removed during the early stage of a PD exchange. It is important to take this into consideration when using rapid fluid exchanges, such as in APD. The sieving effect, particularly of sodium, can have adverse effects on the patient. If rapid exchanges are continually used during the therapy, little sodium will be removed, giving rise to hypernatraemia and its possible effects, such as hypertension, in the longer term.

PROBLEM–SOLVING IN PERITONEAL DIALYSIS

PROTEIN LOSS

Protein is lost through the peritoneal membrane at a rate of 6–12 g day^{-1} in stable patients. To compensate for this loss, patients on PD need to eat between 1.0 and 1.2 g kg^{-1} body weight day^{-1} of dietary protein. This loss is increased during peritonitis, when a patient can lose up to 20 g day^{-1}. Both oral supplements and amino-acid dialysate can successfully improve nutrition in PD. Amino-acid dialysate therapy lowers the phosphorus load, and perhaps the risk of hyperparathyroidism, which offers the patient a benefit to reduce cardiovascular risk (Dasgupta 2002).

CARDIOVASCULAR AND LIPID PROBLEMS

Many patients reach ERF with established left ventricular hypertrophy, coronary ischaemia and vascular disease. However, despite the fact that there have been many advances in the technology and analysis of adequacy of dialysis, cardiovascular morbidity and mortality remain very high in patients on dialysis, and this is the most common cause of death (Fried et al 1999).

Patients experience raised levels of cholesterol and triglycerides within the first year on PD. This is mainly due to the glucose absorbed from PD fluid. Several studies have shown that these changes are not long-lasting and peak levels are usually reached within 3–12 months of starting dialysis. Guidelines on the treatment of lipid disorders were published by Fried et al (1999).

RAISED INTRA-ABDOMINAL PRESSURE PROBLEMS IN PD PATIENTS

Raised intra-abdominal pressure is caused by the pressure of high volumes of fluid in the peritoneal cavity. This pressure is further increased when the patient carries out strenuous exercise or suffers excessive coughing. Continuous raised intra-abdominal pressure can increase the risk of abdominal hernias, such as inguinal, incisional, diaphragmatic or umbilical, and of dialysate leakage around the catheter exit site.

Oedema of the labia in females, and the scrotum and penis in males is a distressing complication caused by dialysate leakage through soft tissues. Usually, it is easily rectified by stopping PD for a short period (usually up to 1 week). Hernias and persistent leaks require surgical repair, while stopping PD for a time to allow the site to heal. If haemodialysis is not an alternative form of treatment for the patient during this temporary interruption to treatment, PD may be continued so long as the patient is lying down, therefore decreasing the intra-abdominal pressure (i.e. by using some form of APD).

In the event of dialysate leakage at the exit site, PD must be ceased immediately, as the presence of a glucose-rich solution at a wound site gives rise to a markedly increased risk of infection. Leakage can be identified by using urine test sticks or blood glucose reagent strips at the exit site. The normal healing time for dialysate leakage is 1 week, but this may be increased in diabetic, severely uraemic or malnourished patients.

CAPD patients with previous vertebral disease may experience back pain owing to the raised intra-abdominal pressure incurred in an upright position. In this situation, APD may be the preferred therapy.

DRAINAGE PROBLEMS

These usually have a minor cause, which can be rectified by the patients themselves at home, with proper patient training and education. The reasons for poor inflow or outflow of dialysis fluid, and the relevant treatments are outlined below.

Kinks in the tubing

The most common cause of poor drainage or inflow of PD fluid is tubing kinks or closed clamps. Patients should be taught to check the tubing for kinks and closed clamps as a first line of action in the event of poor inflow or outflow of dialysis fluid. Catheter kinks sometimes occur due to malpositioning during surgical insertion. This will become apparent shortly after insertion, if not during the insertion procedure, and can be confirmed by X-ray (the PD catheter has a radio-opaque stripe along its length). This problem is usually rectified by surgical intervention; however, it can occasionally be improved if the patient has a bowel motion.

Constipation

Constipation should be avoided in patients on PD, not only because it causes problems with dialysate outflow but also because diverticulosis of the colon increases the risk of peritonitis. Constipation prevention is achieved by encouraging the patient to take a diet high in fibre along with a mild laxative, if appropriate. Regular exercise is also recommended. If constipation does occur, treatment can be with laxatives, glycerine suppositories or a saline enema. The use of phosphate-containing enemas should be avoided owing to the absorption of phosphate through the bowel during their administration.

Fibrin formation

Fibrin strands or plugs (a protein formed from fibrinogen in blood plasma in the process of clotting) in dialysate effluent are a common cause of poor drainage. The blockage, usually in the catheter or tubing, can normally be removed by 'milking' the tubing. Heparin may be added to the dialysis fluid (200–500 units L^{-1}) as a prophylactic measure, as it prevents the formation of fibrin.

If 'milking' the tubing does not remove the obstruction, a fibrolytic agent can be used. Both streptokinase (250 000 IU) and urokinase (5000 IU) in 2–3 mL sodium chloride 0.9% for i.v. injection are available, and should be infused into the catheter under aseptic conditions; the catheter should then be clamped and the drug left to infuse for 2 h. The catheter can then be checked for patency.

Malpositioned catheter

If catheter obstruction is not relieved by any of the above techniques, the problem may be due to obstruction caused by omentum attached to the catheter tip. The omental attachment usually causes the catheter to migrate out of the pelvic cavity. In such cases, it often proves difficult to resolve this problem without surgery.

It is possible to remove omentum from the catheter whilst leaving it in place during the surgical procedure. It is common for the surgeon to perform a local omentectomy at the same time to prevent further obstructions by omentum. If it proves impossible to rectify the obstruction or position of the catheter by surgical methods, the final option is to remove the catheter completely and replace it with a new one.

Shoulder pain

Occasionally, patients complain of shoulder pain following the infusion of fresh dialysis solution. This is thought to be a referred pain caused by intra-abdominal pressure or air under the diaphragm. Although it usually resolves within 10–20 min from onset, the patient may find relief by taking a mild analgesia such as paracetamol 1 g. Bicarbonate/lactate-containing PD solutions have also been shown to reduce pain on infusion of dialysis (Tranaeus et al 1998). This solution is discussed above.

Blood-stained effluent

This is a comparatively rare complication occurring most commonly in menstruating females. It may be due to endometriosis or retrograde bleeding through the fallopian tubes. The bleeding is usually mild and self-rectifies within a day or two without specific intervention.

More severe i.p. bleeding causing darkly blood-stained fluid can be caused by haemorrhage. This could be due to the patient straining whilst lifting a heavy object or suffering trauma to the abdomen and should be investigated.

INFECTIOUS COMPLICATIONS OF PERITONEAL DIALYSIS

Peritonitis is a common clinical problem that occurs in patients with ERF treated by PD. It contributes to the failure of PD and hospitalisation. Severe and prolonged peritonitis can lead to peritoneal membrane failure (Piraino et al 2005). In the past, guidelines have focused on the treatment of peritonitis, but more recent guidelines focus on the prevention of infection as this is one of the keys to success in PD.

PREVENTION OF PD-RELATED INFECTIONS

Peritoneal dialysis programmes should carefully monitor the rate of infections – both peritonitis and exit-site infections. The cause of the infections should also be recorded as part of a continuous quality improvement programme. The incidence of relapsing peritonitis should be recorded and appropriate action taken for patients with recurrent infections. This might involve retraining or examining the PD catheter for signs of colonisation.

Rates of infection are expressed as episodes per patient month and are calculated by dividing the total number of episodes by the number of patients treated each month. For example if 100 patients were being treated with PD in January and four had an episode of peritonitis, the rate would be one episode in 25 or 1:25. Cumulative rates should be calculated over the course of a year. In this way, interventions can be implemented if infection rates are rising to unacceptably high levels. The current recommended acceptable rate for peritonitis is 1:18 patient months (Piraino et al 2005).

The Advisory Committee (Piraino et al 2005) recommends the use of an assist device for all spiking procedures. Some cyclers require a cassette; if reused, there is a high risk of peritonitis with water-borne organisms, so cassette reuse should be avoided (Chow et al 2000). The use of double-bag systems is preferred because they are more efficient in preventing peritonitis due to the flush-before-fill procedure (European Best Practice Guidelines 2005).

The prevention of catheter exit-site infections is the primary goal of exit-site care. Once the catheter is placed, and until healing is completed, the dressing should be changed by a dialysis nurse using sterile technique. The exit site should be kept dry until well healed, which means that showers or baths should not be taken for this period, which can take up to 2 weeks. Once the exit site is well healed, the patient should be taught how to do routine exit-site care. Antibacterial soap and water are recommended by many centres. Use of an antiseptic to clean the exit site is preferred in some programmes (Piraino et al 2005).

Training methods can influence the risk of PD infections (Hall et al 2004). In general, patients must be taught aseptic technique, with emphasis on proper hand-washing techniques. If the water the patient uses is thought to have a high bacterial count, then use of an alcohol hand rub should be encouraged, although this is used routinely in many centres. The hands must be completely dried using a clean towel after washing, before starting the exchange. The place where dialysis exchanges are done must be clean, free from animal hair, dust and fans. All patients must be taught what contamination is and what to do in the event of contamination (they should go to their dialysis unit for a tubing set change if the end of the tubing is touched accidentally).

The PD nurses are central to a successful PD programme with low infection rates. Unfortunately, there are few if any studies on nurse–patient ratios that lead to the best outcomes. Overburdening the nurse with excessive numbers of patients will result in shortened training times and difficulty in retraining as needed. The Advisory Committee (Piraino et al 2005) recommends home visits. These may be very useful in detecting problems with exchange technique, but can only be carried out if the nurses have sufficient time.

CAUSES OF PERITONITIS

Most episodes of peritonitis are caused by organisms that form the normal skin and nasal flora, for example, *Staphylococcus epidermidis* and *S. aureus*. Occasionally, water-borne organisms, such as *Pseudomonas*, may also cause this infection.

There are five main routes of infection causing peritonitis, each one giving rise to common organisms.

Intraluminal (contamination at the solution bag and transfer set connection site)

This contamination occurs most frequently when poor techniques have been used to make the connection. Good patient training and education regarding bag-exchange procedure techniques and hand-washing are essential. The incidence of this cause of infection has reduced in recent years owing to the use of disconnect systems. These systems incorporate a 'flush-before-fill' into the procedure, which has been shown to remove organisms caused by touch contamination (Kubey et al 1998).

Periluminal (infection introduced via the catheter tunnel from the exit site)

Bacteria present on the skin surface can enter the peritoneal cavity via the catheter tunnel. This infection can occur if there is infection present at the exit site or in the subcutaneous tunnel, which has migrated into the peritoneal cavity. The most common organisms seen when periluminal contamination has occurred are *S. epidermidis, S. aureus, Pseudomonas, Proteus* and yeast. *S. aureus* nasal carriage is known to cause an increased risk of *S. aureus* exit-site infections, tunnel infections, peritonitis and catheter loss.

Prophylaxis with intranasal mupirocin, exit-site mupirocin or oral rifampin has been shown to be effective in reducing *S. aureus* exit-site infections (European Best Practice Guidelines 2005). The use of mupirocin ointment at the exit site, however, should be avoided in patients with polyurethane catheters (Cruz catheters), as structural damage to the catheter has been reported. All patients at an increased risk for

S. aureus infections, including *S. aureus* carriers, diabetics and immuno-compromised patients should be provided with prophylaxis. A practical approach is to prescribe exit-site mupirocin for all at-risk PD patients and so routine nasal swab tests are therefore not necessarily required in these patients.

Transmural (infection through the gut wall)

There is an association between both severe constipation and enteritis and peritonitis due to enteric organisms (Singharetnam & Holley 1996). The most common organism seen as a transmural cause of peritonitis is *Escherichia coli*, although multiple contamination with anaerobes and fungi may also be isolated.

Haematogenous (infection via the bloodstream)

This is a rare cause of peritonitis, and it may be the peritonitis itself which causes septicaemia. The most common organisms associated with this cause of peritonitis are *Streptococcus* and *Mycobacterium*.

Vaginal (ascending through the vagina)

This is thought to be from bacteria entering the peritoneum via the fallopian tubes. The most common causative organisms seen here are *Candida* and *Pseudomonas*.

DIAGNOSIS OF PERITONITIS

Early diagnosis of peritonitis, allowing prompt treatment, is essential in minimising damage to the peritoneal membrane. Diagnosis is when two or more of the following conditions are present:

- cloudy PD effluent containing > 100 white blood cells μL^{-1} (more than 50% of which are neutrophils)
- abdominal pain, and tenderness and pyrexia
- identification of micro-organisms in the PD effluent by positive Gram stain or culture.

The process of diagnosis of peritonitis is summarised in Fig. 8.23.

OBTAINING A PD EFFLUENT SPECIMEN

CAPD

After disconnecting the drainage bag containing the effluent from the patient's transfer set, the bag should be inverted several times to mix the contents. Using strict aseptic technique, a sample is taken by sterile needle and syringe from the sample port on the bag (Fig. 8.24).

APD

A sample may either be taken from the day-time dwell, if the patient utilises a 'wet day' (i.e. dialysate in the peritoneum during the day), by attaching a drainage set and bag to the patient's extension set. The sample is then taken in the same way as for a CAPD patient. Alternatively, if the patient is usually 'dry' during the day (i.e. no dialysate in the peritoneum during the day), there are a number of options. Some APD machines have a sample bag that can be attached to the drainage tubing. Alternatively,

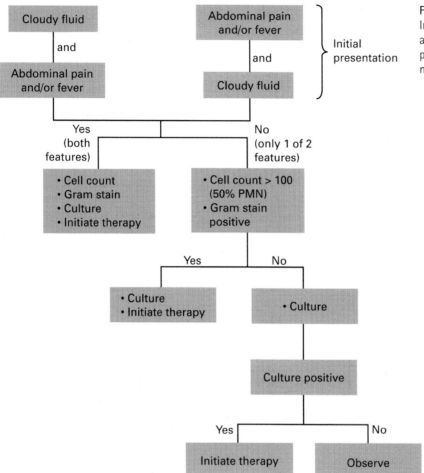

Figure 8.23
Initial clinical and laboratory assessment of a patient for peritonitis. PMN, polymorphic neutrophils.

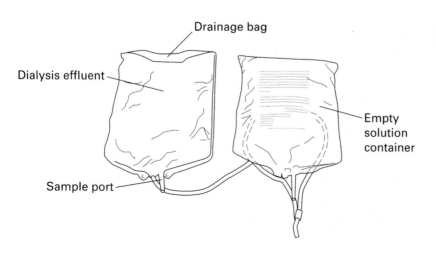

Figure 8.24
Sample port on drainage bag.

the patient may be taught how to take a sample from the drainage solution containers. If this is not possible, the patient may be asked to detach the drainage solution container from the machine following treatment and take this into the unit.

There are many different protocols for the treatment of PD peritonitis. An *ad hoc* advisory committee has reviewed experiences reported in the literature and devised recommendations based upon these assessments. These recommendations were published in *Peritoneal Dialysis International* most recently in 2005 (Piraino et al 2005). Antibiotics have been administered i.p., i.v. or orally, and a number of different dosing regimes have been utilised. The ISPD recommendations (Piraino 2005) include advice on treating peritonitis due to the most common organisms, such as coagulase-negative *Staphylococcus*, *Streptococcus*, *Enterococcus*, *Staphylococcus aureus*, *Pseudomonas aeruginosa*, polymicrobial peritonitis, fungal peritonitis, mycobacteria and culture-negative peritonitis. As always, individual clinical situations and variability in patient populations may necessitate modification of these recommendations.

TREATMENT OF PERITONITIS

Many peritonitis episodes are mild and can be treated at home. Usually the incubation period from time of contamination for bacterial peritonitis is 24–48 h. Any symptoms should resolve quickly following the initiation of therapy. If the infection shows either a slow response or no response to treatment, the choice of antibiotics could be inappropriate.

Those on PD should be taught how to recognise the signs and symptoms of peritonitis during their initial training period and at regular intervals. Ideally, the patient, if on CAPD, should complete the bag exchange at home (the presence of PD fluid in the peritoneum may provide some pain relief from inflammation of the peritoneal membrane) and bring the bag of cloudy dialysate effluent into the clinic for sampling. Treatment can then be initiated immediately.

There is current debate as to the necessity to perform peritoneal lavage immediately after the diagnosis of peritonitis, as it is thought to reduce the number of phagocytes present in the peritoneum that are available to fight infection. Peritoneal lavage is therefore thought by some to be of benefit only to patients with purulent effluent and abdominal pain as a pain-relieving exercise. There is no evidence to suggest that a transfer-set change performed at this time is of any benefit. On admission to the PD clinic, the usual fill volume for the patient is medicated with antibiotics. The patient or carer can be taught how to add the antibiotics to the dialysis fluid to facilitate self-care. Heparin (200–500 units L^{-1}) may also be added to the fluid to prevent the formation of fibrin, which is more likely in the presence of infection.

APD patients may receive antibiotics intraperitoneally by adding the antibiotics to the daytime dwell dialysis solution. Little is known about intermittent dosing requirements in patients treated with APD. In intermittent dosing, the antibiotic-containing dialysis solution must be allowed to dwell for at least 6h to allow adequate absorption of the antibiotic into the systemic circulation. Most antibiotics have significantly enhanced absorption during peritonitis (e.g., i.p. vancomycin is about 50% absorbed in the absence of peritonitis, but closer to 90% in the presence of peritonitis), which permits subsequent re-entry into the peritoneal cavity during subsequent fresh dialysis solution exchanges (Piraino et al 2005).

Peritonitis is monitored closely and dialysate effluent should be clear within 48h of commencing treatment. If the peritonitis resolves, antibiotics are discontinued 7–10 days after the start of therapy. Absorption of antibiotics into the serum through the peritoneum from the dialysate is rapid. Therefore, in most cases, administration of intravenous antibiotics is unnecessary.

PERMEABILITY CHANGES DURING PERITONITIS

The peritoneal membrane permeability tends to increase during episodes of peritonitis, perhaps due to increased blood flow through the peritoneum. Clearances of both large and small molecules increase, as does the absorption of glucose. This can result in marked increases in protein loss through the peritoneum and poor ultrafiltration. Patients need to be educated as to the need to increase dietary protein intake during episodes of peritonitis and to care for their fluid balance ensuring that, if they have no residual renal function, fluid intake is kept to a minimum. Rarely, patients are severely ill with peritonitis and need to be treated in hospital.

CULTURE-NEGATIVE PERITONITIS

Occasionally (less than 20%), cultures may be negative for a variety of technical or clinical reasons. Duration of therapy should be 2 weeks but, if no clinical improvement occurs within 96h, repeat cultures should be taken with consideration of mycobacteria or fungi, and catheter replacement or removal should be considered.

FUNGAL PERITONITIS

Catheter removal is indicated immediately after fungi are identified by microscopy or culture (Wang et al 2000).

RELAPSING PERITONITIS

Relapsing peritonitis is diagnosed as a recurrence of the same organism within 4 weeks of completion of the course of antibiotics. These infections should be treated in the same way as the initial peritonitis; however, the reason may be due to abscess formation, colonisation of the catheter or subcutaneous catheter tunnel infection. If there is no response to the antibiotics within 96h, consideration should be given to catheter removal and replacement at a later date.

EXIT-SITE INFECTION

An exit-site infection is defined by the presence of purulent drainage with or without erythema of the skin at the catheter-epidermal interface (Piraino et al 2005).

A culture of the drainage from around the exit site should be obtained. Antibiotic therapy may be initiated immediately, if the infection looks severe, or delayed until the results of the culture are available. Therapy should be continued until the exit site appears completely normal. Prolonged antibiotics may be necessary. If 3–4 weeks of antibiotics fails to resolve the infection, the catheter may need to be replaced.

Redness and swelling around the catheter exit site without purulent drainage are sometimes an early indication of infection. If infection is suspected, then therapy should be initiated: this may be either intensified local care, a local antibiotic ointment or an oral antibiotic that covers Gram-positive organisms. An alternative approach is careful observation for additional signs of infection.

TUNNEL INFECTION

Tunnel infection can present as an extension of the exit-site infection into the catheter tunnel: swelling, pain and redness over the subcutaneous tunnel may be observed. Tunnel infections do not often respond well to antibiotic treatment and it is usual to remove the PD catheter in these cases, reinserting a new one after about 1 month. Antimicrobial therapy should be given to the patient in the interim to resolve the infection, preventing migration of the organisms into the peritoneum and, therefore, predisposing to peritonitis.

EDUCATION AND TRAINING FOR THOSE ON PERITONEAL DIALYSIS

It is essential that effective education takes place before patients can be expected to treat themselves at home. Upwards of 90% of the care received by home dialysis patients is self-administered in the home. 'It is a common but erroneous belief that anyone can teach PD, but ... success depends upon the approach adopted' (Uttley & Prowant 2000). Literature is scarce regarding PD training programmes. Lauder & Zappacosta (1998) described components of a successful CAPD education programme based on adult learning principles. Adults are usually motivated to learn and are often learning from choice. They bring a wealth of life experiences with them that influence their learning and response to teaching. However, there are often many challenges for nurses, including working with patients who are ill and have to self-care; this poses many problems and barriers to learning.

BARRIERS TO LEARNING

People who are just about to start dialysis are often frightened – the prospect of dialysing oneself at home may not appeal. Many new patients are uraemic; symptoms may include nausea, vomiting, sleep disturbances and confusion. Some patients feel so physically unwell by the time they are to commence dialysis that they lack the motivation to learn, feeling that they will never recover. Teaching this group of patients can be made all the more difficult when other barriers to learning become apparent.

A fundamental barrier is language. In the UK, for instance, there is a growing ethnic population, giving rise to a growing proportion of people who speak little English. There are limited resources available for translation and it is frequently the responsibility of a younger member of the family, often a son or daughter, to act as translator during training. It may thus be difficult to assess who is learning, and with no knowledge of the language that is being translated, the trainer finds it difficult to ascertain just who has grasped the concept or answered the question – the patient or the translator? Language may also become a barrier when speaking to patients with no previous medical knowledge. Jargon and clinical terminology can be frightening and confusing.

Many older patients have to learn PD, and having to learn new concepts and procedures on which their life will depend may seem an overwhelming task. This sometimes makes learners feel vulnerable and inadequate, particularly if they are slow to learn. Short-term memory loss is a problem suffered by many elderly patients, and is a source of great frustration to both learner and trainer. These patients frequently have added physical barriers to learning, such as poor vision or lack of manual dexterity. Varying levels of deafness may also be a problem – the learner is trying not only to understand what has been said but is also straining to hear.

The 'Skills for life national needs and impact survey' (Department for Education and Skills, 2003) found that the literacy levels in England were quite poor, with 16% of the population between 16 and 65 being below entry level (Entry level 3 is the level expected by an 11 year old). If we consider this problem in relation to the concepts and procedures that need to be taught to patients on dialysis, it becomes apparent that the information given must be clear, unambiguous and readily understood, particularly if the patient's literacy difficulty is paired with a second or even a third barrier to learning.

THE LEARNING ENVIRONMENT

The PD training setting was discussed by Hoffman et al (2000) who described increased patient, nurse and physician satisfaction with home administered PD training. When training was individualised to the patient, Davies et al (2000) saw in-home patient training as more efficient than in-centre training as measured by time required to train.

TRAINING MATERIALS

Keeping et al (2001) examined informal learning in CAPD patients and found that learning increased when learners were asked to discuss their experiences or answer direct questions. This concept has been further developed by Hall et al (2004). The group set out to develop a PD training programme based on what the learner needed to know rather than on what the teacher needs to teach. Although their curriculum took on average 28% longer than traditional methods, this was offset by a reduction in re-training time, exit-site infections and peritonitis, and better fluid balance compliance.

RECOMMENDATIONS FOR TRAINING WITHIN RENAL UNITS

- Set aside an area specifically for teaching purposes. The area should preferably be away from the ward, and be non-clinical and quiet. A television and video can be used in this area for teaching.
- Designate a team of nurses for training duties only. Establish some continuity of care by allocating each patient to a designated nurse.
- Invite family members or partners to participate in the teaching programme.
- Use a wide variety of training materials. Five points to good presentation of these materials are:
  - teach the smallest amount possible for the job required
  - make the point as vividly as possible
  - review repeatedly
  - ask the learner to restate and demonstrate material
  - the subject matter should be relevant.
- Any material should be presented in a way that is comprehensible to the learner.
- Despite the fact that the readability of the material can be measured by the same formula, readers' skills may vary with their interest and background of experience in a particular topic area (Doak et al 1985).
- Training materials are most effective when presented in an interesting and appropriate manner. Both the language used and the material's degree of complexity need to be taken into account.
- The material should be presented in a memorable fashion. Any visual aids need vivid, simple messages that are easy for patients to remember.
- Finally, but perhaps most importantly, it is essential that the patients want to learn what is being taught.

The training programme should be designed to prepare patients fully for return to the community. The aim of a training programme is to educate patients to a standard whereby they can confidently care for themselves and perform PD in the community. For some learners this may mean that they learn only how to perform PD, troubleshoot and manage their renal diet. For others, much more detail may be desired, for example, learning how dialysis works.

Group teaching is an excellent way for patients to learn. This not only enables patients to learn from each other, but also helps the teacher, as many patients can be taught the same subject at the same time. The bulk of the training programme should focus on the patients themselves, relating all they are learning to their disease, treatment and, ultimately, their lifestyle. Sessions should be designed to last for no longer than 20 min and visual aids, such as flipcharts, acetates and videos, are used to make the material interesting and varied.

The internet is a useful tool in the education of people with kidney failure. It provides many advantages in that the information is available 24 h a day 7 days a week. There are now many websites dedicated solely to the education of patients with kidney failure. The following list proves a useful addition to any training programme:

- www.renalinfo.com/uk
- www.kidneypatientguide.org/uk
- www.kidney.org/uk
- www.nkrf.org/uk.

WHAT TO TEACH PATIENTS

It is important that new patients to PD are discharged from the renal unit with enough knowledge to care for themselves safely on dialysis. Broadly speaking, when each patient is taught, priority should first be given to what they must know, then to what they should know, and finally to what they could know. However, all learning objectives should be patient-centred.

The following topics should be included in a PD training programme:

- Medication. The patient's own medicines can be used as the central focus for this session. The aim is to ensure that the patient knows how often and why each medicine is taken.
- *Normal functions of the kidney.* This session can be given in groups using visual aids to explain in a simple way the basic functions of the kidney, relating these to the symptoms they suffer when kidneys fail.
- *CAPD and APD procedures.* These are most easily taught on a one-to-one basis. Demonstration techniques can be used to explain the procedure. A PD simulator (plastic torso with a PD catheter) is an excellent tool on which patients can practise their exchanges.
- *Catheter and catheter exit-site care.* This can be taught to the patient on a one-to-one basis. The PD simulator can be used to practise exit-site dressing technique, as can getting the patient to practise the technique in front of a mirror. Photographs are useful to help explain visually the difference between a healthy and an infected exit site.
- *How PD works.* Osmosis and diffusion can be explained using simple experiments or diagrams.
- *Diet.* Eating is an activity which most people enjoy and which therefore takes up a rather large part of our lives. Maybe it is for this reason that many patients focus on diet and want to know all there is to be taught. Plastic models of food can be used in training sessions to make the learning fun.
- *Infections.* It has been well documented that peritonitis is a major complication of PD and it is therefore important that peritonitis is explained to patients well, using a purpose-printed flip chart.
- *Fluid balance.* Fluid overload can be associated with excessive fluid intake and poor education. It is a common experience that one of the most difficult aspects of treatment to adhere to is the reduced fluid allowance. This subject can also be taught in groups using a

purpose-printed flip chart. Weighing a jug of fluid can also be useful to demonstrate the difference between fluid weight and flesh weight.

- *Fertility and sexuality.* It is important to discuss sexuality and body image with PD patients. Having the PD catheter present in the abdomen may inhibit some people (either the patient or partner) and it is essential that any anxieties are discussed. Fertility should also be discussed with patients and partners where appropriate, as it is possible for PD patients to conceive.
- *Employment.* Having dialysis is not a reason for giving up work. The training period is a good time to discuss work options with patients.
- *Ordering and delivery of PD supplies.* The practicalities of ordering and delivery of the PD supplies to the patient's home prove a great worry for many patients and their families. This can often be compounded by the problem of where to store this large amount of equipment. Patients can be encouraged to talk amongst themselves to gain ideas from each other as well as utilising the experience of nurses.
- *Holidays and travel.* It is possible to travel whilst being treated with PD and many patients go on holiday frequently. The practicalities of travel and holidays should be discussed during the training period and on a continuing basis if appropriate.
- *Exercise for PD patients.* The nurse's role is to promote a healthy lifestyle for patients. The training period is an ideal opportunity to discuss what types of activity are best suited to the individual patient.

To complement the training programme, reading materials should be made available, along with posters and videos. Many training materials have been translated into other languages for use by those patients whose first language is not English.

Assessment of how much information the patient has retained is difficult to make accurately. Testing can be seen as a threatening procedure, even though it is essential. Games, therefore, make a valuable contribution to the task of assessing learning and can be used in a variety of forms. Simple homemade crosswords, word searches and quizzes can be fun for patients and relatives to do at the end of their training.

SUMMARY

There have been considerable advances in the delivery of PD, resulting in a cost-effective therapy, which now has equivalent – if not better – outcomes as compared with HD (Gokal 2002). Technologic advances (APD, solutions), the ability to deliver adequate dialysis (both solute and fluid removal) and the minimisation of damage to the peritoneal membrane (biocompatible solutions, less peritonitis) are bound to improve the outcome of patients.

References

Armstrong A, Cunningham J. The treatment of metabolic bone disease in patients on peritoneal dialysis. Kidney Int 1994; 46(Suppl 48): S51–S57.

Ash SR. Chronic peritoneal dialysis catheters: Overview of design, placement and removal procedures. Semin Dial 2003; 16: 323–334.

Ash SR, Daugirdas JT. Peritoneal access devices. In: Daugirdas JJ, Ing TS, eds. Handbook of Dialysis. Boston: Little, Brown, 1994: 275–300.

Ash SR, Nichols WK. Placement, repair, and removal of chronic peritoneal catheters. In: Gokal R, Nolph KD, eds. Textbook of Peritoneal Dialysis. Dordrecht: Kluwer Academic, 1994: 315–333.

Bailie G, Johnson C, Mason N, St Peter W. Peritoneal dialysis. a guide to medication use. Nephrology Pharmacy Associates. www.nephrologypharmacy.com (2005).

Bargman JM, Thorpe KE, Churchill DN for CANUSA study group. Relative contribution of residual renal function and peritoneal clearance to adequacy of dialysis: a reanalysis of the CANUSA study. J Am Soc Nephrol 2001; 12: 2158–2162.

Baxter Healthcare. UK PET Survey. Thetford, Norfolk: Baxter Healthcare, 1992.

Bender K, Swartz MD. The role of nephrology nurses and technicians in the implementation of NKF-DOQI. Nephrol News Issues 1999; 13: 21–23.

Bernardini J, Piraino B, Holley J et al. A randomized trial of Staphylococcus aureus prophylaxis in peritoneal dialysis patients: mupirocin calcium ointment 2% applied to the exit site versus cyclic oral rifampin. Am J Kidney Dis 1996; 27: 695–700.

Brown EA, Davies SJ, Rutherford P et al on behalf of the EAPOS group. Survival of functionally anuric patients on automated peritoneal dialysis: The European APD outcome Study. J Am Soc Nephrol 2003; 14: 2948–2957.

Chow J, Munro C, Wong M et al. HomeChoice automated peritoneal dialysis machines: the impact of reuse of tubing and cassettes. Perit Dial Int 2000; 20: 336–338.

Churchill DN, Taylor DW, Keshaviah PR and the CANUSA Peritoneal Dialysis Study Group. Adequacy of dialysis and nutrition in continuous peritoneal dialysis: association with clinical outcomes. J Am Soc Nephrol 1996; 7: 198–207.

Consensus Conference on Biocompatibility Review. Nephrol Dialy Transplant 1994; 9(Suppl 2): 1–186.

Danielsson A, Blohme L, Traneus A, Hylander B. A prospective randomised study of the effect of a subcuteneously 'buried' peritoneal dialysis catheter technique versus standard technique on the incidence of peritonitis and exit site infection. Perit Dial Int 2002; 22: 211–219.

Dasgupta MK, Kerr L, Kennedy M et al. Randomized crossover study of aminoacids dialysate or oral nutritional supplements for correction of malnutrition in peritoneal dialysis. J Am Soc Nephrol 2002; 13: 2A.

Davies SJ, Tatchell S, Davies D, Fallon M, Coles G. Routine peritoneal dialysis training in the home: extending community treatment. Perit Dialy Int 2000; 20: S83.

Davies SJ, Woodrow G, Donovan K et al. Icodextrin improves the fluid status of peritoneal dialysis patients. Results of a double blind randomised controlled trial. J Am Soc Nephrol 2003; 14: 2338–2344.

Davies SJ, Philips L, Naish PF, Russel GI. Peritoneal glucose exposure and changes in membrane solute transport with time on peritoneal dialysis. J Am Soc Nephrol. 2001; 12: 1046–1051.

Davies SJ, Brown EA, Frandsen NE et al. Longitudinal membrane function in functionally anuric patients treated with APD; Data from EAPOS on the effects of glucose and icodextrin prescription. Kidney Int 2005; 67: 1609–1615.

Department for Education and Skills. The skills for life survey: a national needs and impact survey of literacy, numeracy and ICT skills. Research brief, RB 490. London: Department for Education and Skills, 2003.

Detsky AS, Mclaughlin JR, Baker JP. What is subjective global assessment of nutritional status? J Parenteral Enteral Nutr 1987; 11: 458–482.

Di Paolo N, Garosi G, Petrini G et al. Peritoneal dialysis solution biocompatibility testing in animals. Perit Dial Int 1995; 15(suppl): S61–S70.

Doak CC, Doak LG, Root JH. Teaching patients with low literacy skills. Philadelphia: Lippincott, 1985.

Esson ML, Quinn MJ, Hudson EL, Teitelbaum I. Subcutaneously tunnelled peritoneal dialysis catheters with delayed externalization: long term follow-up. Adv Perit Dial 2000; 16: 123–128.

European Best Practice Guidelines. Nephrol Dial Transplant 2005; 20(Suppl 9): ix1-ix37.

Farina J. Peritoneal dialysis and intraperitoneal insulin: how much? Nephrol Nurs J 2004 March–April; 31(2) 225–226.

Flanigan MJ, Gokal R. Peritoneal catheters and exit site practices towards optimum peritoneal access: a review of current developments. Perit Dial Int 2005; 25: 132–139.

Fried L, Hutchison A, Stegmayr B et al. Recommendations for the treatment of lipid disorders in patients on peritoneal dialysis. Perit Dial Int 1999; 19: 7–16.

Gadallah MF, Ramdeen G, Mignone J et al. Role of preoperative antibiotic prophylaxis in preventing post operative peritonitis in newly placed PD catheters. Am J Kidney Dis 2000; 36: 1014–1019.

Gadallah MF, Pervez A, El-Shahawy M et al. Peritoneoscopic versus surgical placement of peritoneal dialysis catheters: a prospective randomized study on outcome. Am J Kidney Dis 1999; 33: 118–122.

Gokal R, Ash SR, Holfrich BG et al. Peritoneal catheters and exit site practices. Toward optimum peritoneal access. 1998 Update. Perit Dial Int 1998; 18: 29–39.

Gokal R. Peritoneal dialysis in the 21st century: an analysis of current problems and future developments. J Am Soc Nephrol. 2002; 13: S104–S116, 20.

Golper TA, Tranaeus A. Vancomycin revisited. Perit Dial Int 1996; 16: 116–117.

Gotch FA, Sargent JA. A mechanistic analysis of the National Co-operative Dialysis Study (NCDS). Kidney Int 1985; 28: 526–534.

Gotch FA, Sargent JA, Parker TJ et al. National co-operative dialysis study: comparison of the study groups and a description of morbidity, mortality, and patient withdrawal. Kidney Int 1983; 26(Suppl 23): S42–S49.

Hall G, Bogan A, Dreis S et al. New directions in peritoneal dialysis patient training. Nephrol Nurs J 2004; 31: 149–154, 159–163.

Hofmann M, Ciligianan S, Owen R, Conick M, Bloom M, Marion R, Brase J. Peritoneal dialysis training in the home. Perit Dial Int 2000. 20: S84.

Hutchison A. Peritoneal dialysis solutions for the future. Do we have the solution? Dial Transplant 1992; 21: 57–63.

Jacobs C, Issad B, Allouache M et al. The crucial role of medical and nursing staff in the care of chronic peritoneal dialysis patients. Perit Dial Int 1997; 17: 23–28.

Johnson DW, Arndt M, O'Shea A et al. Icodextrin as a salvage therapy in peritoneal dialysis patients with refractory fluid overload. BMC Nephrology 2001; 2: 2.

Jones S, Holmes CJ, Kredeit RT et al. Bicarbonate/lactate-based peritoneal dialysis solutions increases cancer antigen 125 and decreases hyaluronic acid levels. Kidney Int 2001; 59: 1529–1538.

Keeping L, English L, Fleming-Couts M. Informal and incidental learning with patients who use CAPD. Nephrol Nurs J 2001; 28: 313.

Kelman B. The roles of the peritoneal dialysis nurse. Perit Dial Int 1995; 15: 114–115.

Keshaviah PR, Nolph KD, van Tone JC. The peak concentration hypothesis: a urea kinetic approach to comparing peritoneal and haemodialysis. Perit Dial Int 1989; 9: 257–260.

Khanna R. Applied peritoneal physiology. Semin Dial 1999; 12: 32–37.

Konings CJAM, Kooman JP, Schonck M et al. Effect of icodextrin on volume status, blood pressure and echocardiographic parameters: A randomized study. Kidney Int 2003; 63: 1556–1563.

Krediet RT, Pannekeet MM, Zemel D et al. Markers of peritoneal membrane status. Perit Dial Int 1996; 16 (Suppl 1): S42–S49.

Kubey W, Straka P, Holmes CJ. Importance of product design on effective bacterial removal by fluid convection in Y-set and twin-bag systems. Blood Purif 1998; 16: 154–161.

Lauder S, Zappacosta A. Components of a successful CAPD education programme. ANNA J 1998; 15: 243–247.

Lee H, Chung S, Chu W, Kim J, Ha H. Peritoneal dialysis in diabetic patients. Am J Kidney Dis 2001; 38: 200–203.

Lye WC, Lee EJ, Tan CC. Prophylactic antibiotics in the insertion of Tenckhoff catheters. Scand J Urol Nephrol 1992; 26: 177–180.

Mactier RA, Sprosen TS, Gokal R et al. Bicarbonate and bicarbonate/lactate peritoneal dialysis solutions for the treatment of pain on infusion. Kidney Int 1998; 53: 1061–1067.

Marshall J, Jennings P, Scott A et al. Glycaemic control in diabetic CAPD patients assessed by continuous glucose monitoring system (CGMS). Kidney Int 2003; 64: 1480–1486.

McEnzie R, Holmes C, Moseley A et al. Bicarbonate/lactate and bicarbonate buffered peritoneal dialysis fluids improve ex vivo peritoneal macrophage TNFα secretion. J Am Soc Nephrol Dial Transplant 1998; 9: 1499–1506.

Moist LM, Port FK, Orzol SM et al. Predictors of loss of residual renal function among new dialysis patients. J Am Soc Nephrol 2000; 11: 556–564.

Mujias S, Nolph K, Gokal R et al. Evaluation and management of ultrafiltration problems in peritoneal dialysis. Perit Dial Int 2000; 20(Suppl): S5–S21.

Mupirocin Study Group. Nasal mupirocin prevents Staph. aureus exit-site infection during peritoneal dialysis. J Am Soc Nephrol 1996; 7: 2403–2408.

Nielsen PK, Hemmingsen C, Friis SU et al. Comparison of straight and curled Tenckhoff peritoneal dialysis catheters implanted by percutaneous technique: a prospective randomised study. Perit Dial Int 1995; 15: 18–21.

Paniagua R, Amato D, Mujais S, Ramos A, Vonesh E. Summary results of the Mexican adequacy (ADEMEX) clinical trial on mortality and morbidity in peritoneal dialysis. J Am Soc Nephrol 2001; 12: 235A.

Park MS, Lee HB, Lim AS et al. Effect of prolonged subcutaneous implantation of peritoneal catheter on peritonitis rate during CAPD: a prospective randomised study. Perit Dial Int 1996; 16(Suppl 2): S54.

Park MS, Yim AS, Chung SH et al. Effect of prolonged subcutaneous implantation of peritoneal catheter on peritonitis rate during CAPD: a prospective randomised study. Blood Purif. 1998; 16: 171–178.

Piraino B, Bailie GR, Bernardini J et al. ISPD Guidelines/Recommendations. Peritoneal dialysis related infections recommendations: 2005 Update. Perit Dial Int 2005; 25: 107–131.

Plum J, Hermann S, Fussholler A et al. Peritoneal sclerosis in peritoneal dialysis patients related to dialysis settings and peritoneal transport properties. Kidney Int 2001; 59(Suppl 78): S42–S47.

Prowant BF, Twardowski ZJ. Recommendations for exit care. Perit Dial Int 1996; 16(Suppl 3): S94–S99.

Renal Association. Treatment of adult patients with renal failure. London: Royal College of Physicians and the Renal Association, 2002.

Renal Competency Framework. www.skillsforhealth.org.uk (2005).

Selgas R, Bajo MA, Paiva A et al. Stability of the peritoneal membrane in long-term peritoneal dialysis patients. Adv Renal Replace Ther 1998; 5: 168–178.

Singharetnam W, Holley JL. Acute treatment of constipation may lead to transmural migration of bacteria resulting in gram-negative, polymicrobial, or fungal peritonitis. Perit Dial Int 1996; 16: 423–425.

Tranaeus AP, Mactier RA, Sprosen TS et al. Bicarbonate and bicarbonate/lactate peritoneal dialysis solutions for the treatment of pain on infusion. Kidney Int 1998; 53: 1061–1067.

Twardowski ZJ, Nolph KD, Khanna R et al. Peritoneal equilibration test. Perit Dial Bull 1987; 7: 138–147.

UK Renal Association Clinical Practice Guidelines. Peritoneal Dialysis, 5th edition, 2007, www.renal.org/guidelines

Uttley L, Prowant B. Organisation of a CAPD programme-the nurse's role. In: Gokal R, Khanna R, Krediet R et al, eds. Textbook of peritoneal dialysis. Dordrecht: Kluwer, 2000: 363–386.

Venturoli D, Rippe V. Validation by computer simulation of two indirect methods for quantification of free water transport in peritoneal dialysis. Perit Dial Int 2005; 25: 77–84.

Wang AY, Yu AW, Li PK et al. Factors predicting outcome of fungal peritonitis in peritoneal dialysis: analysis of a 9-year experience of fungal peritonitis in a single center. Am J Kidney Dis 2000; 36: 1183–1192.

Wikdahl AM, Engman U, Stegmayr B et al. One-dose cefuroxime i.v. and i.p. reduces microbial growth in PD patients after catheter insertion. Nephrol Dial Transplant 1997; 12: 157–160.

Williams JD, Craig KJ, Topley N, Williams GT. Peritoneal dialysis: changes to the structure of the peritoneal membrane and potential for biocompatible solutions. Kidney Int 2003; 63(Suppl 84), S158–S161.

Williams P, Marriot J, Coles G, Stead R, Tranæus A. Insulin efficacy with a new bicarbonate/lactate peritoneal dialysis solution. Perit Dial Int 2000; 20: 467–469.

Wolters J, Van Der Sande FM, Leunissen KML. Effect of icodextrin on volume status, blood pressure and echocardiographic parameters: a randomized study. Kidney Int 2003; 63: 1556–1563.

Woodrow G, Stables G, Oldroyd B et al. Comparison of Icodextrin and glucose solutions for the daytime dwell in automated peritoneal dialysis. Nephrol Dial Transplant 1999, 14: 1530–1535.

Chapter 9

End of life care

Frances Coldstream and Fliss Murtagh

LEARNING OUTCOMES FOR THIS CHAPTER

- To understand which patients require consideration of their end of life needs
- To describe the different domains of palliative and end of life care for patients with stage 5 chronic kidney disease (CKD):
  - following the conservative management pathway
  - withdrawing from dialysis
- To understand the range of symptoms patients with CKD experience towards the end of life, and how to assess and address these symptoms
- To analyse the role of the renal nurse in providing palliative and end of life care

INTRODUCTION

This chapter considers the needs of patients, their partners, carers and families at a sensitive time – towards the end of life. Gunda et al (2005) consider that there is a significant and growing need for palliative care within nephrology. The focus of the chapter is on those who choose not to dialyse and follow a conservative pathway, but those who withdraw from dialysis will also be mentioned. Both groups of patients present specific challenges to the nurses caring for them.

NUMBERS OF PATIENTS

Chronic kidney disease (CKD) is a disease that is found across the age spectrum but is more commonly seen in older people. A recent survey suggests that there are approximately 23 000 patients with stage 4 or 5 CKD in the UK who are under the care of nephrologists and not yet on dialysis (Renal Registry 2005). Over the last 40 years there have been many changes that have increased our understanding and improved life expectancy for people with CKD. Medical and technological advances have led to increased availability of treatment for renal problems and an ability to treat older people who have other illnesses (Department of Health (DOH) 2005). Predictions are often difficult to make, but it is necessary to make them to help to plan effective services for both nephrology and palliative care. The Renal Registry report for 2004 (Ansell, 2005) suggests that the number of people on renal replacement therapy (RRT) will continue to rise for the next 20 years until a steady state is achieved, and that older patients treated by haemodialysis will make up a disproportionate amount of the growth in the acceptance rate for RRT. This currently stands at 104 per million population (pmp) for adults. The need for RRT will also be influenced by demographic changes, particularly those predicted with the overall ageing of the population and the ageing of the ethnic minority populations. These groups have a higher rate of renal problems; a study undertaken in the Thames region showed a three times higher acceptance rate and prevalence for RRT in the black and Asian population than in the white population (Roderick et al 1994). The Department of Health has produced similar data suggesting that the numbers of those receiving treatment for established renal failure will increase by 50% over the next 10 years, and that this increase will be particularly noticeable within the black and minority ethnic groups and older people. In addition, treatment rates in England are noted to be lower than in other comparable countries and this is thought to be another indicator of unmet need (DOH 2005).

WHY END OF LIFE CARE IS IMPORTANT

Twenty-two per cent of all patients beginning dialysis are over the age of 75 years (Renal Registry 2005). There are many factors that can influence the treatment choices of these older patients. With increased age, there is usually increased co-morbidity: 67% of those over 65 have one or more co-morbidities when commencing dialysis. For those over 85, 28% die within the first 90 days of commencing dialysis, and treatment withdrawal is the commonest cause of death after the first 90 days of dialysis in those over 75 (Renal Registry 2005). However, it is important to remember that dialysis therapy, and indeed transplantation, have never been considered as cures for CKD, but as therapeutic interventions to sustain life (Taylor 2000). Indeed, Rich (2000) presents an argument that dialysis could be seen as a palliative treatment from the start. Treatment for CKD has uncertain benefit in those with high co-morbidity and this, combined with an ageing population, has led to the development of conservative management pathways (where dialysis is not commenced) and consideration of how to manage, appropriately, people who express a wish to withdraw from dialysis. A recent audit in the Thames region suggested that 8% of new patients were opting for conservative management (Pan Thames Predialysis Audit 2004), but this represents considerable variation between different renal units. Smith et al (2003) showed that approximately 20% of patients assessed were recommended to follow a palliative (conservative) pathway. These patients were more likely to be diabetic and have higher co-morbidity scores that those for whom dialysis or transplantation were recommended.

THE PALLIATIVE APPROACH

Palliative care is a relatively new discipline, emerging in the 1960s, through the inspiration of Dame Cicely Saunders and others (Rich 2000). The World Health Organisation (WHO) definition (2002) is widely accepted (see Box 9.1).

It is important to recognise that this definition is not disease orientated but patient focused, and also reflects changes made to move away from a disease-specific definition, i.e. cancer, to an understanding that palliative care should be available to all with a life-threatening illness. It also encompasses early introduction of a palliative approach, while enabling a person to continue with life-prolonging therapies, such as dialysis.

A much shorter description of the aims of palliative care is given by Rich (2000). She suggests that palliative care 'aims for an holistic approach to patients whose disease is incurable; encompassing physical, spiritual and psychosocial aspects – and employing a multi-disciplinary approach to achieve total care'. Neither the WHO nor Rich focus on palliative care as exclusive to people who have cancer. This reflects the growing recognition that palliative and end of life care should be provided on the basis of need, not diagnosis (Addington-Hall 1997, Addington-Hall & Higginson 2001). It is not yet clear what model of palliative care provision should be adopted; whether it should be provided by renal professionals, by specialist palliative care professionals, or by primary care professionals, or (most likely) by some combination of these three groups.

Box 9.1   Definition of palliative care (WHO 2002)

Palliative care is an approach that improves the quality of life of patients and their families facing the problem associated with life-threatening illness, through the prevention and relief of suffering by early identification and impeccable assessment, and the treatment of pain and other problems psychosocial and spiritual. Palliative care:

- Provides relief from pain and other distressing symptoms
- Affirms life and regards dying as a normal process
- Intends neither to hasten or postpone death
- Integrates the psychological and spiritual aspects of patient care
- Offers a support system to help patients live as actively as possible until death
- Offers a support system to help the family cope during the patient's illness and in their own bereavement
- Uses a team approach to address the needs of patients and their families, including counselling, if indicated
- Will enhance quality of life, and may also positively influence the course of illness
- Is applicable early in the course of illness, in conjunction with other therapies that are intended to prolong life, such as chemotherapy or radiation therapy, and includes those investigations to better understand and manage distressing clinical complications

Palliative care is at different stages of development throughout the world, as Meghani indicates (2004). She describes palliative care as a dynamic concept that all practitioners should be integrating into their daily practice. It may be inappropriate to move a person to a different group of healthcare professionals just because of their stage of life. Hine (1998) suggests that the nephrology nurse should act as the coordinator of care, thereby maintaining continuity and allowing the principles of palliative care to be incorporated into nephrology practice. One of the big influences on and challenges to practice, therefore, is the integration of the extensive knowledge and experience in end of life care from the specialist palliative care field into the expertise of nephrology practice, for the benefit of patients. Until evidence supporting different models of care is available, clinical practice is likely to be influenced by local resources and the availability of both nephrology and specialist palliative care services.

RECENT GOVERNMENT AND OTHER INITIATIVES

Recent political and national developments in the UK have given considerable impetus to development of clinical services for those approaching the end of life. The National Service Framework (NSF) for Renal Services (DOH 2005) gives the following as a quality requirement:

> People with established renal failure receive timely evaluation of their prognosis, information about the choices available to them, and for those near the end of life a jointly agreed palliative care plan, built around individual needs and preferences.

The UK CKD guidelines (Renal Association 2005) recommend referral to the nephrology services of all people who have stage 4 or 5 CKD, even if it is anticipated that RRT will not be appropriate. However, most specialist palliative care resources are still devoted to patients with cancer. The National Council for Palliative Care (2005) estimates that 95% of specialist palliative care is devoted to cancer sufferers. Department of Health policy publications reflect this (National Institute for Clinical Excellence 2004), but there is growing recognition that survival rates of adults with CKD stage 5 are comparable with or worse than those for people with many types of cancer (Moss et al 2004), and therefore needs may be as great in CKD.

It is important to distinguish between end of life care and palliative care. Meghani (2004) cautions against using the terms synonymously; end of life care is palliative care, but not all palliative care will be end of life care. This is an important distinction that should help to guide practice. There appears to be interest at governmental level in improving care for the dying, with investment in initiatives designed for use at the end of life, such as the Liverpool Care Pathway (LCP) for the dying patient. The LCP is seen as a model of good care, which encourages the use of best practice as developed within the hospice movement, and translates this into other settings (Ellershaw et al 2001). An LCP specific to the last days of life of renal patients is currently being developed; further information is available via www.mcpcil.org.uk.

COMMUNICATION, DECISION-MAKING AND PLANNING

PATIENT COMMUNICATION

As the end of life approaches, skilled communication becomes increasingly important in the delivery of effective patient care. Communication between patient and nurse is important; patients want to know what to expect as their illness advances, and they value professionals who can talk openly about death and dying (Steinhauser et al 2001). Information needs to be delivered in amounts, and at a pace, that each individual patient can cope with. It is important to ensure there is the time and conditions for difficult questions to be asked and answered, since many factors will prevent such questions being explored.

Communication between the patient and their family also becomes increasingly important to patients as death approaches (Singer et al 1999), and nurses have a key role in facilitating this. Sometimes, understandably, family members adopt a protective attitude towards each other, shielding each other from bad news, but this is not always helpful, particularly if the patient is seeking openness and honesty.

Although most patients with a life-threatening illness prefer as much information as possible, a small proportion prefers not to know the details (Jenkins et al 2001). Information needs to be carefully matched to each patient's preference for information and for involvement in decisions (NHS Centre for Reviews and Dissemination 2000). At the same time, the patient's choices about end of life care need to be explored. If open communication does not occur, choices are likely to be more limited. An example of this is the preference to die at home if possible; this cannot be facilitated if initial communication and discussions about the implications of the illness have not taken place.

For patients dying with CKD, some specific considerations are important. Firstly, some patients will be 'long-term', living with their renal condition over a long period of time. It can be more difficult then for both patient and professional to perceive the change from living with a long-term condition to a decline in health towards death. If health professionals do not see this change, they may well deny the patient and their family the opportunities they need to understand their illness, and address and plan for their remaining time.

Secondly, the pattern of decline may be more uncertain than for other terminal conditions, such as cancer. The limited available evidence suggests that prognosis in conservatively managed patients varies considerably, depending partly on the underlying cause of the renal failure and on which other co-morbid conditions co-exist (Davies et al 2002, Smith et al 2003). Dealing with this uncertainty is hard for both patient and professional, and it needs to be honestly acknowledged in any communication.

Thirdly, renal professionals rightly focus on active disease management. End of life care requires a change of focus from a primarily disease-centred approach to a more patient-centred approach. Disease management takes a much lower priority, particularly as the end of life approaches. Controlling symptoms, attending to psychosocial and spiritual needs, and anticipating future care needs all become as important, or more important, than renal expertise. Nurses may feel uncertain about their skills in this area, particularly if they work with patients at the end of life infrequently.

FAMILY COMMUNICATION

Effective end of life care cannot be delivered without good family communication. However, the ethical and legal responsibilities of the nurse are predominantly to the patient, so it is important to seek patient agreement *before* any communication with their family, particularly if that communication takes place away from the patient. In the final days of life, increasing uraemia may mean that patients are confused, and increasingly lack the ability to make decisions for themselves. It is important therefore to ensure from the beginning that relevant family members are involved in any management decisions (if the patient wishes) and that they are aware of the patient's end of life preferences, before the patient becomes less well. The work of Holley (2005) highlights the importance of the patient–family relationship, rather than the patient–professional relationship, as a better context for exploring preferences and undertaking advance care planning.

COMMUNICATION WITHIN THE TEAM

A number of key decisions will be made with any patient as they approach the end of their life. These include decisions around withholding or withdrawing dialysis, decisions around preferred place of care and death, and cardiopulmonary resuscitation (CPR) decisions, among others. Each of these needs to be communicated to the whole renal team. Patients will often see different professionals at each clinic visit or hospital admission, and it is important that patient and family are given clear and consistent messages.

A wide variety of non-renal healthcare professionals may also be involved in end of life care; ranging from the general practitioner and district nurses, to specialist palliative care professionals (who may be community, hospital or hospice based). Time and energy, therefore, need to be devoted to communicating any decisions made to *all* members of the team, including those providing care out of hours, and those who may be called in a crisis, both at home or in hospital.

DIALYSIS DECISION-MAKING

Towards the end of life, decisions are made either to withdraw dialysis, or to follow a conservative pathway. This raises complex and challenging issues. These issues have been reviewed (Rothenburg 1993), and guidelines have been developed to inform decision-making (Moss 2001). The guidelines are built on shared decision-making, recognising that patients are individuals and have their own history, perspectives and preferences. Renal patients are known to have widely differing preferences for involvement in decisions, but generally receive less information than they want and have less involvement in decisions than they prefer (Orsino et al 2003). Work by Cohen and colleagues (1993) also suggests that there is considerable difference between dialysis patients' hypothetical considerations for the future and their actual decisions when the time comes.

Some nephrologists feel that most, if not all, patients requiring RRT should receive dialysis, but there is growing recognition that, for some patients, dialysis may not greatly increase survival while adding a considerable treatment burden. For these patients, conservative management (care without dialysis, but with management to minimise disease progression, and full supportive and palliative care) may be a better option, although any final decision will depend on patient preferences as well as professional advice. Work by Chandna et al (1999) and others has shown that patients with poor functional status and high levels of co-morbidity do not do well on dialysis. Munshi and colleagues (2001) describe poor survival in the very elderly (> 75 years) on dialysis, but recognised that survival alone is an insufficient measure of outcome; they also recorded hospitalisations and rates of dialysis complications (both high in the elderly).

Following a conservative management pathway sometimes demands especially difficult decision-making, since it requires weighing up patient preferences, estimated survival on or off dialysis, anticipated quality of life on or off dialysis, and the treatment burden with dialysis. Estimating survival and quality of life is difficult for the individual patient. These factors have been studied in dialysis patients, but symptom burden, survival and quality of life have rarely been studied in conservatively-managed patients (Joly et al 2003). Smith and colleagues (2003) measured survival in patients recommended for conservative management, and found little difference in survival between those following this pathway and those who were in fact dialysed.

ADVANCE PLANNING

Effective and appropriate care can only be delivered by planning ahead and anticipating future care needs. It is, therefore, important to explore sensitively with patients (and their family, if desired) what their wishes are for future care, or in the event of a sudden deterioration or crisis. Relatively few patients choose to write a formal advance directive, but all should be offered the chance to discuss preferences for future care and management. These discussions should be carefully documented and revisited regularly (since preferences may change).

Advance directives are written documents which specify patients' preferences, in anticipation of loss of the capacity to make their own decisions, when they are less well. In the UK, the Mental Capacity Bill (expected to become law in 2007) will clarify the legal status of such documents, and also make provision for a person to be named to represent the patients' preferences in their place. Where a patient has made such a directive, the evidence suggests that these facilitate dialysis decision-making and reduce the chance of inappropriate interventions (Holley et al 1991, Moss et al 1993). They may also increase the chance of a 'good' death (Swartz and Perry 1993).

There are other ways to facilitate planning, including use of tools such as the Preferred Place of Care document (Pemberton et al 2003). This was developed to promote discussion around patients' preferred place of care and death. It provides an accessible patient-held record that records their preferred wishes, and has been recommended by the NSF for Renal Services (DOH 2005). Anticipating and planning for acute admissions is also particularly important for some renal patients, especially those with cardiac disease, who may be more liable to develop fluid overload or acute pulmonary oedema.

Whether specific documents or advance directives are used or not, every patient should, as their disease progresses, have the chance to discuss their future care, concerns, hopes and preferences. The responsibility lies with the professional to ensure that these opportunities arise. These issues should be addressed early and systematically, remembering that both patients and professionals find it hard to introduce and address such matters. Quill (2000) aptly describes unaddressed end of life issues as the 'elephant in the room', and suggests useful questions to initiate such discussions (see Box 9.2).

Careful consideration should be given to resuscitation status, since this may be an issue during hospital admission. CPR in this group of patients may be inappropriate, depending on prognosis and co-morbidity. It is important to recognise that there is no ethical obligation to

Box 9.2   Suggested questions to initiate discussion about end of life issues, based on work by Quill (2000)

- What is most important for you to achieve?
- What are your most important hopes?
- What are your biggest fears?
- What are your thoughts about balancing quality and length of life?
- What do you feel about your quality of life at present?
- What would most improve your quality of life at present?
- How is your family handling your illness?
- Have you given any thoughts to what treatments you might or might not want?

discuss CPR with terminally ill patients if this treatment is judged to be futile and, therefore, would not be provided.

CARE OF PATIENTS MANAGED WITHOUT DIALYSIS

Conservatively-managed patients need much more than just symptom management (see Box 9.3).

Achieving these goals requires a shift from a predominantly disease-focused approach towards more patient-centred management (the disease itself, while it must not be neglected, is less important than overall quality of life, and the patient themselves should be encouraged to decide what treatment they can or cannot tolerate as the illness progresses). Careful judgements need to be made as to when to discontinue onerous treatments; these will often depend on perceived burden and patient preference.

Box 9.3   The needs of patients managed conservatively (Czapla 2003)

- Skilled communication to facilitate the 'not for dialysis' decision, to explain disease progression and prognosis, and to facilitate future management decisions, in accordance with the patient's information preferences
- Regular review(s) of the 'not for dialysis' decision
- Continuing disease management to maximise and maintain residual renal function
- Continuing disease management to minimise symptoms
- Regular and detailed assessment of symptoms
- Proactive intervention to control symptoms

- Advance planning as the illness progresses:
  - to avoid inappropriate acute admissions
  - to avoid inappropriate reversal of 'not for dialysis' decision
  - to enable place of care preferences to be met if possible
- Ongoing psychological and social care
- Involvement and support of family as appropriate
- Spiritual care, especially as the end of life approaches
- Detailed and expert end of life care in the final days or weeks

SYMPTOMS TOWARDS THE END OF LIFE

The most common physical symptoms that patients with CKD report are lack of energy or fatigue, itching or pruritus, pain, sleep disturbance and restless legs (see Box 9.4; Curtin et al 2002, Parfrey et al 1987, 1988).

A number of studies report fatigue as extremely common (70–90%; Curtis et al 2002, Merkus et al 1999, Parfrey et al 1987). Pruritus has been studied extensively; some of the larger studies suggest that 40–70% of patients may be troubled by this symptom (Curtin et 2002, Curtis et al 2002, Zucker et al 2003). Pain has been infrequently studied, but the few studies undertaken suggest more than 50% of patients have pain (Davison 2003, Weisbord et al 2003). Sleep disturbance, and the related symptom of restless legs, has been studied more often and appears to affect 30–52% of patients (Holley et al 1992, Locking-Cusolito et al 2001, McCann and Boore 2000, Sabbatini et al 2002).

Anxiety and depression may also be experienced by some patients. Reports of how common these problems are depend on how they are defined and sought. Screening questionnaires are positive in 26–58% of patients (al Hihi et al 2003, Craven et al 1988, Rodin and Voshart 1987, Smith et al 1985, Watnick et al 2003, Wuerth et al 2005), but fewer patients (12–26%) have depression diagnosed at formal psychiatric interview (Farmer et al 1979, Hinrichsen et al 1989, O'Donnell and Chung 1997, Smith et al 1985).

A variety of other less common symptoms have been described, including anorexia, constipation, cough, dyspnoea, nausea and vomiting (Barrett et al 1990, Parfrey et al 1989). Most evidence comes from patients on dialysis; some symptoms (such as muscle cramps, pruritus, restless legs) may be dialysis-related, and will occur less often in conservatively managed patients, while other symptoms are disease-related and will worsen with declining renal function.

As the illness progresses, symptoms may worsen. Symptoms in the last days of life, in both the conservatively managed patient and the patient withdrawing from dialysis, may follow different patterns, but

---

Box 9.4 Symptoms commonly experienced in stage 5 CKD

- Fatigue or lack of energy
- Itching (pruritus)
- Pain
- Sleep disturbance
- Restless legs
- Anxiety and/or depression
- Anorexia
- Constipation
- Cough and dyspnoea
- Nausea and vomiting

there have been very few studies of symptoms in either group at the end of life. Cohen et al (2000) carried out one of the few studies on dialysis withdrawal, and they describe pain, agitation, myoclonus (involuntary jerking of muscles), fatigue and dyspnoea, each occurring in at least one in four patients in the last day of life.

SYMPTOM ASSESSMENT

The most important step is to identify symptoms when they are present. This is best done by asking the patient about potential symptoms, in a systematic way. Symptom questionnaires, such as the Dialysis Symptom Index (Weisbord et al 2004), may be helpful. There is evidence that symptoms may go unrecognised in CKD (Davison 2003). This may partly be because the focus has been on the disease itself, and not the symptoms. Also, symptoms may be related to other co-existent illnesses (co-morbidity), not to the renal disease. Many of these patients will have several co-morbid conditions and management of symptoms may fall to a variety of health professionals. However, these patients will have an estimated glomerular filtration rate (eGFR) < 15 mL min^{-1}, and non-renal health professionals may be both unskilled and unconfident in, for example, using appropriate medications for symptom management. The key to good symptom control is proactive, detailed and thorough symptom assessment at regular intervals, without waiting for the patient to report a symptom.

Careful attention must be given to the underlying cause of each symptom. For example, pain may more likely be due to co-morbid conditions than the renal disease itself, with ischaemic pain from peripheral vascular disease, neuropathic pain from polyneuropathy (often related to diabetes mellitus), bony pain from osteoporosis, or musculoskeletal pains from a variety of causes, all common. There may less often be specific pains related to the renal disease, such as bone pain from renal osteodystrophy, cyst pain in polycystic kidney disease, or the infrequent but acute pain of calciphylaxis (Angelis et al 1997, Rich et al 2001).

SYMPTOM MANAGEMENT

Management of symptoms in CKD is complex, because of the altered pharmacology of drugs in advanced renal impairment, and high risk of toxicity and side effects. Symptoms are also commonly due to conditions other than the renal disease, although it is nevertheless important to recognise and treat them. A brief outline of the most frequent or challenging symptoms is given here, but more detail can be found elsewhere, such as in Levy et al (2004).

Constipation

This is common, and usually multifactorial. Fluid restriction, poor mobility and drug side effects are common contributors. A stool softener, such as lactulose or docusate, often needs to be used in combination with a stimulant laxative, such as senna or bisacodyl.

Fatigue or lack of energy

This is one of the commonest problems and difficult to alleviate. Measures (such as erythropoietin replacement and iron supplementation) to maintain haemoglobin between 11 and $12\,g\,dL^{-1}$ should be taken, and probably continued even when prognosis is short because of the symptom improvement they provide. Nutrition should be carefully considered, and megestrol acetate may have a role for some patients.

Nausea and vomiting

It is important to try to identify the cause, if effective management is to be achieved; history often provides the best clues. Gastroparesis (reduced gastric motility, usually presenting with early fullness, vomiting after eating and relief of nausea with vomiting) responds to metoclopramide. Uraemic nausea is often more constant and less closely related to eating; haloperidol is a more appropriate treatment. Persistent nausea or vomiting near the very end of life can be treated with levomepromazine; this is very effective but doses may be limited by sedation. Ondansetron or granisetron may also be used, especially if nausea is drug-related, but severe constipation is a common side effect, and should be proactively managed by co-prescription of a laxative.

Pain

Pain management needs to be tailored, both to the individual patient, and to the specific cause of the pain. If the cause cannot be removed or reduced, then pain medication should be given according to the WHO 'analgesic ladder'. This consists of three steps: Step 1 is essentially paracetamol, Step 2 is opioids for mild to moderate pain, and Step 3 is opioids for moderate to severe pain. Initial analgesia should start with the lowest appropriate step. It is important to understand that, if the full dose is insufficient for relief, then using another medication from the same 'step' does not usually provide any better relief, and it is better to move up to the next step. Tramadol is probably the optimal Step 2 opioid, although it should be used at a reduced dose and at an increased dose interval in stage 5 CKD (Broadbent et al 2003). Use of Step 3 opioids in stage 5 CKD is highly problematic (Davies et al 1996): morphine and diamorphine in particular accumulate and readily cause toxicity. Fentanyl is probably safer, although evidence is limited, and available formulations are restrictive (Mercadante & Arcuri 2004). According to the cause of the pain, additional (adjuvant) medication may need to be used alongside opioids. This is particularly true of neuropathic pain.

Pruritus

Dry skin is very commonly associated with pruritus, and should be actively managed with liberal regular emollients (such as aqueous cream). High serum levels of calcium, phosphate, magnesium and parathyroid hormone have all been associated with pruritus to a greater or lesser extent (Lugon 2005), and should be sought and actively managed, if present. Oral antihistamines are often used, although there is little evidence for benefit. If pruritus disturbs sleep, a sedative antihistamine (such as chlorpheniramine) given at night may be useful. Other treatment options include naltrexone (not with opioids), capsaicin cream (especially if pruritus is localised) or thalidomide (caution with handling; Lugon 2005).

These two symptoms frequently co-exist. Simple measures, such as avoiding caffeine, avoiding alcohol in the evenings and reducing day-time sleep, are important in facilitating sleep. Hypnotics, such as zolpidem, zopiclone or temazepam, can be used, although doses should be reduced in stage 5 CKD without dialysis, and the risk of dependence should be considered carefully if prognosis is months or more.

Restless legs should be managed specifically with reduction in caffeine and any aggravating medications (such as tricyclics), and active treatment of anaemia and low ferritin (which are both associated with restless legs). Clonazepam or dopaminergic agents are most often prescribed, although if these are effective, then symptoms often recur after an interval. For this reason, the lowest possible doses should be used; intermittent rather than continuous use may be helpful.

Restless legs and sleep disturbance

PSYCHOLOGICAL, SOCIAL AND SPIRITUAL ISSUES

As seen earlier when considering the definition of palliative care, it considers the whole person and his or her family. Gunda et al (2005) indicate clearly the need to incorporate palliative care, including the psychosocial and spiritual issues, into nephrology care when starting, withholding or withdrawing dialysis. As Davison (2005) identifies, unless the psychological, social and spiritual components of pain are addressed, pain will never be relieved adequately. This chapter now moves on to consider some of these issues which are most important within the context of conservative management.

PSYCHOLOGICAL AND SOCIAL ISSUES

There are many psychological and social implications of living and dying with CKD, many of which are similar to other life-threatening or chronic diseases. Both the patient and their carer or family face many potential changes and these can be related to, for example, role change, appearance, sexuality, financial challenges and becoming more physically dependent on someone. It is important that timely discussions occur to ensure that patients and their families are prepared for potential changes, and aware of services and benefits that may help. Reiter & Chambers (2004) feel that failure to address psychosocial issues can lead to technical treatment without healing. They also indicate how important it is to provide support to the carer and family; by doing this the patient is also supported.

The involvement of the multidisciplinary team is essential. The timely intervention of, for example, an occupational therapist can help promote independence and safety, which gives a boost to both patients and carers. The provision of a bereavement service is also seen as essential by Gunda et al (2005). Some renal units offer an annual memorial service; see for example, the report by Ormandy (1998). Families of renal patients who have died in the previous year are invited to the service, as well as renal professionals. It is an opportunity for all to acknowledge the loss, to continue to provide support and often helps families progress in their bereavement journey.

SPIRITUAL CARE

The term 'spiritual' is ill-defined and can mean very different things to different people (Davies & Byock 2004). To add to the confusion, the terms spiritual and religious are frequently used interchangeably, which is unhelpful. Spirituality is to do with meaning, not necessarily through formal religious beliefs, while religion is an expression of spiritual beliefs through a more formal framework (Speck et al 2004). Davies & Byock (2004) consider that for people with CKD, spiritual care should be integrated into practice to ensure that the whole person is considered within the context of their care. Illness, and the end of life in particular, involves mind and spirit, not just what happens to the body, and it is therefore important that care of mind and spirit are included in overall care. Spiritual care is often neglected until the end of life is perceived as being very near, leaving little time for spiritual care or resolution of issues.

The closeness of death, and the prospect of facing mortality, can have significant effects on both patient and family, as well as on professionals. Sometimes people look for meaning in what is happening, or ask the question 'why me?' There may be issues of guilt, or some families may be facing multiple losses or another recent bereavement. Knowledge and discussion of spiritual needs should help to address these issues as death approaches, although as Davies & Byock indicate, listening is frequently the most important skill in spiritual care.

SUMMARY

The needs of patients with kidney disease (and their families) as they approach the end of life are complex. They need skilled and open communication from an early stage, advance planning, high quality symptom control, and good psychological and spiritual care. Their families may also need bereavement care. Effective delivery of such care also requires communication with, and coordination of, the network of professionals who may be involved, including primary care, renal and specialist palliative care professionals, as well as families and informal carers.

It is imperative that nephrology nurses develop generic palliative care skills to ensure that appropriate care, including good symptom relief, is given to patients and their families at all stages of their disease trajectory. In addition, partnerships with specialist palliative care providers need to be nurtured to ensure that their timely intervention can be of full benefit, and that there is maximum sharing of expertise and experience. The overall aim is to enable the last months and days of each patient's life to be lived as fully as possible, and for them to achieve a good death. It is a challenging area for nephrology nursing practice, but one which cannot and must not be ignored.

References

Addington-Hall J. Reaching out: specialist palliative care for adults with non-malignant diseases. Occasional Paper 14. London: National Council for Specialist Palliative Care and Hospices, 1997.

Addington-Hall JM, Higginson IJ, eds. Palliative care needs for non cancer patients. Oxford: Oxford University Press, 2001.

al Hihi E, Awad A, Hagedorn A. Screening for depression in chronic hemodialysis patients. Missouri Med 2003; 100: 266–268.

Angelis M, Wong LL, Myers SA, Wong LM. Calciphylaxis in patients on hemodialysis: a prevalence study. Surgery 1997; 122: 1083–1089.

Ansell D, Feest T, Rao R, Williams A, Winearls C. UK Renal Registry Report 2005. Bristol, UK: Renal Registry; 2005.

Barrett BJ, Vavasour HM, Major A, Parfrey PS. Clinical and psychological correlates of somatic symptoms in patients on dialysis. Nephron 1990; 55: 10–15.

Broadbent A, Khor K, Heaney A. Palliation and chronic renal failure: opioid and other palliative medications – dosage guidelines. Prog Palliative Care 2003; 11: 183–190.

Chandna SM, Schulz J, Lawrence C, Greenwood RN, Farrington K. Is there a rationale for rationing chronic dialysis? A hospital based cohort study of factors affecting survival and morbidity. BMJ 1999; 318: 217–223.

Cohen LM, Germain M, Poppel DM, Woods A, Kjellstrand CM. Dialysis discontinuation and palliative care. Am J Kidney Dis 2000; 36: 140–144.

Cohen LM, Germain M, Woods A, Gilman ED, McCue JD. Patient attitudes and psychological considerations in dialysis discontinuation. Psychosomatics 1993; 34: 395–401.

Craven JL, Rodin GM, Littlefield C. The Beck Depression Inventory as a screening device for major depression in renal dialysis patients. Int J Psychiatry Med 1988; 18: 365–374.

Curtin RB, Bultman DC, Thomas-Hawkins C, Walters BA, Schatell D. Hemodialysis patients' symptom experiences: effects on physical and mental functioning. Nephrol Nurs J J ANNA 2002; 29: 562, 567–574, 575, 598.

Curtis BM, Barret BJ, Jindal K et al. Canadian survey of clinical status at dialysis initiation 1998–1999: a multicenter prospective survey. Clin Nephrol 2002; 58: 282–288.

Czapla K. Management of chronic renal insufficiency in frail older patients who are unfit for renal replacement therapy. Rev Clin Gerontol 2003; 13: 25–37.

Davies C, Byock I. Spiritual care in the renal patient. In: Chambers EJ, Germain M, Brown E, eds. Supportive care for the renal patient. Oxford: Oxford University Press, 2004: 15–26.

Davies G, Kingswood C, Street M. Pharmacokinetics of opioids in renal dysfunction. Clin Pharmacokinet 1996; 31: 410–422.

Davies SJ, Phillips L, Naish PF, Russell GI. Quantifying comorbidity in peritoneal dialysis patients and its relationship to other predictors of survival. Nephrol Dial Transplant 2002; 17: 1085–1092.

Davison SN. Chronic pain in end-stage renal disease. Adv Chronic Kidney Dis 2005; 12: 326–334.

Davison SN. Pain in hemodialysis patients: prevalence, cause, severity, and management. Am J Kidney Dis 2003; 42: 1239–1247.

Department of Health. National service framework for renal services – Part 2. London: HMSO, 2005.

Ellershaw J, Smith C, Overill S, Walker SE, Aldridge J. Care of the dying: setting standards for symptom control in the last 48 hours of life. J Pain Symptom Manage 2001; 21: 12–17.

Farmer CJ, Snowden SA, Parsons V. The prevalence of psychiatric illness among patients on home haemodialysis. Psychol Med 1979; 9: 509–514.

Gunda S, Smith S, Thomas M. National survey of palliative care in end-stage renal disease in the United Kingdom. Nephrol Dial Transplant 2005; 20: 392–395.

Hine J. Standards of palliative care in a renal care setting. EDTNA-ERCA J 1998; 24: 27–29, 35.

Hinrichsen GA, Lieberman JA, Pollack S, Steinberg H. Depression in hemodialysis patients. Psychosomatics 1989; 30: 284–289.

Holley JL. Palliative care in end-stage renal disease: focus on advance care planning, hospice referral, and bereavement. Semin Dial 2005; 18: 154–156.

Holley JL, Foulks CJ, Moss AH. Nephrologists' reported attitudes about factors influencing recommendations to initiate or withdraw dialysis. J Am Soc Nephrol 1991; 1: 1284–1288.

Holley JL, Nespor S, Rault R. A comparison of reported sleep disorders in patients on chronic hemodialysis and continuous peritoneal dialysis. Am J Kidney Dis 1992; 19: 156–161.

Jenkins V, Fallowfield L, Saul J. Information needs of patients with cancer: results from a large study in UK cancer centres. Br J Cancer 2001; 84: 48–51.

Joly D, Anglicheau D, Alberti C et al. Octogenarians reaching end-stage renal disease: cohort study of decision-making and clinical outcomes. J Am Soc Nephrol 2003; 14: 1012–1021.

Levy JB, Chambers EJ, Brown EA. Supportive care for the renal patient. Nephrol Dial Transplant 2004; 19: 1357–1360.

Locking-Cusolito H, Huyge L, Strangio D. Sleep pattern disturbance in hemodialysis and peritoneal dialysis patients. Nephrol Nurs J J ANNA 2001; 28: 40–44.

Lugon JR. Uremic pruritus: a review. Hemodialysis International 2005; 9: 180–188.

McCann K, Boore JR. Fatigue in persons with renal failure who require maintenance haemodialysis. J Adv Nurs 2000; 32: 1132–1142.

Meghani S. A concept analysis of palliative care in the United States. J Adv Nursing 2004; 46: 152–161.

Mercadante S, Arcuri E. Opioids and renal function. J Pain 2004; 5: 2–19.

Merkus MP, Jager KJ, Dekker FW, de Haan RJ, Boeschoten EW, Krediet RT. Physical symptoms and quality of life in patients on chronic dialysis: results of The Netherlands Cooperative Study on Adequacy of Dialysis (NECOSAD). Nephrol Dial Transplant 1999; 14: 1163–1170.

Moss AH. Shared decision-making in dialysis: the new RPA/ASN guideline on appropriate initiation and withdrawal of treatment. Am J Kidney Dis 2001; 37: 1081–1091.

Moss AH, Holley JL, Davison SN et al. Core curriculum in nephrology – palliative care. Am J Kidney Dis 2004; 43: 172–173.

Moss AH, Stocking CB, Sachs GA, Siegler M. Variation in the attitudes of dialysis unit medical directors toward decisions to withhold and withdraw dialysis. J Am Soc Nephrol 1993; 4: 229–234.

Munshi SK, Vijayakumar N, Taub NA, Bhullar H, Lo TC, Warwick G. Outcome of renal replacement therapy in the very elderly. Nephrol Dial Transplant 2001; 16: 128–133.

National Institute for Clinical Excellence. Improving supportive and palliative care for adults with cancer. London: National Institute for Clinical Excellence, 2004.

National Council for Palliative Care. Minimum data sets project update. London, National Council for Palliative Care, 2005.

NHS Centre for Reviews and Dissemination. Informing, communicating and sharing decisions with people who have cancer. Effective Health Care 6[6]. York: NHS Centre for Reviews and Dissemination, 2000.

O'Donnell K, Chung JY. The diagnosis of major depression in end-stage renal disease. Psychother Psychosom 1997; 66: 38–43.

Ormandy P. A memorial service for renal patients. EDTNA/ERCA J 1998; 24: 22–24.

Orsino A, Cameron JI, Seidl M, Mendelssohn D, Stewart DE. Medical decision-making and information needs in end-stage renal disease patients. Gen Hosp Psychiatry 2003; 25: 324–331.

Pan Thames Audit Group 2006. Audit of pre-diaylsis care. Accessed from nww.esussex.nhs.uk/aian (can only be accessed from an NHS computer).

Parfrey PS, Vavasour H, Bullock M, Henry S, Harnett JD, Gault MH. Symptoms in end-stage renal disease: dialysis v transplantation. Transplant Proc 1987; 19: 3407–3409.

Parfrey PS, Vavasour HM, Henry S, Bullock M, Gault MH. Clinical features and severity of nonspecific symptoms in dialysis patients. Nephron 1988; 50: 121–128.

Parfrey PS, Vavasour H, Bullock M, Henry S, Harnett JD, Gault MH. Development of a health questionnaire specific for end-stage renal disease. Nephron 1989; 52: 20–28.

Pemberton C, Storey L, Howard A. The Preferred Place of Care document: an opportunity for communication. Int J Palliat Nurs 2003; 9: 439–441.

Quill TE. Perspectives on care at the close of life. Initiating end-of-life discussions with seriously ill patients: addressing the 'elephant in the room'. JAMA 2000; 284: 2502–2507.

Reiter GS, Chambers EJ. The concept of supportive care for the renal patient. In: Chambers EJ, Germain M, Brown E, eds. Supportive care for the renal patient. Oxford: Oxford University Press, 2004: 15–26.

Renal Association. 2005 Guidelines for the identification, management and referral of adults with chronic kidney disease. Internet communication, accessed on 21/01/06 at www.renal.org/CKDguide/full/CKDprintedfullguide.pdf

Renal Registry. Eighth annual renal registry report. Bristol: Renal Registry, 2005 (www.renalreg.com).

Rich A. The role of palliative care in patients with renal failure. Br J Renal Med 2000; 5: 6–8.

Rich A, Leach A, Ellershaw J. A case of difficult pain in a patient with chronic renal failure and calciphylaxis. J Pain Symptom Manage 2001, 22: 617–21

Roderick PJ, Jones I, Raleigh VS, McGeown M, Mallick N. Population need for renal replacement therapy in Thames regions: ethnic dimension. BMJ 1994; 309: 1111–1114.

Rodin G, Voshart K. Depressive symptoms and functional impairment in the medically ill. Gen Hosp Psychiatry 1987; 9: 251–258.

Rothenberg LS. Withholding and withdrawing dialysis from elderly ESRD patients: Part 2 – ethical and policy issues. Geriatr Nephrol Urol 1993; 3: 23–41.

Sabbatini M, Minale B, Crispo A et al. Insomnia in maintenance haemodialysis patients. Nephrol Dial Transplant 2002; 17: 852–856.

Singer PA, Martin DK, Kelner M. Quality end-of-life care: patients' perspectives. JAMA 1999; 281: 163–168.

Smith C, Silva-Gane M, Chandna S, Warwicker P, Greenwood R, Farrington K. Choosing not to dialyse: evaluation of planned non-dialytic management in a cohort of patients with end-stage renal failure. Nephron Clin Pract 2003; 95: c40–c46.

Smith MD, Hong BA, Robson AM. Diagnosis of depression in patients with end-stage renal disease. Comparative analysis. Am J Med 1985; 79: 160–166.

Speck P, Higginson I, Addington-Hall J. Spiritual needs in health care. BMJ 2004; 329: 123–124.

Steinhauser KE, Christakis NA, Clipp EC et al. Preparing for the end of life: preferences of patients, families, physicians, and other care providers. J Pain Symptom Manage 2001; 22: 727–737.

Swartz RD, Perry E. Advance directives are associated with 'good deaths' in chronic dialysis patients. J Am Soc Nephrol 1993; 3: 1623–1630.

Taylor K. Renal dialysis – does the burden of treatment outweigh the benefit? Nephrol News 2000; Summer: 4–5.

Watnick S, Kirwin P, Mahnensmith R, Concato J. The prevalence and treatment of depression among patients starting dialysis. Am J Kidney Dis 2003; 41: 105–110.

Weisbord SD, Carmody SS, Bruns FJ et al. Symptom burden, quality of life, advance care planning and the potential value of palliative care in severely ill haemodialysis patients. Nephrol Dial Transplant 2003; 18: 1345–1352.

Weisbord SD, Fried LF, Arnold RM et al. Development of a symptom assessment instrument for chronic hemodialysis patients: the Dialysis Symptom Index. J Pain Symptom Manage 2004; 27: 226–240.

World Health Organisation. Definition of palliative care. 2002. Internet communication, accessed on 21/01/06 at www.who.int/hiv/topics/palliative/care/en/

Wuerth D, Finkelstein SH, Finkelstein FO. The identification and treatment of depression in patients maintained on dialysis. Semin Dial 2005; 18: 142–146.

Zucker I, Yosipovitch G, David M, Gafter U, Boner G. Prevalence and characterization of uremic pruritus in patients undergoing hemodialysis: uremic pruritus is still a major problem for patients with end-stage renal disease. J Am Acad Dermatol 2003; 49: 842–846.

Chapter 10

Renal care in infancy, childhood and early adulthood

Diane Blyton and Shelley Jepson

- To gain an understanding of the physiological differences between children and adults
- To develop an appreciation of the psychosocial impact of chronic kidney disease and renal replacement therapies on children and their families
- To identify the key differences in the management of chronic kidney disease, dialysis, transplantation and acute renal failure in children
- To be able to identify important issues around transition, and the transfer of young people to adult services

LEARNING OUTCOMES FOR THIS CHAPTER

INTRODUCTION

The aim of this chapter is to address the unique needs of infants, children and young adults who have renal insufficiency. The challenge is to meet the needs of the patients and their parents within each of these age groups. Infants and young children are dependent upon their parents/carers for their global needs, and as they mature, they are increasingly able to become self-caring.

The Renal National Service Framework (NSF) for children and young people emphasises the need for families to be partners in their child's care (Department of Health 2006). Therefore, the approach taken with this client group needs to be flexible, and the multiprofessional team needs to be diverse to support this. Specialist units will commonly comprise not only medical staff and specialist nurses, but also specialist dieticians, social workers, nursery nurses/hospital play specialists, hospital school teachers, psychologist and, where possible, youth workers.

Key concerns are the psychosocial impact of the condition, which will often be long-term, on both the children and their families (Department of Health 2006). The prevention of complications that may have an impact on the health of the child throughout his or her future, on transfer to adult services, is also important.

The following sections will highlight both the physiological and psychosocial differences between children and adults, and how renal replacement therapies need to be adapted accordingly.

PHYSIOLOGY IN CHILDHOOD – IMPACT ON RENAL CARE

There are several key areas where physiology in childhood differs from that in adulthood.

GROWTH

A major difference is that children are continually growing, with accelerated growth spurts during infancy and adolescence. Normal birth weight is 3.5 kg and, during infancy, growth varies between 50 and 200 g a week, with an expected 25 cm length increase in the first year. This gradually declines to 2 kg per year with 6 cm height increase until the pubertal growth spurt (Shaw & Lawson 2001). Body proportions also change: the head changes from a proportion of 1:4 in infancy to 1:8 in adulthood (MacGregor 2000).

Several factors have an influence in growth, including diet, genetic inheritance and growth hormone production, which are discussed further below.

FLUID BALANCE

Water comprises 70–80% of the body in infants, decreasing to 60% in adults. There is also a greater proportion of extracellular water in infants, therefore water is more easily lost, particularly during pyrexia (MacGregor 2000, Willock and Jewkes 2000).

RENAL ANATOMY

Neonates' kidneys are affected by the removal of blood flow from the placenta, leading to a reduction in glomerular filtration rate (GFR) and renal blood flow. Newborns have immature kidneys with small underdeveloped glomeruli, short loops of Henle and an underdeveloped renal cortex. The main consequences of this are a reduced GFR of $30\,mL\,min^{-1}\,m^{-2}$ at birth reaching $100\,mL\,min^{-1}\,m^{-2}$ by 9 months of age.

There is a reduced ability to concentrate urine and also to secrete hydrogen ions. This becomes particularly important if the infant enters into a state of metabolic acidosis. There is rapid development particularly in the first 6 months of age, and normal levels for GFR are usually reached by around one year of age (MacGregor 2000). However, these should be adjusted according to surface area, as standard GFR is based upon $1.73\,m^2$.

Careful consideration is needed when monitoring children that age-appropriate parameters are used.

- Infants in particular are expected to have higher levels for many electrolytes. They also have a reduced serum creatinine as a result of smaller muscle mass. Age-appropriate reference ranges should be consulted for biochemistry results throughout childhood, as other variations are seen (see Table 10.1).
- Blood pressure increases with size/age. As children with renal dysfunction are often short in stature, height centile charts should be used to monitor blood pressure rather than those based on chronological age.
- Minimum urine output decreases with age: $1-2\,mL\,kg^{-1}\,h^{-1}$ should be used when monitoring children and infants and $0.5\,mL\,kg^{-1}\,h^{-1}$ for young adults.

CHRONIC KIDNEY DISEASE

The common causes of chronic kidney disease (CKD) in children are different from those experienced in later life, as indicated in Table 10.2. In comparison with the numbers seen in the adult population, it is difficult to gain accurate figures. In 2004, data suggested that the incidence of established renal disease (ERD) was 51.3 pmcp (per million child population) and 10.4 pmp (per million population) as a whole. This rate was estimated to be 626 pmp in the adult population (UK Renal Registry 2004).

The presenting symptoms of CKD commonly seen in children are:

- failure to thrive or anorexia
- nausea, vomiting and loss of appetite
- lethargy
- headaches and high blood pressure
- reduced urine output or polyuria/polydipsia, possibly wetting.

Table 10.1
Biochemistry reference
ranges for children.

Sodium (mmol L⁻¹)	132–142
Potassium (mmol L⁻¹)	
< 1 month	3.0–6.6
> 1 month	3.0–5.6
Bicarbonate (mmol L⁻¹)	22–32
Urea (mmol L⁻¹)	2.5–6.5
Albumin (g L⁻¹)	34–45
Calcium (mmol L⁻¹)	
< 1 year	2.4–2.8
1–2 years	2.3–2.7
3–16 years	2.2–2.6
Phosphate (mmol L⁻¹)	
< 4 weeks	1.2–3.1
5 weeks–6 months	1.5–2.4
6 months–1 year	1.5–2.1
1–3 years	1.2–2.0
3–6 years	1.0–1.8
6–15 years	1.0–1.7
Adult	0.8–1.4
Creatinine (μmol L⁻¹)	
< 5 years	< 44
5–6 years	< 53
6–7 years	< 62
7–8 years	< 71
8–9 years	< 80

Table 10.2
Common causes of
established renal failure in
children.

Renal dysplasia	22.9%
Glomerulopathies	22.9%
Obstructive uropathies, e.g. posterior urethral valves	14.6%
Reflux nephropathy	10.9%

Source: UK Renal Registry 2004

Children can present at any age and at different stages of renal disease. It is important that investigations are undertaken to determine the cause and, therefore, the interventions required. Dialysis may be necessary in some cases; however, many children can be treated conservatively.

Some conditions are familial and so siblings may also need to be assessed, even if they are asymptomatic. In rare cases, a parent and one or more children may be dialysis dependent, and a thorough plan of psychosocial support is a necessity in this situation.

CONSERVATIVE MANAGEMENT

Providing the biochemistry is stable, children can be maintained without dialysis for some time. Several interventions can be incorporated into conservative management. These interventions continue into the established phase of chronic kidney disease, and may be temporarily used to support children in an acute phase of renal disease.

Diet

Poor appetite, gastrointestinal reflux and vomiting are common problems seen in children and infants with chronic kidney disease. Parents often see feeding their child as an important aspect of their role and, therefore, this is potentially an area of great stress (Coleman 2001).

It is important that a paediatric renal dietitian is involved in the management of children with renal disorders, providing support in this area of anxiety (Department of Health 2006). Dietary control can assist in delaying the need for dialysis, and all of the medical and psychosocial problems associated with it, as discussed further below. Adequate nutrition is also important for growth and neurological development.

Energy requirements should be based upon EAR (estimated average requirement) for chronological age, or height age if the child falls below the 2nd percentile (Coleman 2001). Modified milk formulas may be necessary for infants, dependent upon biochemistry, as standard formulations may have inappropriate protein and electrolyte concentrations.

Individualised dietary guidance is needed for each family, based on the child's biochemistry. Negotiation with food allowances is often needed with older children to improve adherence to the nutritional plan. Clear education is needed for these children and their parents, to ensure understanding of the necessity of restricting many of the favourite childhood foods, such as chips and pizza. Sodium, potassium and phosphate intakes often need to be altered. A small number of patients with tubular disorders may require supplementation (Sedman et al 1996). Protein intake may also need to be modified to balance growth requirements against potential uraemia (Coleman 2001).

High-energy food and drinks are encouraged, as it can be difficult to achieve EAR when on an altered diet. Good nutrition is very important in reaching the minimum weight to be placed on the transplant list (commonly 10 kg).

It is common for younger children and infants in particular, to refuse to eat, and enteral feeding via the nasogastric or gastrostomy route is often required. Gastrostomy feeding in particular has been shown to be a valuable tool in nutritional support (Coleman et al 1998).

Socialisation with food is still important, with the end goal of transplantation in mind. Feeding problems can remain following a successful transplant, and speech and language therapy can be required. Conversely, in older children, advice is often needed to prevent excessive weight gain, particularly when taking corticosteroids as immunosuppression.

Fluid management

The approach to fluid management will be dependent upon whether the child concerned has a reduced urine output or is polyuric. Patients who have a reduced urine output will usually be given a fluid allowance and placed on a diuretic regimen. The common guideline used is to add $400\,mL\,m^{-2}$ surface area day^{-1} to the average daily urine output, to allow for insensible losses (Coleman 2001). Some patients are polyuric and great care needs to be taken to ensure that fluid intake is sufficient to prevent dehydration.

Along with dietary changes, it is the reduction in fluid allowance that older children often find the most difficult to adhere to. It is important to give advice on ways of managing fluid. Fluid overload is a contributor to hypertension in many patients and, therefore, can impact on cardiovascular health (Wright 2004).

Blood pressure

As with adults, hypertension is a complication children with renal disease may experience. It is essential that accurate measurements are taken to enable effective treatment of hypertension. Cardiovascular complications are a major cause of mortality and morbidity in adult patients (Hingorani & Watkins 2000, UK Renal Registry 2004). Prevention of early complications is essential, with hypertension being one of the most modifiable. Hypertension has also been associated with acceleration of renal disease.

Blood pressure increases with age, and there are reference guidelines to assist in patient management. As children with renal insufficiency are often short in stature, their height should be used as a reference, rather than chronological age. It is recommended that systolic blood pressure should be maintained below the 90th percentile for height and sex (UK Renal Registry 2004). There are charts based upon gender, age and height that should be used (National High Blood Pressure Education Program Working Group 2004).

The British Hypertension Society has guidelines on blood pressure measurement, which include some guidance on children. Mercury sphygmomanometers are identified as the gold standard method; however, because of health and safety guidance, these are difficult to obtain (Dillon 1998). Non-mercury sphygmomanometers are available and are more accurate than standard aneroid devices, and many units are now using these. The issue of automated blood pressure versus manual blood pressure measurement is controversial. Care needs to be taken when using automated machines as very few are validated for use in children (O'Brien et al 2001). The cuff used should also be selected carefully so it is important to have a wide selection of cuffs available in paediatric areas. Box 10.1 provides a summary of blood pressure measurement guidelines.

There are other issues to consider in very small children. Firstly, they can be uncooperative. It can also be difficult to hear Korotkoff sounds in small children using a stethoscope. As a result, Doppler devices are recommended in children under 2 years of age.

Single readings should not be used to direct management, because 'white-coat hypertension' can be particularly problematic in children. Ambulatory blood pressure monitoring is often used to assist in the treatment of hypertension enabling monitoring away from the hospital environment (Sorof & Portman 2000).

Box 10.1   Key principles in blood pressure measurement

- The bladder in the cuff should cover 80–100% of arm circumference
- Doppler devices are the recommended method in children under 2 years
- Inflate to 30 mmHg above the estimated systolic pressure
- Deflate the cuff at 2–3 mmHg s^{-1}
- Record the reading to the nearest 2 mmHg
- Blood pressure should be compared to centile charts for height, age and gender

---

Anaemia

Anaemia is also associated with an increased risk of cardiac morbidity and mortality, and also affects growth and development (Szromba et al 2002, UK Renal Registry 2004). Haemoglobin should be maintained above or equal to 11 g dL^{-1}, ferritin 100–500 ng mL^{-1} and TSATS (Transferin Saturation) > 20%. Initially oral iron supplementation with nutritional management is sufficient in managing anaemia. However, as renal function deteriorates, recombinant erythropoietin may need to be introduced. Most children with established renal failure require treatment. Darbopoietin is also now being used in older patients with good effect.

Intravenous iron sucrose (Venofer®) can be beneficial if the oral supplementation is unsuccessful (Tenbrock et al 1999). This is usually given on an as-required basis; however, weekly doses for children on haemodialysis can be effective in counteracting the blood loss experienced. Whenever possible, blood transfusions are avoided.

Growth and bone health

Growth problems are common in children with renal disease, and monitoring is essential. Height, length, weight and head circumference in the under 2s should be measured and recorded on a growth chart (Coleman 2001).

Renal bone disease is a major contributor to growth problems. Close monitoring of phosphate levels and parathyroid hormone is essential. Non-dominant hand and wrist x-ray is also used to monitor growth, enabling bone age to be compared to chronological age.

Diet has a major impact, including control of calcium and phosphate levels. Phosphate binding medication is often required (Miller et al 2004). In infants and young children this is added as a suspension into feeds, whereas older children follow similar regimes to adults. Again adherence can be a problem, and education and negotiation is essential to identify a regime that is realistic. The UK Renal Registry (2004) report suggests that over 30% of all patients have hyperphosphataemia.

Vitamin D analogue treatments may also be required. Combining these treatments can control serum calcium levels and prevent the development of hyperparathyroidism (Miller et al 2004). Progression to tertiary hyperparathyroidism can make long-term treatment very difficult, and may ultimately lead to the need for a parathyroidectomy. Vascular calcification is also a major concern, and can be a contributing factor in cardiovascular complications (Klaus et al 2006, UK Renal Registry 2004).

Growth problems in children with renal disorders have been associated with deranged secretion of growth hormone and resistance. Recombinant growth hormone can be effective, and this treatment should be considered. However, normalisation of calcium, phosphate and parathyroid hormone levels should be achieved first, as there is a possibility of abnormal growth of long bones with growth hormone treatment (Klaus et al 2006).

NEPHROTIC SYNDROME

Nephrotic syndrome is an uncommon childhood condition with an annual incidence of 2 per 100 000 in the UK (Moore et al 1994). However, children with nephrotic syndrome are regularly seen in paediatric renal units and therefore warrant discussion in this chapter.

Nephrotic syndrome is a term used to describe a collection of symptoms: hypoalbuminaemia, oedema, proteinurea and hyperlipidaemia. In this syndrome, the glomeruli become permeable to plasma proteins, resulting in loss of protein in the urine (Bell 2002). Protein loss is generally in excess of $2\,g\,24\,h^{-1}$, which is represented as 3–4+ of protein on dipstick. Serum albumin levels are less than $25\,g\,L^{-1}$. This leads to a decrease in the plasma oncotic pressure, water leaks into the interstitial space and there is resulting oedema.

Minimal-change nephrotic syndrome is the most common cause of nephrotic syndrome in childhood, affecting 70–80% of children with the disease. The cause is unknown, although onset is often triggered by a viral illness or allergy.

The treatment of nephrotic syndrome is with corticosteroids, $60\,mg\,m^{-2}\,day^{-1}$ for 28 days, followed by $40\,mg\ m^{-2}\,day^{-1}$ for a further 28 days. The child is considered to be in remission when the urine has been negative of protein for 3 consecutive days. Relapse occurs when there is proteinurea of 2+ or more on dipstick for 3 consecutive days after remission (Bell 2002). Renal biopsy is only indicated if remission is not achieved within 28 days of commencing treatment.

NURSING CARE

Accurate monitoring of fluid balance is essential along with daily weight and regular blood pressure measurement. Frequent assessment of oedema is necessary and mobilisation should be encouraged to disperse oedema. Children with nephrotic syndrome often have a fluid allowance of 750 mL daily (under 5 years of age) and 1000 mL daily (over 5 years). Although oedema may be present, hypovolaemia may occur due to the shift of fluid into the interstitial space. Diuretics are therefore not routinely prescribed.

In severe cases of oedema or hypovolaemia, albumin infusions may be prescribed. Albumin should be administered with caution and frequent observations made during and after the infusion. Urine should be checked for protein daily and a teaching programme arranged for children and carers so that they can continue urinalysis at home following discharge.

Referral to a paediatric renal dietician is recommended. A healthy eating plan should be observed with a no-added salt diet. Monosaturated or polyunsaturated fats should be used to prevent hyperlipidaemia.

Minimal-change nephrotic syndrome has a favourable prognosis. Children who present with this syndrome between 1 and 8 years of age are likely to respond to steroid treatment. The disease usually burns out before adulthood leaving no residual renal damage (Hodson et al 2002)

CONGENITAL NEPHROTIC SYNDROME

This is a rare disorder that usually presents antenatally or within the first 3 months of life. It is an inherited disorder that affects 1:10 000 infants. Referral to a paediatric nephrology unit is essential. Daily albumin infusions are necessary and ultimately nephrectomy and renal replacement therapy is required.

RENAL REPLACEMENT THERAPY

TRANSPLANTATION

Transplantation is the treatment of choice for children with established renal failure. Normal renal function provides children with better opportunities for growth and development. In addition, successful transplantation maximises the opportunities for education and normal childhood activities, which may be compromised during dialysis.

Allocation of deceased donor transplants currently gives priority to paediatric recipients (under 18 years of age). This was agreed as children are likely to require more than one kidney transplant in their lifetime and a good match at first transplant will mean less difficulty in finding a suitable donor in the future (UK Transplant 2006)

It is possible to transplant kidneys from adult donors depending on the size of the child's abdominal cavity. If the donor kidney is disproportionately large, it may be placed intraperitoneally. There is a concern that, intraoperatively, a large shift of blood into the transplanted kidney may occur, following release of vascular clamps (El-Mekresh 2000). Intraoperative fluid management is, therefore, essential to prevent hypovolaemia. However, intraperitoneal placement is avoided where possible in order to maintain the peritoneum for subsequent dialysis.

Transplantation into very small children is rarely successful. Most transplant surgeons require children to weigh approximately 10 kg or have reached at least 22 months of age before transplantation is considered. This is due to the risk of infarction in small vessels postoperatively. Children receiving renal replacement therapy from birth, therefore, require the maintenance of dialysis access up until this time. This places a significant burden on the carers and a challenge for professionals.

Living donor transplantation

With the decrease in the number of deceased donors, living donor transplantation is on the increase and is now routinely considered as an early option. In children, the donor is most frequently a parent, although donation from grandparents has been reported. UK law prohibits minors from donating a kidney and, therefore, siblings under 18 years of age are not considered. For children placed on the deceased donor waiting list, the avoidance of parental antigens will allow living related transplantation to be considered in the future.

Living related donation (LRD) is advantageous in that families are able to plan the timing of the transplant, which allows them to consider employment, education and family arrangements. It is recommended that children receiving kidney transplants must be cared for within a paediatric unit (Department of Health 2004) therefore there is the potential for the recipient and the donor to have surgery at different hospitals simultaneously. Professionals need to pay attention to the psychosocial needs of the family during this time, as often the non-donating parent must divide their time between the two sites. Supportive care could be provided in terms of video links and assistance with transport.

Pre-emptive transplantation

Transplantation prior to the need for dialysis is increasing. A total of 22% of children in the UK receive pre-emptive transplantation, of which the majority are from a living related donor (UK Transplant 2005). The benefits of transplant before dialysis include less interruption of schooling and family life, preservation of the peritoneum and vessels for future dialysis treatments, improved growth and development, and reduction in the symptoms of established renal failure.

A child is generally considered for transplantation once the GFR has fallen below $10–15 \, mL \, min^{-1} \, 1.73 \, m^{-2}$, and dialysis is anticipated within 12–24 months and/or a significant complication of growth failure is present (Webb et al 2003). In addition, pre-emptive transplantation should be considered if the child exhibits symptoms of established renal disease, i.e. renal bone disease, poor growth, fatigue and inability to take part in normal childhood activities.

Care of the child post-kidney transplant

Nursing care of the child following renal transplant must be in a designated high dependency nursing area. One to one nursing care is required for 48 h so that careful monitoring of fluid balance, blood pressure and psychosocial support can be delivered (British Association of Paediatric Nephrologists 2003). After the first 48 h recovery is generally fast and, if there are no complications, children can be discharged 7–10 days following transplant.

Close monitoring of kidney function and immunosuppression levels is necessary, and children are usually seen as outpatients several times a week in the first 4 weeks. Owing to the long travelling distances often necessary, close collaboration with local health centres and district hospitals is encouraged so that blood tests can be taken locally and results sent to the tertiary centre.

Children can return to school within 4–6 weeks of a successful transplant. School liaison is recommended in order to reassure teaching staff (Royal College of Nursing (RCN) 2000).

Immunosuppression

There is currently no standard immunosuppression regimen for children and young people undergoing renal transplantation. However, most children in the UK receive triple therapy with a calcineurin inhibitor (tacrolimus), a DNA proliferation inhibitor (azathioprine) and a corticosteroid (National Institute for Health and Clinical Excellence 2006). Research studies are ongoing to guide optimum treatment, whilst minimising potential side effects.

Complications

There are several potential complications following paediatric renal transplant: Hypertension is common, and occurs in 80% of deceased donor transplants and 61% of LRD recipients in the immediate postoperative period (Baluarte et al 1997) Other complications include urinary tract infection, rejection and recurrence of primary disease.

Poor concordance to treatment regimen is a common problem, particularly in young people and those with family instability. The development of a youth work programme with increased peer support has demonstrated some success in dealing with this problem (Hilton et al 2004)

PREPARATION FOR DIALYSIS AND TRANSPLANT

Prior to commencing renal replacement therapy, children, young people and their carers need to be given information regarding treatment options. In order for them to make an informed choice, information that is appropriate to age and understanding must be available. Hospital play specialists, who are trained to prepare children for procedures, are invaluable members of the paediatric multi-professional team. Evidence shows that appropriate preparation for family members prior to treatment may prevent trauma later (Waby et al 2005). Consideration must also be given to siblings who may feel distressed by the treatment and are concerned about family separation (Batte et al 2006).

Home visits are an important tool in this process, both in assessing the home environment and also in promoting open discussion about the therapies. This can be difficult in busy clinical environments (RCN 2000).

There are a number of investigations that are required within the preparation period, which are summarised in Box 10.2.

IMMUNISATION

Live vaccines should not be given in immunosuppressed children. In order to receive optimal protection against infectious diseases children should be given a full course of primary immunisations prior to transplant listing. In addition to routine immunisation, hepatitis B, bacilli Calmette–Guérin (BCG) and varicella zoster vaccine should be given to non-immune children (Royal College of Paediatrics and Child Health 2002).

DIALYSIS

Although every attempt is made to transplant pre-emptively and hold off dialysis, this is not always possible. Peritoneal dialysis is often the dialysis of choice; however, some families prefer haemodialysis. It is important that children and their families are aware of all of the options available, and that they are actively involved in the decision-making process.

Other professionals often require information when children progress on to dialysis. General practitioners and community health staff should be informed of changes in the child's treatment. School and nursery visits are also often required to inform teaching staff about the impact dialysis has on the child, and also for health and safety reasons (RCN 2000).

Peritoneal dialysis

In 2004, 14% of paediatric patients with ERD were on peritoneal dialysis (PD). The benefit of peritoneal dialysis in paediatric patients is the reduced disruption to normal life. In many paediatric units, automated PD is the most frequent mode of delivery (77.5% of all PD patients in 2004). This is usually carried out overnight reducing the impact on schooling in particular. Machines can deliver fill volumes as low of 60 mL with reduced recirculation of fluid using specialised sets; therefore, enabling most infants to be dialysed in this way. Another advantage of this method is that it reduces the number of times the catheter is accessed, lowering the potential for contamination and therefore infection. Fill volumes are usually calculated based on surface area ($1.1 \, \mathrm{L\,m^{-2}}$), or weight $30–50 \, \mathrm{mL\,kg^{-1}}$.

Ambulatory peritoneal dialysis is less frequently used for younger patients. Young adults may choose this method, as it gives them more freedom during the evenings. At present it is estimated that less than 30% of paediatric patients use this mode of PD.

It is proposed that peritoneal membrane permeability changes with age, and mode of delivery should be modified accordingly (Mendley & Majkowski 1995). However, it is suggested that, as in adults, the best way to identify the optimum treatment is to perform peritoneal equilibrium tests (PETs; Warady et al 1996).

There are two main problems experienced with this type of dialysis.

- Parental/carer burnout is always an issue. Whenever possible, young adults are taught to do their own dialysis, with the support of another family member. However, with young patients there is a reliance on their relatives/carers to provide this treatment. Respite care provision should be made available, where possible.

- Infection is a major concern in the paediatric population. Peritonitis can quickly lead to systemic illness in very young children. There is also the long-term treatment of the child/young person to consider. Even if they are successfully transplanted, this patient group will usually face a return to dialysis at a later date. Therefore, it is very important to prevent sclerosis of the peritoneum due to either repeated or single severe peritonitis episodes, increasing the longevity of this type of dialysis. Changes in treatment modality may be required if a child has repeated peritonitis episodes (Andreoli et al 1999). Research into prevention and treatment is continuing as a result.

Periodic updating of families on technique may be required to prevent peritonitis, or repeated episodes. Young people and their families are trained to recognise early symptoms of infection to enable prompt treatment (RCN 2000).

A great difficulty can be in maintaining hygiene in infants wearing nappies, who do not understand that their catheter/line should be kept clean. Fasten-through vests and Tubigrip can be useful tools in preventing them from tampering with any type of access.

Haemodialysis

Haemodialysis is often the second choice, because of the disruption it causes. Less than 9% of children with ERD were treated with haemodialysis in 2004 (UK Renal Registry 2004). Children should be cared for in a specialist paediatric renal unit (Renal Association 2002). However, because of the very small numbers of children requiring this treatment, there are only 13 paediatric renal units in the UK. This inevitably leads to children travelling to receive this treatment. As a result, the psychosocial impact of haemodialysis can be considerable for children and their families.

Older children and young adults who dialyse 3–4 times a week are unable to attend school with their peers on dialysis days, so schooling should be provided for them whilst on dialysis. Pre-school children need distraction as well as play programmes to promote their global development.

Families need support, particularly those with children under 16, who must be transported with an escort each time they attend the hospital.

There can also be technical difficulties when using haemodialysis for children.

Venous access

Central lines are frequently used as a form of chronic access, particularly in children awaiting transplantation for which dialysis will hopefully be a relatively short-term treatment. A range of sizes is required for the patient group cared for in paediatric renal units. As with PD catheters, these lines can become infected (Shroff et al 2003) and can also become thombosed.

Arteriovenous fistulas are used, more for older patients with a longer-term need for dialysis. Play preparation and the use of anaesthetic creams are very important in these patients, as this is a painful procedure (Wright 2004). However, patient choice is important. Grafts are rarely used in paediatric patients in the UK.

The challenge in children is maintaining access sites for the future, which can become very problematic in children receiving renal replacement therapies from a very early age. Prevention of complications is very important, as indicated in the Renal NSF for children and young people (Department of Health 2006).

Prescribing dialysis and adequacy

Standardised treatment regimens cannot be used in patients on paediatric programmes. Guidelines on prescribing haemodialysis safely must be adhered to, to ensure adequate dialysis whilst preventing complications of overefficient dialysis such as disequilibrium. Common guidelines are a pump speed of 6–8 $mL\,min^{-1}\,kg^{-1}$, whilst not exceeding urea clearance of 3–5 $mL\,kg^{-1}$ (RCN 2000). It is also important to use a circuit of < 10% of the child's total circulating volume (Table 10.3). Therefore, a variety of line volumes and dialysers need to be available to meet these requirements.

Guidelines recommend initial treatment should use a dialyser with a surface area no more than 75% of the child's own surface area (Wright 2004). This is usually increased in size to achieve a urea reduction rate (URR) of at least 75%. *Kt/V* is a controversial measurement in children, although many units do use these tests as a measure of dialysis efficiency.

Careful consideration is also needed in guiding fluid removal on dialysis; 0.2 $mL\,min^{-1}\,kg^{-1}$ of fluid is the upper limit commonly used for guiding fluid removal whilst dialysing (RCN 2000). Additional fluid removal is undertaken via isolated ultrafiltration, sequentially followed by the prescribed dialysis. However, greater than a 10% reduction in fluid in one session is not advised (Fischbach et al 2005). Blood volume monitoring can be used to guide fluid removal and can be a useful tool in assessing dry weight (Michael et al 2004). Owing to the continual growth of children, it can be difficult to establish dry weight. Regular reviews are required to prevent frequent hypotensive episodes during dialysis.

ACUTE RENAL FAILURE

Acute renal failure (ARF) in childhood is less common than in adults. The incidence in childhood decreases with age and it is most common

Table 10.3 Blood volume calculation. (From Willock & Jewkes 2000)	
Neonates	90 $mL\,kg^{-1}$
Infants and children	80 $mL\,kg^{-1}$
Adults	65 $mL\,kg^{-1}$

in the neonatal period. ARF is recognised when renal excretory function declines rapidly. Rising urea and creatinine is usually accompanied by oliguria ($< 1\,mL\,kg^{-1}h^{-1}$) or occasionally polyuria (Strazdins et al 2004).

CAUSES

The causes of acute renal failure in childhood are commonly divided into three groups: prerenal, intrinsic and postrenal.

- *Prerenal disorders* are those that compromise renal perfusion, such as renal vein or renal artery thrombosis, shock and hypovolaemia. Cardiac insufficiency is the most common cause of ARF in infancy and is responsible for a mortality rate of 51% of infants following cardiac surgery (Renal Association 2002).
- *Intrinsic renal disorders* are those that occur following damage to renal parenchymal cells. These include malignancy, congenital malformation, glomerulonephritis, and the haemolytic–uraemic syndrome, which is the most common cause of ARF in older children.
- *Postrenal disorders* include urethral obstruction (valves, phimosis), ureteral obstruction and neurogenic bladder. These conditions require intervention by a paediatric urologist with nephrology liaison.

TREATMENT

There is no evidence for an optimum level of renal function for starting dialysis in children with acute renal failure, or for an optimum dialysis modality. The choice of renal replacement therapy depends on the circumstances, the skill of the nursing staff and the therapies available. Whilst not all children with ARF are referred to a paediatric renal centre, discussion with a paediatric nephrologist is recommended (Department of Health 2006). Indications for referral include oliguria, anuria, hyperkalaemia, hyponatraemia, acidosis or the need for blood transfusion (Strazdins et al 2004). Children with multiorgan failure should be transferred to a paediatric intensive care facility with nephrology support at the earliest opportunity.

Traditionally, peritoneal dialysis has been the treatment of choice for children with ARF. The advantage of PD is that it can be provided as a continuous therapy, which does not require vascular access. In addition, PD does not rely on specialist nursing expertise, although prior experience with this therapy is advisable if using an automated machine. For units without this expertise, manual PD sets for infants and children are available. Bicarbonate dialysis solutions should be considered for use in infants or children who have lactate intolerance.

Peritoneal dialysis in ARF must be commenced as soon as possible and there is a consequent risk of leakage. Small volumes of $10–20\,mL\,kg^{-1}$ ($300–600\,mL\,m^{-2}$) of continuous cycling therapy are recommended to prevent complications.

Haemodialysis is commonly used to treat children with ARF cared for within paediatric renal centres, when PD has failed or is contraindicated. Haemodialysis is suitable for rapid fluid and toxin removal. The disadvantages of this therapy are the need for vascular access, a water supply that is often only available within paediatric nephrology units, and the need for specialist nurses.

Haemofiltration is frequently used in intensive care units in children with multiorgan failure. However, the need for this therapy in children is rare compared with use in adults. The provision of this therapy in very small children can be technically challenging and skilled nursing staff are essential. In order that nurses maintain their skills in delivering this therapy, a continuous programme of nurse education is recommended (Harvey et al 2002).

Continuous venovenous haemofiltration (CV-VH) and continuous venovenous haemodiafiltration (CVVHDF) can be delivered to children using machinery that is adapted to provide low blood-pump speeds and ultrafiltration rates. Children require vascular access of a sufficient size to deliver appropriate blood flow through the filter. A dual-lumen central venous line of a minimum 6.5fg is recommended. Equipment must be calibrated to deliver blood-pump speeds as low as 20 mL min^{-1}. Recommended fluid removal should not exceed 0.02 mL kg^{-1}min^{-1}. As in haemodialysis, the extracorporeal circuit size should not exceed 10% of the child's circulating blood volume. In infants, regular blood priming is necessary if the line volume exceeds the child's extracorporeal volume.

HAEMOLYTIC–URAEMIC SYNDROME

The commonest cause of ARF in childhood is the haemolytic–uraemic syndrome (HUS). This disease is characterised by thrombocytopenia, haemolytic anaemia and renal failure. *Escherichia coli* (*E. coli*) 0157 bacteria cause approximately 90% of HUS cases. Children usually present with bloody diarrhoea, nausea and vomiting. Consequently, children with HUS are often misdiagnosed with surgical problems. Early investigation of renal function and blood film is essential, and transfer to a tertiary referral centre is recommended.

Approximately 50% of children with HUS require dialysis during the acute stage of the illness. Supportive treatment such as blood transfusion and treatment of hypertension is also required. A total of 70% of children with HUS recover renal function; however, approximately 25% need treatment for high blood pressure and chronic kidney disease management.

Atypical HUS may occur during childhood. This is associated with factor H deficiency (Fremeaux-Bacchi et al 2005). Children may present with the symptoms of renal failure but there is often no preceding diarrhoeal illness. Treatment is with regular plasma exchange or plasma infusion to prevent established kidney disease. The outlook for atypical HUS is poor, with disease recurrence in transplant kidneys (Bresin et al 2005). Liver and kidney transplant is considered an option.

TRANSITION TO ADULT SERVICES

Transition is a process preparing for the movement to adult services, of which transfer should be seen as the end-point. The concerns of both the young person and their family should not be underestimated. Many young people have been cared for in the paediatric unit since infancy, and it can be very difficult to face the move to a new team and unit (Watson 2006).

Transition can be approached using a number of models, including the use of joint clinics with both adult and paediatric staff present. A checklist can also be beneficial in ensuring that key issues are addressed in the preparation process (RCN 2004). Youth work input is invaluable in the transition process and can assist in the development of health- and non-health-related competencies such as sexual health.

It is especially stressful when the young adult is dialysis dependent, particularly on haemodialysis. The differences in adult and paediatric units are not just in approach and focus of care, but also in physical size and number of patients. Patients on haemodialysis benefit from prior visits to the adult unit, so they are able to adjust to this in advance.

There is no 'gold standard' model for transition and transfer. However, it is important that these are well planned, and completed in partnership with the young adults and their family.

CONCLUSION

As this chapter has highlighted, providing treatment for children with renal disorders has different challenges from those for the adult population. In addition to treating the renal-associated complications, there are the additional issues around growth, development and the psychosocial impact on the whole family.

The Renal NSF 'Working for Children and Young People' (Department of Health 2006) identifies standards for care and markers for good practice in the service provision for these patients. The challenge for all paediatric nephrology services is to ensure that these standards are achieved, and that the highest quality of care is provided for these children and young people.

References

Andreoli SP, Leiser J, Warady BA, Schlichting L, Brewer ED, Watkins SL. Adverse effects of peritonitis on peritoneal membrane function in children on dialysis. Pediatr Nephrol 1999; 13: 1–6.

Baluarte HJ, Graskin AB, Inglefinger JR, Stablein D, Tijani A. Analysis of hypertension in children post renal transplantation: a report of North American Renal Transplant Cooperative Study. Paediat Nephrol 1997; 8: 570–573.

Batte S, Watson AR, Amess K. The effects of chronic renal failure on siblings. Pediatr Nephrol 2006; 21: 246–250.

Bell F Assessment and management of the child with nephrotic syndrome. Paediatr Nurs 2002; 14: 37–42.

Bresin E, Daina, E, Noris, M et al. Outcome of renal transplantation in patients with non-shiga toxin-associated hemolytic uremic syndrome: prognostic significance of genetic background. Clin J Am Soc Nephrol 2005; 1: 88–89.

British Association of Paediatric Nephrologists (BAPN). Review of multi-professional paediatric nephrology services in the UK – towards standards and equity of care. BAPN, Bristol, 2003.

Coleman J. The kidney. In: Shaw V, Lawson M, eds. Clinical paediatric dietetics, 2nd edn. Oxford: Blackwell Science, 2001: 158–181.

Coleman J, Watson A, Rance C, Moore E. Gastrostomy buttons for nutritional support in chronic dialysis. Nephrol Dial Transplant 1998; 13: 2041–2046.

Department of Health The national service framework for renal services: working for children and young people. London: Department of Health, 2006.

Department of Health. Department for Education and Skills: national service framework for children, young people and maternity services. Core standards. London: Stationery Office, 2004.

Dillion MJ. Blood pressure. Arch Dis Child 1998; 63: 347–349.

El-Mekresh M. Renal transplantation in children. Br J Urol 2000; 85: 979–986.

Fischbach M, Edefonti A, Schröder C, Watson A. Hemodialysis in children: general practical guidelines. Pediatr Nephrol 2005; 20: 1054–1066.

Fremeaux-Bacci V, Kemp E, Goodship J et al. The development of atypical HUS is influenced by susceptibility factors in factor H and membrane cofactor protein – evidence from two independent cohorts. JMG online. 2005. Available from http://jmg.bmjjournals.com/cgi/content/abstract/jmg.2005.030783v1 (accessed August 2006).

Harvey B, Watson AR, Jepson S. A renal critical care educator: The interface between paediatric intensive care and nephrology. Intensive Crit Care Nurs 2002; 18 (40): 250–254.

Hilton D, Watson AR, Walmsley P, Jepson S. Youth work in hospital. Paediatr Nurs 2004; 16: 36–39.

Hingorani S, Watkins SL. Dialysis for end-stage disease. Curr Opin Pediatr 2000; 12: 140–145.

Hodson EM, Knight JF, Willis NF, Craig JC. Corticosteroid therapy for nephrotic syndrome in children (Cochrane review). The Cochrane Library 2002; Issue 3. The Oxford Update.

Klaus G, Watson A, Edefonti A et al. Prevention and treatment of renal osteodystrophy in children on chronic renal failure: European guidelines. Pediatr Nephrol 2006; 21: 151–159.

MacGregor J. Introduction to the anatomy and physiology of children. London: Routledge, 2000.

Mendley SR, Majowski NL. Peritoneal equilibrium test results are different in infants, children, and adults. J Am Soc Nephrol 1995; 6: 1309–1312.

Michael M, Brewer ED, Goldstein SL. Blood volume monitoring to achieve target weight in pediatric hemodialysis patients. Pediatr Nephrol 2004; 19: 432–437.

Miller D, Macdonald D, Kolnacki K, Simek T. Challenges for nephrology nurses in the management of children with chronic kidney disease. Nephrol Nurs J 2004; 31: 287–294.

Moore E, Collier J, Evans J, Watson AR. The need to know: information needs of parents of children with nephrotic syndrome. Child Health 1995; 2(4): 147–149.

National High Blood Pressure Education Program. Working Group on High Blood Pressure in Children and Adolescents: The fourth report on the diagnosis, evaluation and treatment of high blood pressure in children and adolescents. Pediatrics 2004; 114: 555–576.

National Institute for Health and Clinical Excellence (NICE). Immunosuppressive therapy for renal transplantation in children and adolescents. London: NICE, 2006.

O'Brien E, Waeber B, Parati G, Staessen J, Myers MG. Blood pressure measurement devices: recommendations of the European Society of Hypertension. BMJ 2001; 322: 532–536.

O'Brien ET, Petrie JC, Littler WA et al. Blood pressure measurement: recommendations of the British Hypertension Society, 3rd edn. London: BMJ Publishing Group, 1997.

Renal Association. Treatment of adults and children with renal failure. Standards and audit measures. London: Royal College of Physicians, 2002.

Royal College of Nursing (RCN). Paediatric nephrology nursing: guidance for nurses. London: RCN, 2000.

Royal College of Nursing (RCN). Adolescent transition care: guidance for nursing staff. London: RCN, 2004.

Royal College of Paediatrics and Child Health (RCPCH). Immunisation of the immunocompromised child: best practice statement. London: RCPCH, 2002.

Sedman A, Friedman A, Boineau F, Strife CF, Fine R. Nutritional management of the child with mild to moderate chronic renal failure. J Pediatr 1996; 129: 14s–18s.

Shaw V, Lawson M. Principles of paediatric dietetics. In: Shaw V, Lawson M, eds. Clinical paediatric dietetics, 2nd edn. Oxford: Blackwell Science, 2001: 3–18.

Shroff R, Wright E, Ledermann S, Hutchinson C, Rees L. Chronic hemodialysis in infants and children under two years of age. Pediatr Nephrol 2003; 18: 378–383.

Sorof J, Portman RJ. Ambulatory blood pressure monitoring in the pediatric patient. J Pediatr 2000; 136: 578–586.

Strazdins V, Watson AR, Harvey B. Replacement therapy for acute renal failure in children: European Guidelines. On behalf of the European Peritoneal Dialysis working group. Pediatr Nephrol 2004; 19: 199–207.

Szromba C, Thies MA, Ossman SS. Advancing chronic kidney disease care: new imperatives for recognition and intervention. Nephrol Nurs J 2002; 29: 547–559.

Tenbrock K, Muller-Berghaus J, Michalk D, Querfeld U. Intravenous iron treatment of renal anemia in children on hemodialysis. Pediatr Nephrol 1999; 13: 580–582.

UK Renal Registry. UK Renal Registry report 2004: the seventh annual report. London: The Renal Association & UK Renal Registry, 2004.

UK Transplant. Kidney allocation 2006. Available from: www.uktransplant.org.uk/ukt/about_transplants/ organ_allocation/kidney (accessed August 2006).

UK Transplant. Pre-emptive transplantation 2005. Available from: www.uktransplant.org.uk/ukt/about_transplants (accessed March 2006).

Waby K, Helm K, Watson AR. Preparing children for kidney transplantation through play. Bri J Renal Med 2005; 10: 9–11.

Warady BA, Alexander SR, Hossli S et al. Peritoneal membrane transport function in children receiving long-term dialysis. J Am Soc Nephrol 1996; 7: 2385–2391.

Watson AR. Transition from paediatric to adult renal care. Business briefing: European kidney and urological disease. London: Touch Briefings, 2006.

Webb NJA, Johnson R, Postlethwaite R. Renal transplantation. Arch Dis Child 2003; 88: 844–847.

Willock J, Jewkes F. Making sense of fluid balance in children. Paediatr Nurs 2000; 12(7): 37–42.

Wright E. Assessment and management of the child requiring chronic haemodialysis. Paediatr Nurs 2004; 16(7): 37–41.

Chapter 11

Renal nutrition

Barbara Engel

LEARNING OUTCOMES FOR THIS CHAPTER	■ To describe the historical background to renal nutrition and dietetics ■ To evaluate nutritional management in the predialysis phase ■ To identify the dietary principles of haemodialysis and peritoneal dialysis ■ To discuss the role of the nurse in giving dietary advice as part of the multiprofessional team

INTRODUCTION

Dietary treatment has always been regarded as an important part of treating patients with established renal failure (ERF), before and during renal replacement therapy (RRT). During the 1960s many patients were treated with diet alone. The renal diet was adapted to dialysis and transplantation once these modes of RRT became available during the 1970s and early 1980s. Nowadays, chronic fluid overload, hyperphosphataemia and protein energy malnutrition are amongst the most common problems. These can lead to long-term complications if not resolved, and adversely affect outcome of treatment and the quality of life of patients with renal diseases on decades of chronic treatment. This chapter will address the important issues of dietary management and the role it plays in the overall treatment of ERF.

HISTORICAL REVIEW OF DIETARY MANAGEMENT

PRE-DIALYSIS TREATMENT (1960–2000)

Haemodialysis (HD) was only accepted as a regular form of RRT for selected patients at the end of the 1960s. Prior to this period, patients approaching ERF with gastrointestinal symptoms were advised to follow a very low protein diet (VLPD). The best known diet was the Giovanetti diet, containing 20 g protein of high biological value to cover essential amino acid requirements. An intake of 50 kcal kg^{-1} body weight (BW) was recommended to prevent loss of muscle and maintain nitrogen balance (Berlyne 1968). This diet was prescribed to selected patients with a creatinine clearance of 3 ml min^{-1} or a plasma urea level of 33 mmol L^{-1} (200 mg dL^{-1}) and was the only treatment available to improve the well-being of patients, until regular HD treatment became available.

It became apparent in later years that a badly managed protein-restricted diet contributed to malnutrition before starting HD, and that this prolonged the rehabilitation period and also contributed to the outcome of treatment, with an increased morbidity and mortality.

During the 1980s there was a renewed interest in protein allowance as partially nephrectomised rats showed protein restriction delayed the progression of renal disease. This was the hyperfiltration/hyper-perfusion hypothesis (Brenner 1983). It was more difficult to prove the same effect in humans. High-energy diets containing no more than 0.6 g protein kg^{-1} BW were prescribed during the early stages of chronic renal disease to asymptomatic patients who not surprisingly found this difficult to follow for extended periods of time.

In the United States, the National Institutes of Health (NIH) stated in 1993 that the nutritional health of a patient prior to dialysis was an important indicator of outcome and that all patients were entitled to receive a nutritional assessment by a trained renal dietitian. In the absence of obvious malnutrition, a moderate low-protein diet of up to 0.7–0.8 g protein kg^{-1} BW day^{-1} should be prescribed. When malnutrition was present, the amount of energy was increased and the amount of protein raised to 1.0–1.2 g kg^{-1} to allow for nutritional repletion or to counter the catabolic effects of stress. Dietary prescriptions should also include guidelines for energy, fat and carbohydrate, fluid, sodium, phosphate and potassium as well as other nutrients and micronutrients (NIH 1993) – a comprehensive review in fact. The NIH had also commissioned a large multicentre study to ascertain once and for all the efficacy of low-protein diets. The Modification of Diet in Renal Disease (MDRD) study compared diets with different levels of protein restriction at different levels of renal impairment. The diets ranged from usual intake to VLPD supplemented with ketoacids and combined with phosphorus restriction. The results of this 2-year study, which had been launched in 1985, were finally published in 1994 (Klahr et al 1994).

The MDRD study showed that, in the absence of severe proteinuria and hypertension, a reduction of protein intake by 0.2 g kg^{-1} BW resulted in a modest reduction in the rate of progression. There appeared to be no further advantage in using a VLPD supplemented with essential amino acids. However, it did reveal that subjects accustomed to a 'western' diet containing typically > 1.2 g protein kg^{-1} found it very difficult to achieve the designated protein restrictions of < 0.6 g protein kg^{-1} day^{-1}. The report cautioned that, while lowering blood pressure and protein intake appears to be safe, both must be carefully monitored.

Several meta-analyses were subsequently conducted, which included studies such as the MDRD study. Fouque et al (2000), Pedrini et al (1996) and Ginn et al (1999) concluded that dietary protein restriction effectively slows the progression of diabetic and non-diabetic renal disease (see also ongoing Cochrane reviews: www.cochrane-renal.org). On the basis of these analyses as well as expert opinion, the NKF/DOQI published the 'Clinical practice guidelines for nutrition in chronic renal failure' (Kopple et al 2000) and the European Dialysis and Transplant Nurses Association/ European Renal Care Association (EDTNA/ERCA; 2002) also published guidelines shortly afterwards. The suggested protein and energy requirements for patients with advanced chronic kidney disease (CKD), not on dialysis, are summarized in Table 11.1. These take the patient's ideal body weight (IBW; see Appendix 11.1 for calculation) as well as the residual renal function into consideration.

The debate about whether to restrict protein and how low to go continues to this day. In support of protein restriction, a low-protein diet will reduce the burden of waste products that have to be removed: nitrogen compounds, acids, phosphate and also potassium. This potentially has beneficial effects on reducing symptoms of uraemia and controlling the development of problems such as acidosis and renal bone disease (Mandayam & Mitch 2006).

The main deleterious effect of the low-protein diet is the risk of malnutrition; energy requirements are difficult to meet (although not impossible) without resorting to sources of carbohydrate and fat, which may have an impact on cardiovascular disease (CVD). Vitamin and mineral intakes also have to be monitored closely. Those clinicians not in favour of low-protein diets argue that the risk of malnutrition outweighs any benefits that may be gained from the (very moderate) reduction in the rate of decline in kidney function (Johnson 2006). Even the most recent Cochrane review concluded that the optimal level of protein prescription could still not be confirmed (Fouque et al 2006).

As there are many different elements to patient care prior to starting dialysis, a more realistic approach to protein recommendations is usually taken which is described below.

Table 11.1 Suggested protein and energy requirements versus degree of renal function

GFR (mL min⁻¹)	Protein (g kg⁻¹ IBW)[a]	Energy (kcal kg⁻¹ IBW)
> 50	Normalise	30–35
25–50	0.6–1.0[a]	30–35
< 25	0.6–0.75[a]	30– 35
< 10 start dialysis		

GFR glomerular filtration rate; IBW, ideal body weight.
[a] Protein should contain at least 50% sources of high biological value: 35 kcal kg⁻¹ IBW for active patients and 30 kcal kg⁻¹ IBW for sedentary or older patients, i.e., > 65 years of age.

CURRENT CONCEPTS OF PREDIALYSIS DIETARY INTERVENTION

The nutritional content of the diet should be specifically adapted to each patient's individual needs and personal circumstances. This should result in the reduction of accumulated metabolic waste products, which can be controlled as chronic disease progresses. The following are important in the dietary therapy of conservative management and are, in fact, identical to the list drawn up by the NIH (1993; Box 11.1):

Box 11.1   Dietary aspects of conservative management of chronic renal failure: daily intake

Protein	0.75–1.0 g kg^{-1} IBW 50% HBV
Energy	30–35 kcal kg^{-1} IBW or use Schofield equations with activity factor if weight changes are desirable
Fat	< 35% energy reduce SFA, increase PUFA and MUFA
Carbohydrate	50% of energy: decrease monosaccharides, increase sources of soluble and insoluble fibre
Phosphorus	19–31 mmol (600–1000 mg)
Sodium	80–110 mmol (1800–2500 mg)
Potassium	Approx. 1.0 mmol kg^{-1} IBW (with hyperkalaemia)
Minerals	Calcium, iron, zinc
Vitamins	Water-soluble vitamin supplements if needed

HBV, high biological value; MUFA, monounsaturated fatty acids; PUFA, polyunsaturated fatty acids; SFA, saturated fatty acids.

The Renal Association Guidelines (2002) include the following in their 'key elements of care' for the management of patients approaching ERF, all of which have dietary implications:

- malnutrition
- hypertension
- anaemia
- prevention of disordered calcium/phosphate metabolism
- acidosis
- hyperlipidaemia
- glucose control in diabetics
- hyperkalaemia (included for completeness).

MALNUTRITION

Irrespective of whether a therapeutic diet is recommended to treat any of the other problems listed above, all patients at CKD 4–5 should receive a dietary assessment and be screened for malnutrition. This is because a spontaneous decrease in protein intake has been measured in patients with renal diseases as the disease progresses (Ikizler et al 1995). A patient with poor nutritional status at the start of dialysis will have a poor outcome in terms of survival (Churchill 1997) and therefore it is important to prevent malnutrition from occurring at the outset (Walters et al 2002). Some expert nephrologists have recommended that if the patient's protein intake has fallen below $0.8\,g\,kg^{-1}\,day^{-1}$, dialysis should be initiated (Hakim & Lazarus 1995).

Regular dietary follow-up in clinic or by telephone should help to maintain optimal nutritional status by ensuring that a balanced diet is being achieved, i.e. containing adequate macronutrients (protein, fat, carbohydrate) and micronutrients (vitamins and minerals). If specific dietary restrictions are advocated, it is important that the impact of these restrictions on the intake of other nutrients and the social effects are fully evaluated. The diet should provide sufficient dietary freedom and enable the patient to lead a near-normal life. This means that dietary flexibility must be incorporated, and relatives or friends involved while educating the patient to promote maximum dietary compliance.

PROTEIN

Protein is an important nutrient for the repair and maintenance of tissue and for growth.

Quantity

The level of dietary protein intake should maintain nitrogen balance (in a well-nourished adult) or be sufficient for growth (in children) and repair (in patients recovering from malnutrition or illness). For instance, if a patient consumes a high-protein diet ($>1.2\,g\,kg^{-1}$ IBW), a reduction to $1.0\,g\,kg^{-1}$ IBW may initially be sufficient, which can be reduced to $0.8\,g\,kg^{-1}$ IBW if renal function deteriorates at a later stage. This is an acceptable degree of protein allowance for long-term use and it meets the maintenance requirement of $0.66\,g\,kg^{-1}$ advised by World Health Organisation (WHO)/Food and Agriculture Organisation (FAO) (Millward & Jackson 2003). The Renal Association (2002) recommended that a protein intake of no less than $0.75\,g\,kg^{-1}$ is realistic and needs to be combined with an energy intake of $35\,kcal\,kg^{-1}\,day^{-1}$ to prevent malnutrition.

Quality

The quality of protein is affected by its digestibility and amino-acid content. Meat, fish, eggs and milk score highly for content of the essential amino acid lysine, and are usually referred to as containing high biological value (HBV) protein. Soy protein is also considered HBV. The quality of an UK vegetarian diet is affected by digestibility but the amino-acid content is comparable with UK omnivores. Rice-based vegetarian diets have poorer amino-acid content (compared to wheat-based diets) as well as lower digestibility. In order to ensure a reduced-protein diet contains adequate levels of all the amino acids, it is particularly important for vegetarians to have proteins from a variety of sources including cereals, pulses and legumes (Millward & Jackson 2003).

In addition to the slightly slower rate of progression discussed above, an improvement in well-being has been noted, often with a corresponding decrease in serum urea and creatinine levels (urea is the breakdown product of the amino acids, and creatinine is the breakdown product of creatine). Some patients notice that mild symptoms like 'morning sickness' and a 'metallic taste' in the mouth disappear. Surprisingly perhaps, quality of life is maintained and perceived energy levels have been noted to improve (Hart et al 1992).

The effect of a reduced protein diet

ENERGY

Protein, fat, carbohydrate and alcohol all contribute to a person's energy intake.

Insufficient energy intake will lead to protein catabolism, which may present as muscle wasting. Fat stores will also be used to provide energy, which initially may not be a problem, particularly if the patient is obese. The advantages of not having excess body fat include a decreased risk of CVD, hypertension and diabetes. Formation of a fistula or insertion of a Tenckhoff is also more difficult in obese patients. However, fat is used to insulate the body, provide cushioning for bones and has hormonal roles. Recent evidence has shown that, while being underweight increases mortality in dialysis patients, being overweight may actually confer some advantage, at least in the first few years of dialysis (Friedman 2006). This is reflected in the Kidney Disease Quality Outcomes Initiative (K/DOQI) guidelines (2003a), which have stated that a body mass index (BMI) of up to $28 \, kg \, m^{-2}$ is acceptable.

Quantity

Example:

To calculate energy requirements for a 70 kg person (IBW):

$$70 \times 30\text{--}35 \, kcal \, (126\text{--}150 \, kJ) = 2100\text{--}2450 \, kcal \, (8.8\text{--}10.3 \, MJ)$$

The range of energy requirements ($30\text{--}35 \, kcal \, kg^{-1}$) is similar to the result obtained using the Schofield equations for basal metabolic rate and assumes a physical activity level of 1.3–1.4, which is low (Todorovic & Micklewright 2004). Patients with increased metabolism due to infection, injury or increased activity levels should have their requirements calculated using equations such as Schofield with appropriate stress and activity factors added.

Quality

The quality of foods providing energy is as important as the quantity. Cardiovascular disease and some cancers are associated with a high proportion of saturated fat in the diet. Hypertriglyceridaemia (common in patients with renal diseases) is associated with high intakes of rapidly absorbable carbohydrates and alcohol. The ideal balance of the macronutrients is described in Box 11.1. If a protein restriction has been advised, there has to be an increase in calories to make up the deficit. This could take the form of monounsaturated fat (olive oil) and carbohydrates with a medium to low glycaemic index (pasta, basmati rice, new boiled potatoes, some fruits).

MICRONUTRIENTS: VITAMINS AND MINERALS

Vitamins and minerals regulate metabolic pathways and some of the most observable clinical features of uraemia (anaemia and renal bone disease) are caused or at least exacerbated by vitamin and mineral deficiencies. Metabolism of protein, carbohydrate and fat will be affected by deficiencies of vitamins and minerals. These can arise because uraemia alters their serum levels and body stores and also interferes with their function. Drug interactions can affect the absorption of minerals (such as calcium, iron, zinc and magnesium) and the activity of vitamins (such as B6, folate and B12). Requirements for these three vitamins may be higher in renal disease in order to treat hyperhomocysteinaemia, which is a risk factor for CVD (Hong et al 1998). Dietary restrictions which limit protein, phosphate and potassium intake will inevitably limit the intake of various micronutrients. A low-protein diet can contain low levels of B vitamins (B1, B2, B6, B12), iron, calcium and zinc (Hadfield 1992). A low-potassium diet will limit intake of folic acid, vitamins C and E as well as phytochemicals, such as fructo-oligosaccharides, phytosterols and polyphenols.

On the other hand, there may be reduced renal losses of some nutrients. Vitamin supplements containing the fat-soluble vitamins A, D, E and K are contraindicated in patients with renal failure. Vitamin A metabolites are less well excreted and accumulate over time; toxicity has been reported in patients receiving total parenteral nutrition containing a high dose of vitamin A (Muth 1991). High-dose vitamin E supplementation may potentially disrupt the clotting mechanisms. Vitamin K supplementation is also contraindicated unless a patient is on chronic antibiotic treatment (Rocco & Makoff 1997). It is recommended that vitamin and mineral status should be part of a patient's regular nutritional assessment.

HYPERTENSION

Sodium (Na) and fluid retention occurs in most types of renal disease and contributes to high blood pressure. The Renal Association guidelines (2002) recommend that to improve blood pressure control, patients should be advised to reduce dietary salt and alcohol intake, stop smoking and take regular exercise. Medication such as diuretics and angiotensin-converting enzyme (ACE) inhibitors control fluid retention by increasing urinary Na and fluid excretion.

A moderate salt-reduced diet (about 80–120 mmol Na) will facilitate the action of antihypertensive medication. In practice this is not simple, as many people rely on the purchase of processed foods (Appendix 11.2). About 80% of our salt intake is hidden in processed foods, including staple food items such as bread and breakfast cereals. Patients should be advised as follows.

- Prepare meals using fresh ingredients.
- Use spices and herbs to add flavour to food.
- Only use a little salt in meal preparation.
- Avoid adding salt to food after preparation.
- Avoid excessive amounts of salty foods, such as cured and processed foods: this includes take-away meals (see Appendix 11.2).
- Avoid using salt substitutes containing potassium salts, such as potassium chloride (KCl): see 'Hyperkalaemia' section.
- Avoid meals prepared with monosodium glutamate. This is added to enhance the taste of food in restaurants, take-away outlets and ready-to-eat meals sold in supermarkets.
- Read food labels and check for additives, such as monosodium glutamate and salt substitutes. (NB 1 mmol Na = 23 mg Na; 2 g (2000 mg) Na = 5 g NaCl = 90 mmol Na).

Some patients are 'salt losers' (i.e. they lose salt easily) and need to add salt to their meals and/or use salt supplements such as slow sodium.

ANAEMIA

Anaemia can impact on general nutritional status by causing general lethargy, taste changes and a poor appetite. It is also involved in the pathogenesis of left ventricular hypertrophy (LVH) and therefore increases the risk of CVD. A serum ferritin of $< 100\,ng\,mL^{-1}$ or a transferrin saturation of $< 20\%$ indicates relative iron deficiency. It is important to ensure an adequate intake of iron, B12 and folate. Vitamins B6 and C also have important roles in erythropoiesis. The consumption of foods that are high in iron, such as red meat, offal and pulses may be reduced in a renal diet, particularly if protein- or phosphate-restricted diets have been prescribed. A potassium lowering diet may result in a decrease of iron, folate and vitamin C.

If oral iron supplements are used, $200–300\,mg$ Fe day^{-1} is required to restore iron status. These can cause side-effects such as constipation and black stools. They can also interact with other medication, such as the calcium-containing phosphate binders. In order to obtain a rapid improvement in iron status, intravenous preparations are more often used. This is discussed in more detail in Chapter 5.

CALCIUM, PHOSPHATE AND VITAMIN D METABOLISM

The pathophysiology of renal bone disease (RBD) is discussed in Chapter 2 and overall management is discussed in Chapter 5. As shown in Table 11.2, the first signs of impaired calcium (Ca) and phosphate (P) homeostasis arise early in renal impairment (CKD 2) as parathyroid hormone levels start to rise. This is due to phosphate retention and impaired hydroxylation (activation) of vitamin D, which results in reduced absorption of Ca

Table 11.2 Stages of renal dysfunction. (Reproduced from CKD: management strategies: MS Parmar: www.uninet.edu/cin2003/conf/parmar/parmar.html)

Stage	Description	Creatinine clearance (≈GFR) (mL min^{-1} 1.73 m^{-3})	Metabolic components
1	Normal or increased GFR Persons at *increased risk* or with *early renal damage*	> 90	
2	Early renal insufficiency (ERI)	60–89[a]	Parathyroid hormone level starts to rise (GFR ≈ 60–80)
3	Moderate renal failure (CRF)	30–59	Decrease in calcium absorption (GFR < 50) Lipoprotein activity falls Malnutrition Onset of left ventricular hypertrophy Onset of anaemia (erythropoietin deficiency)
4	Severe renal failure (pre-ESRD)	15–29	Triglyceride levels start to rise Hyperphosphataemia Metabolic acidosis Hyperkalaemia tendency
5	ESRD (uraemia)	< 15	Azotaemia develops

GFR, glomerular filtration rate.
[a] May be normal for age.

from food in the gut. The ensuing hypocalcaemia stimulates an increased release of parathyroid hormone, which, in an attempt to normalise plasma calcium levels, releases calcium and phosphate from the bone (eventually causing weakened bones). As renal disease progresses, the release of calcium and phosphate from the bone and reduced excretion of phosphate in the urine leads to hyperphosphataemia.

Treatment at these various stages can include the use of: calcium supplements, activated forms of vitamin D (alfacalcidol and calcitriol), dietary phosphate restriction and phosphate binders (Sexton & Vincent 2004).

Calcium supplements

The recommended daily Ca intake for predialysis patients is 1000–1500 mg. If this is not being reached (particularly if protein intake is low), calcium supplements may be needed but should be taken in between meals, preferably at bedtime to maximize Ca absorption.

'Active' vitamin D

Vitamin D is a fat-soluble vitamin and is obtained from food and also from exposure to sunlight (this may be reduced in the elderly and certain ethnic groups). It needs to be converted to an active form by hydroxylation in the liver and kidney. The use of active forms of vitamin D, alfacalcidol and calcitriol, can be a double-edged sword. On the one hand, they reduce parathyroid hormone (PTH) levels (which will reduce the negative effects on bone) but simultaneously calcium and phosphate absorption from the gut increases, which can lead to hypercalcaemia and hyperphosphataemia if not monitored closely. The precipitation of this excess calcium and phosphate in the soft tissues (blood vessels, coronary arteries and aortic valves) is considered to be one of the major causes of morbidity and mortality in adults, particularly young adults, with renal failure (Block et al 1998, Goodman et al 2000).

Dietary phosphate restriction

The Renal Association has advised that 'patients need dietary advice to restrict dietary phosphate'. Although the optimal time to start phosphate restriction/binders has not been established, the K/DOQI (2003) guidelines recommend that:

> Dietary phosphorus should be restricted to 800 to 1000 mg day^{-1} (adjusted for dietary protein needs) when the serum phosphorus levels are elevated (1.49 mmol L^{-1} (> 4.6 mg dL^{-1})) at Stages 3 and 4 of CKD, and > 1.78 mmol L^{-1} (5.5 mg dL^{-1}) in those with kidney failure (Stage 5).

A reduction in dietary phosphate allowance should also be initiated when levels of intact PTH are elevated above the target range of the CKD stage. The aim is to maintain serum phosphate < 1.8 mmol L^{-1}.

Calcium and phosphate are obtained from most foods with a high-protein content. Examples are milk and its products: cheese and yogurt. Phosphorus also appears in high-fibre cereal products and fish with edible bones, offal, pulses and nuts.

Appendix 11.3 lists high-phosphorus foods, not all of which have alternatives with comparable nutrient content and, therefore, total elimination from the diet is not feasible. Hyperphosphataemia is difficult to control by dietary manipulation alone and needs to be combined with phosphate binders. A moderate protein restriction will also tend to reduce phosphate intake, which is one of the arguments in favour of a protein restriction in the predialysis population. However, the impact on other nutrients must always be considered. For example, wholemeal products contain more phosphorus as well as fibre. Fibre improves bowel habits and the general well-being of patients. Serum phosphate levels may rise (0.25 mmol L^{-1}) with a high-fibre diet (Pender 1989); however, the benefits of a high-fibre intake outweigh the risk of hyperphosphataemia and, if necessary, phosphate binding agents can be increased.

Phosphate binders

Phosphate binding occurs in the stomach and small intestine, and reduces the absorption of phosphate into the body. Calcium and aluminium salts are used as these initially dissolve in the acid environment of the stomach and then form an insoluble precipitate with phosphate. This product is eliminated via the gastrointestinal route. Phosphate binders should be taken with food, particularly as main meals and snacks containing phosphate, and with milk-based nutritional supplements. Ideally, the dose of the binder can be altered to reflect the phosphate content in a particular meal.

A high gastric pH (i.e. less acidic), which is found generally in the elderly and particularly in people taking H2-receptor antagonists, such as ranitidine, can reduce the effectiveness of the binders and hyperphosphataemia can result (Tan et al 1996).

Both the calcium and aluminium in the binder are absorbed to some extent, and this has given rise to worries about aluminium toxicity and calcium overload. Therefore, new phosphate binders are being developed, such as sevelamer hydrochloride (Renagel), which does not contain calcium or aluminium and has an added benefit in that it also binds cholesterol.

HYPERLIPIDAEMIA

Hyperlipidaemia is one of the risk factors contributing to the high incidence of CVD in patients with renal diseases. The other factors include calcium and phosphorus imbalance, hyperhomocysteinaemia, inflammation and anaemia. Recommendations from the K/DOQI (2003a) guidelines were that CKD was a high risk factor for CVD and that 'major findings from randomized trials in the general population are applicable to patients with CKD, until proven otherwise'. In practice, this means that for triglycerides > 5.6 mmol L^{-1} (500 mg dL^{-1}) and low-density lipoprotein (LDL)> 2.6 mmol L^{-1} (100 mg dL^{-1}), therapeutic lifestyle changes (TLC) should be implemented in the first instance for 2–3 months. For high triglycerides, a fibrate or niacin can be considered, for high LDL cholesterol a statin can be started if LDL > 3.4 (130 mg dL^{-1}) or TLC fails to reduce the cholesterol levels. The Renal Association (2002) also recommend lifestyle changes in the predialysis group in order to improve cardiovascular mortality, this includes weight loss where necessary, lower salt intake and regular exercise.

More studies are needed to elucidate the role of diet, exercise and weight reduction in reducing the risk of CVD in patients with CKD.

GLUCOSE CONTROL IN PATIENTS WITH DIABETES

The results of the Diabetes Control and Complications Trial (DCCT), and the UK Prospective Diabetes Study (UKPDS) showed that careful control of blood glucose and hypertension significantly decreases the renal complications of diabetes (Delahanty 1998, UKPDS 1998, Yale 2005). Drugs to control hyperglycaemia will need to be adjusted regularly as requirements may diminish as renal function declines.

A Cochrane review has supported the use of protein restriction to slow down the progression of nephropathy in Type 1 diabetics (Waugh & Robertson 1997), the same level of evidence does not exist for Type 2 diabetes (CARI guidelines 2005). With the rising levels of diabetes in the population there needs to be a concerted effort in primary care to prevent nephrology services from being overwhelmed with patients who have diabetes.

HYPERKALAEMIA

Plasma potassium levels are tightly controlled and, in order to maintain normal levels, 90% of potassium is usually excreted by the kidney with the remainder excreted via the gastrointestinal route. Progressive renal failure is often complicated by hyperkalaemia (plasma potassium > 5 mmol L^{-1}) and may occur when renal function has declined to a GFR of 5 mL min^{-1} despite normal urine output. Hyperkalaemia can also occur at an earlier stage when patients receive ACE inhibitors for blood pressure control. This can be exacerbated if combined with a high intake of potassium-rich foods and is potentially life threatening, particularly as it is not associated with physical warning signs and requires immediate treatment. Dietary and non-dietary causes of hyperkalaemia should be investigated at the same time (Bansal 1992).

Examples of non dietary causes are:

- metabolic acidosis
- increased catabolism (and conditions which cause cell destruction: rhabdomyolysis, gastrointestinal bleed)
- endocrine abnormalities
- drugs such as potassium supplements (i.e. slow K), some laxatives, potassium-sparing diuretics, ACE inhibitors and non-steroidal anti-inflammatory drugs
- constipation (and drugs that exacerbate constipation, e.g. iron tablets).

Dietary management

Dietary sources of potassium are listed in Appendix 11.4. A dietary intake of no more than 60-70 mmol/d (1 mmol/kg IBW) is sufficient to prevent or treat hyperkalaemia in the presence of an adequate urine output or dialysis treatment. However serum K levels, in anuric non-dialysed patients taking a 50 mmol potassium diet, can rise by 1 mmol/d despite gastrointestinal adaptation to increase potassium excretion (Bansal 1992).

Most foods contain potassium, but vegetables and fruits are major sources: some varieties contain more than others. Staple foods such as potatoes, yam, sweet potatoes, green bananas and plantain are high in potassium, but should be included in a potassium-reduced diet. Potassium-containing salts, such as dipotassium phosphate, are used as food additives but in small quantities. Of greater concern is the use of potassium chloride as a substitute for sodium chloride, as part of the food manufacturers' attempt to reduce the sodium content of food.

Patients should receive dietary advice regarding the potassium content of specific foods, avoiding or at least limiting the quantities eaten of those that are high. Cooking techniques such as boiling (and throwing away the water) will remove some of the potassium in vegetables. Cooking methods that *retain* potassium include cooking in a pressure cooker or microwave, stir-frying, roasting and casseroling vegetables.

Potassium and high-fibre foods

Constipation is a common problem for patients on peritoneal dialysis (PD), older and sedentary patients. High-fibre cereal products are recommended to prevent constipation and can have a beneficial effect on hyperlipidaemia. Some high-fibre foods are high in potassium (Pagenkemper et al 1994), although earlier studies showed that the overall effect of a high-fibre diet on serum potassium was not significant – about 0.3 mmol L^{-1} (McKenzie & Henderson 1986).

Potassium exchange resins

Potassium binders, such as calcium or sodium ion-exchange resin (i.e. calcium or sodium resonium), may be used to control hyperkalaemia. Calcium resonium is a gritty textured powder and is best taken with a sweet drink to mask its taste, although it can be administered rectally. Calcium ions (or sodium) are exchanged for potassium ions in the gut and the potassium is then eliminated. The long-term use of calcium resonium can lead to severe constipation unless appropriate laxatives are prescribed and is therefore not used for routine control of plasma potassium levels.

NEPHROTIC SYNDROME

Nephrotic syndrome (NS) is characterised by proteinuria $> 3\,\mathrm{g\,day^{-1}}$, which results in hypoalbuminaemia and generalised oedema. Hyperlipidaemia, clotting problems and hypertension are also present. Loss of immunoglobulins and proteins that bind iron, copper, zinc and vitamins A and D can result in an increased risk of infections and general malnutrition. The syndrome can arise in diseases which primarily cause glomerular damage, such as FSGS (Focal Segmented Glomerulo Sclerosis), MN (membranous nephropathy), MCN (minimal change nephropathy), or secondary to other diseases including diabetic nephropathy and autoimmune disease, such as systemic lupus erythematosus (SLE). Treatment aims to control oedema, reduce proteinuria and treat complications that arise including infections, hyperlipidaemia and clotting problems (Orth & Ritz 1998). Diet therapy has a role to play in several of these areas (Table 11.3).

Protein restriction

Historically, a high-protein diet was advised with the aim of replacing protein losses. This is now thought to cause further damage to the glomerular basement membrane and exacerbate the proteinuria. An intake of 0.8–$1\,\mathrm{g}$ protein $\mathrm{kg^{-1}}$ IBW $\mathrm{day^{-1}}$ has been recommended. This can result in reduced proteinuria and improvements in other

Table 11.3 Management of nephrotic syndrome

Symptom	Dietary management
Hypertension and oedema	Dietary sodium restriction: 80–100 mmol day^{-1}; fluid restriction may also be necessary, depending on the response to medication ACE inhibitors are commonly used (monitor potassium levels)
Proteinuria/hypoalbuminaemia	Moderate protein restriction: 0.8–1 g kg^{-1} IBW day^{-1} Good control of blood glucose in diabetics Medication can include steroids to treat the primary disease
Hyperlipidaemia	Standard lipid lowering advice; 30% calories from fat including 10% calories from PUFA Statins and bile acid sequestrants
Lower immunity	A balanced, nutritious diet will help prevent PEM and maintain micronutrient levels: monitor for signs of vitamin D deficiency

IBW, ideal body weight; PEM, protein energy malnutrition; PUFA, polyunsaturated fatty acids.
* Thromboembolism is increased in NS: 10–30% of adult patients with NS may develop clotting problems.

biochemical parameters, such as fibrinogen[*], phosphate, lipid and renin levels, although not all studies have shown a corresponding increase in plasma albumin levels.

The incidence of myocardial infarction has been reported as 5–6 times greater in NS compared with normal. Increased liver synthesis of lipo-proteins and impaired metabolism of triglycerides results in raised trig-lycerides and cholesterol. Standard lipid-lowering advice can be given as well as the use of lipid-lowering agents, such as 5-hydroxy-3-methyl-glutaryl-coenzyme A (HMG-CoA) reductase inhibitors (statins) and bile acid sequesters.

Hyperlipidaemia

DIETARY MANAGEMENT: DIALYSIS TREATMENTS

HISTORICAL REVIEW

During the past three decades, considerable progress has been made regarding modes and quality of treatment. Regular haemodialysis became available from the mid-1960s onwards.

Patients were initially selected for treatment: they were usually young and free from concomitant disease. HD lasted for 10–15 hours depending on the number of sessions, twice or three times a week. Dietary man-agement was aimed at controlling the patient's fluid balance and bio-chemistry. During these early days of dialysis, a strict diet (by present standards) was followed by many patients, which consisted of a daily intake of: 50 g protein, 50 mmol sodium, 50 mmol potassium, 3500 kcal and 300 mL fluid.

As the quality of dialysis treatment improved during the 1970s and 1980s, dietary restrictions were relaxed to a daily intake of 60 g protein, 60 mmol sodium, 60 mmol potassium, 2500–3000 kcal and 300–500 mL fluid. Even this type of HD diet was impossible to follow without the help of high-energy, low-electrolyte supplements and several books were pub-lished during the following years to promote dietary education (Vennegoor 1982, 1986, 1992).

During the early 1980s CAPD became established as a new chronic dialysis technique, although it had been used since the 1960s for patients who were haemodynamically too unstable for HD. By the mid-1980s, the diet for both HD and PD was similar to that prescribed today: 1–1.2 g pro-tein kg^{-1} IBW day^{-1} for HD patients and 1.2–1.5 g protein kg^{-1} IBW day^{-1} for PD patients (Vennegoor 1986).

CURRENT CONCEPTS OF DIALYSIS DIETARY MANAGEMENT

Most patients will receive some nutrition information in the predialy-sis phase. Specific dietary requirements will need adjusting when the mode of therapy (HD, PD or transplantation) commences or changes. Current recommendations for dietary requirements are shown in Table 11.4 and the biochemical standards for which diet has a role in achieving are shown in Table 11.5.

Table 11.4
Dietary recommendations for
patients on renal replacement
therapy

	HD	PD	TXP
Protein (g kg^{-1} IBW)	1.0–1.2	1.2–1.3	EAR
Energy (kcal kg^{-1} IBW)	35	35	EAR
Na (mmol day^{-1})^a	80–110	80–110	80–110
K (mmol kg^{-1} IBW)	1.0	1.0	Free
P (mmol day^{-1})	31–45	31–45	Free
Vitamins	Yes	Yes	Not required
Phosphate binders	Yes	Yes	Not required

^{a} 80–110 mmol equals 1800–2500 mg sodium.
EAR, estimated average recommendations (national agreement); HD, haemodialysis; IBW, ideal body weight; PD, peritoneal dialysis; TXP, transplantation.
Protein intake for HD and PD based on K/DOQI recommendations (Kopple et al 2000).
Energy intake for HD and PD based on K/DOQI recommendations (Kopple et al 2000).
Sodium, potassium and phosphorus intake for HD and PD based on EDTNA/ERCA nutritional guidelines (2001).

Table 11.5
Nutritional standards for
patients on renal replacement
therapy

	HD	PD
Albumin (g L^{-1})	> 35	> 35
K (mmol L^{-1a})	3.5–6.5	3.5–5.5
P (mmol L^{-1a})	< 1.8	< 1.8
Ca (mmol L^{-1})	2.2–2.6	2.2–2.6 (within locally agreed normal range, corrected for serum albumin)
Urea kinetic	> 1.2 per treatment	> 1.7 per week per modelling treatment (Kt/V)^a
Urea reduction rate (URR)^a	> 65% per treatment	

^{a}Reference: Renal Association (2002).
HD, haemodialysis; PD, peritoneal dialysis.

PROTEIN

During haemodialysis approximately 6–12 g of amino acids are lost per session. For peritoneal dialysis, 8–12 g protein in addition to 3 g amino acids are lost per day. On the basis of these figures alone, the additional dietary protein required to replace these losses can be calculated as 0.1 g kg^{-1} for HD patients and 0.2 g kg^{-1} day^{-1} for PD patients. Some authors have argued that, as the minimum safe protein intake for healthy individuals and in the predialysis phase is approximately 0.75 g kg^{-1} day^{-1} as discussed above, the recommended minimum intake on dialysis should be as follows: 0.9 g kg^{-1} day^{-1} for HD and 1 g kg^{-1} day^{-1} for PD (Lim & Flanigan 2001). These are slightly lower levels than that recorded in Table 11.4 and, for *some* metabolically stable patients (i.e. not catabolic), nitrogen balance studies have shown that intakes at this level can be sufficient. As with any patient, in order to ensure that they are not becoming malnourished, it is important to measure nutritional status using a number of different methods such as those used in subjective global assessment (SGA; McCann 1996; Appendix 11.5).

ENERGY REQUIREMENTS

An intake of 35 kcal kg IBW is recommended to maintain nitrogen (protein) balance in HD and PD patients. For sedentary and older patients, 30–35 kcal kg^{-1} IBW is sufficient. Underweight patients may need additional calories (and supporting micronutrients) to encourage weight gain, while overweight patients may need a calorie adjustment to encourage weight loss if appropriate (K/DOQI 2000, Todorovic & Micklewright 2004).

Dextrose (glucose) is used as an osmotic agent in peritoneal dialysis for the removal of fluid. Up to 70% of this glucose is absorbed through the peritoneum and this can exacerbate hyperglycaemia, hyperlipidaemia and obesity. The amount of glucose absorbed increases as the osmotic strength of the dialysate increases. When calculating energy requirements for peritoneal dialysis patients, the glucose (and hence calories) absorbed from the dialysate need to be included. Glucose absorption may provide approximately 70 kcal for a 2-L 1.36% exchange, 130 kcal for a 2-L 2.5% exchange and 200 kcal for a 2-L 3.86% exchange. Daily intake from this source could be between 100 and 300 g glucose (400–1200 kcal), depending on the strength and size of the exchanges used. Icodextrin is a PD solution that contains glucose polymers with a larger molecular weight than glucose and is an effective osmotic agent. The calorie uptake is only half that of a comparable 3.86% exchange while achieving the same level of ultrafiltration. Some improvements in glycaemic control have been measured in diabetic patients using one icodextrin exchange per day.

SODIUM AND FLUID

Once a patient becomes oliguric and eventually anuric, the intake of salt and fluid will need to be reduced to control interdialytic weight gain (IDWG) with HD and fluid balance with PD.

Excessive IDWG in HD patients contributes to hypertension prior to HD treatments, necessitating antihypertensive medication (Ifudu et al 1997). Longstanding fluid overload also results in left ventricular cardiac hypertrophy (Konings et al 2002).

A reduced fluid allowance is probably the most difficult part of the dialysis diet to cope with. Up to 86% of patients may exceed an IDWG guideline of 1.5 kg and there appears to be no difference between those who have diabetes and those who do not (Halverson et al 1993). Some groups of patients with different ethnic backgrounds appear to have additional problems with IDWG. Indo–Asian patients in particular may often be unable to adhere to their fluid allowances; this is attributed to a higher fluid and salt content of traditional foods and meals (Davidson 2000).

Most renal centres in the UK regard an IDWG ranging from 1.5 to 2.0 kg as acceptable. Considering the differences in size of patients, it may be more appropriate to base IDWG on dry weight using 4% as an acceptable IDWG (EDTNA/ERCA nutrition guidelines 2002). However, an upper limit needs to be set for patients with a BMI > 25.

Sodium intake: the mechanism of thirst

It is important to remember what causes thirst. The sodium level in the body is finely tuned in healthy individuals as well as those with renal failure. Too much dietary salt will cause the plasma sodium level to rise (transiently) and the thirst mechanism in the brain to act. It is then necessary to drink sufficient fluid to normalize the sodium level. A sodium intake of 80–110 mmol day^{-1} can help control thirst; this can be achieved by following the advice listed in the earlier section on hypertension.

Excessive IDWG may not always be due to poor understanding of dietary advice. Even 'solid' food contains some fluid and patients with a good appetite will have higher IDWG; this can be established with a detailed dietary assessment, indicating a high protein and energy intake (Sherman et al 1995).

Fluid includes anything liquid at room temperature (apart from vegetable oils) and includes jelly, ice-cream, ice cubes, gravy, soups, sauces and custard. A daily fluid allowance of 500–750 mL in addition to the average daily urine output is usually sufficient to prevent excess IDWG in those patients on HD. Patients on PD can increase their intake to at least 750 mL plus average daily urine output. This amount may be modified depending on the level of ultrafiltration that is achieved with the lower strength exchanges of PD fluid. The following additional tips can help the patient keep to their fluid allowance.

- Measure the daily fluid allowance in a water jug: take out the equivalent amount after having a drink or if food with a significant amount of fluid is eaten.
- Divide the fluid allowance throughout the day.
- Use a small cup or glass instead of a mug or large glass.
- Drink only half a cup each time, if possible.
- Ice cubes may be more thirst quenching, but each cube contains 30 mL fluid (2 tablespoons): lemon juice or other flavourings can be added.
- Rinse the mouth with water; gargle but do not swallow.
- Stimulate saliva production by sucking a piece of lemon or grapefruit, sherbets or chewing gum.
- Try artificial saliva sprays.
- Take medicines with the meals unless contraindicated.
- When going out, save the allowance of fluid to allow for an extra drink when socialising.
- Keep occupied.
- A daily weight check in the morning before breakfast will reveal the rate of fluid accumulation in between HD treatments and the fluid status on PD.

POTASSIUM

Most patients starting dialysis continue to produce fairly good quantities of urine. This helps to some extent with the excretion of sodium, potassium and, of course, fluid. The urine is often described as 'poor quality' in that the level of these solutes is lower than usual and plasma potassium levels should be monitored closely. The risk of hyperkalaemia is greater in anuric patients. The dietary intake of potassium should be reduced to $1 \, \text{mmol} \, \text{kg}^{-1}$ IBW day^{-1} for patients on HD. Patients on PD, if previously restricted, may be able to relax this, as potassium is constantly removed and hypokalaemia has been observed. A detailed diet history should be taken for all patients so that the main sources of potassium in the patient's diet are known, and the level of restriction and dietary advice given is based on a risk assessment of their usual dietary intake, urine output and plasma potassium levels.

Hyperkalaemia can be a frequent problem, especially on HD, and dietary indiscretion is partly to blame, although the amount of potassium removed during dialysis can vary by as much as 70%. Other reasons for hyperkalaemia should be investigated simultaneously as previously described. Some patients on haemodialysis consume foods with high potassium content during the first couple of hours on dialysis. The transit of food and fluid through the gastrointestinal tract may be slower while the patient is dialysing and so it is advisable to at least put a limit on this consumption as the potassium may not be completely removed.

PHOSPHORUS

The recommended intake varies from 1000 to 1400 mg ($31–45 \, \text{mmol} \, \text{day}^{-1}$) or approximately 0.5 mmol phosphorus per gram of protein up to $45 \, \text{mmol} \, \text{day}^{-1}$. This will help prevent hyperphosphataemia and preserve an adequate and acceptable diet for the patient to follow (EDTNA/ERCA nutritional guidelines 2002). Absorption from the gastrointestinal tract is usually about 80%. Dialysis clears a varying amount depending on the mode of dialysis and the adequacy of the dialysis treatment. Phosphate binders also vary in the amount of phosphate they are able to bind. Dietary phosphorus restriction combined with the appropriate use (type and dose) of phosphate binders and adequate dialysis helps to prevent severe hyperphosphataemia.

VITAMINS AND MINERALS

During dialysis the small molecules, such as water-soluble vitamins, are removed and losses are higher with high-flux HD. The fat-soluble vitamin A is a larger molecule and vitamin A metabolites are therefore more difficult to remove and could lead to toxicity. However, with a functioning kidney there are vitamin losses and so the question is whether dialysis removes greater amounts of vitamins than would normally occur. Evidence of vitamins at risk includes thiamine (B1) in PD patients, pyridoxine (B6) and ascorbic acid (vitamin C) in PD and HD, and folate in HD. Ascorbic acid is easily dialysed in both HD and PD. In some unsupplemented patients, vitamin levels dropped below the normal range (Henderson et al 1984, Ramirez et al 1986) and also in a more recent study, six out of 43 HD and PD patients showed low levels of vitamin C (Wood et al 1998). A high-dose vitamin C supplement should be avoided to prevent hyperoxalosis: 60 mg may be sufficient with a normal dietary vitamin C intake, while a supplement of 200 mg vitamin C may increase serum oxalate levels. Oxalate deposits as crystals in soft tissues such as muscle tissue and vital organs, and may increase the risk of myocardial infarction, muscle weakness and bone disease.

Deficiencies of iron, zinc, copper, manganese and chromium are most likely to occur as a result of dietary restrictions, drug nutrient interactions and protein losses (Rocco & Makoff 1997, Wolk 1993).

Despite the risk of vitamin and mineral deficiencies, routine supplementation does not occur in the UK, as it does in the USA and some European countries. This may change as the results of the Dialysis Outcomes and Practice Patterns Study (DOPPS) showed that water-soluble vitamin supplementation is associated with a 15% decrease in mortality (Fissell et al 2004). Table 11.6 lists the suggested daily recommendations (Makoff 1999).

MALNUTRITION

Protein energy malnutrition (PEM) is a complication of HD and PD, and its consequences have been well documented since these techniques became available. Marckmann (1988) concluded in his cross-sectional study that 53% of HD and 46% PD patients suffered from PEM,

Table 11.6 Suggested daily dosage of vitamins for renal failure patients. (From Makoff 1999, with permission)

Vitamins	Dosage	%RDI (USA)
Vitamin A	0	0
Vitamin E	0	0
Vitamin B1	1.5 mg	100
Vitamin B2	1.7 mg	100
Vitamin B6	10 mg	500
Vitamin B12	6 µg	100
Folic acid	800–1000 µg	200–250
Pantothenic acid	10 mg	100
Niacin	20 mg	100
Biotin	300 µg	100
Vitamin C	60 mg	100

RDI, recommended daily intake.

and some degree of malnutrition was recorded in all patients who had been on dialysis for less than 1 year. A multicentre study of PD patients using a variety of biochemical and anthropometric measures to assess nutritional status identified similar levels of malnutrition: 33% of patients were moderately malnourished and 8% were severely malnourished (Young et al 1991), although there was widespread variation between the centres (20–70% malnutrition). Lowrie & Lew (1990) showed that the relative risk of death increases as the serum albumin of the HD patient falls. These authors also concluded that longer treatment time and better nutritional status improve the clinical outcome of HD treatment.

Later studies revealed that albumin was also a marker for morbidity and mortality in PD patients. Plasma albumin was lower in non-survivors after 30 months on PD (Davies et al 1998) and, as albumin decreased by $10\,g\,L^{-1}$, there was an increased risk of morbidity (hospitalisation), which was five times greater in non-diabetic PD patients and 10 times greater in diabetics on PD (Spiegel et al 1993). The Canada-USA (CANUSA) peritoneal dialysis study group showed the relative risk of death on PD increased with age, insulin-independent diabetes mellitus, cardiovascular disease, low serum albumin and worsening nutritional status. Malnutrition (identified by SGA) correlated strongly with an increase in number of days hospitalised (CANUSA 1996).

It had always been assumed that serum albumin was a reliable marker of nutritional status; however, this relationship has been questioned as other causes of low albumin are also common in renal failure (Fine & Cox 1992, Heimberger et al 1994). The correct diagnosis of the cause of a low albumin is crucial for appropriate medical management.

HYPOALBUMINAEMIA

Hypoalbuminaemia is an important predictor of morbidity and mortality. There are several potential causes as listed below.

- Decreased synthesis owing to PEM – albumin has a half-life of 2–3 weeks, therefore, starvation can take at least this length of time to make an impact on plasma levels.
- Decreased synthesis owing to the acute phase response – this is part of the body's immune response to cell damage, which can arise through trauma, infection or cancer.
- Redistribution of albumin pools, e.g. from vascular spaces to the intervascular space or the peritoneal cavity.
- Albumin losses owing to proteinuria, dialysis losses or peritonitis.
- Dilution – if the patient is fluid overloaded, e.g. before a HD session, or if dry weight needs to be adjusted: e.g. 3 L overload can dilute plasma albumin from $42\,g\,L^{-1}$ to $37\,g\,L^{-1}$.
- Albumin assay methods vary – it is important to use the same method of measurement each time or if comparing patients based at different renal units (Carfray et al 2000).

SYSTEMIC INFLAMMATORY RESPONSE OR ACUTE PHASE RESPONSE

One of the initial stages in the systemic inflammatory response (SIR) is the release of cytokines, e.g. tumour necrosis factor alpha (TNFα; cachexin), interleukin 1 (IL-1) and IL-6. These cytokines affect protein production in the liver: C-reactive protein (CRP) is one of the proteins that increase as part of the acute phase response (APR) or SIR. At the same time, the liver reduces the production of other proteins including albumin and transferrin. The cytokines are also responsible for cachexia seen in chronic illnesses as they cause an increase in metabolic rate, poor tolerance to glucose and increased breakdown of protein (Roubenoff et al, 1997). They may also reduce appetite, as is often found in people with chronic illness, such as AIDS and renal disease (Aguilera et al 1998). Additionally, Chung et al (2003) showed that PD patients with a high CRP were more likely to have a lower total fluid removal and the resulting increase in extracellular fluid could lower plasma albumin through plasma dilution (Jones et al 2002). This inter-relation between CRP and albumin may explain why a low albumin has been associated in so many studies with increased morbidity and mortality.

Nutritional consequences of SIR

The rapid turnover of immune cells, increased antibody production and production of acute phase proteins (such as CRP and fibrinogen) create an increased demand for certain nutrients, such as branch-chain amino acids and glutamine (Grimble 1998). The specific nutritional needs of the stress response are met by breaking down existing proteins, which may partly explain the muscle weakness and wasting seen in renal disease. Conventional nutrition support regimens may not result in an improved nutritional status, nor reduce mortality because they do not supply enough of the relevant nutrients and they may even add to the burden of nutrients that cannot be efficiently utilized at the time.

MALNUTRITION, INFLAMMATION, ATHEROSCLEROSIS (MIA) SYNDROME

There has been increasing evidence of a link between inflammation, malnutrition and atherosclerosis (Kaysen & Kumar 2003). A total of 30–50% of patients with renal disease show evidence of an ongoing inflammatory response. This may be due to dialysis-related factors: clotted grafts, incompatibility of dialysis membranes or simply lower clearance of cytokines (McIntyre et al 1997). However, significant correlations between the presence of malnutrition (defined by low serum creatinine, LBM (lean body mass) and urea nitrogen appearance), inflammation (measured by CRP, TNFα and fibrinogen) and carotid plaques have been demonstrated in predialysis patients (Stenvinkel et al 1999). It is unclear whether the CRP is raised in response to endothelial cell damage or whether CRP and other acute-phase reactants, such as IL-6, are actually involved in the initiation and progression of atherosclerosis

(Stenvinkel 2003). The relationship between the inflammatory response and cachexia was described in the previous section (i.e. the presence of inflammatory cytokines results in appetite loss, muscle breakdown and low albumin). This has led researchers to ask the question 'Are there two types of malnutrition in established renal failure: one type representing "classic" PEM, and the other linked with cytokines and atherosclerosis' (Stenvinkel et al 2000).

Future research will continue to investigate targeted nutrition, which aims to supply essential nutrients, such as glutamine, arginine and DNA precursors, or attempts to attenuate the inflammatory response using omega-3 essential fatty acids in order to reduce catabolism. This research needs further development in patients with kidney disease.

MANAGEMENT OF PROTEIN ENERGY MALNUTRITION

The consequences of PEM are:

- failure to thrive
- increased morbidity
  - delayed wound healing
  - decreased resistance to infection
  - electrolyte imbalance
  - prolonged hospitalisation
  - muscle wasting (skeletal muscle as well as heart/lung, etc.)
  - loss of protective subcutaneous fat
  - lethargy/apathy
- increased mortality.

Prevention and treatment of PEM should be started during the predialysis phase of ERF. Many renal departments hold multidisciplinary education sessions for patients to provide information on treatment options, diet and support from social services. Ideally a specialist renal nurse, dietitian, social worker and consultant should be involved in the sessions, with access to a counsellor available. All patients should also receive individual dietary advice and frequent monitoring is essential to accommodate any changes in renal function.

There are several reasons for PEM in dialysis patients and these are multifactorial as listed below.

1. Reduced dietary intake:
   - reduced appetite (see point 2 below)
   - existing malnutrition at the start of dialysis due to uraemia or unsupervised predialysis dietary restriction
   - conflicting dietary recommendations, e.g. increasing protein whilst decreasing the intake of phosphorus
   - dietary recommendations that decrease the palatability of food – decreased salt intake, decreased fat or sugar intake
   - co-existing gastrointestinal disease (i.e. gastroparesis) or other co-morbidities, such as cardiac failure, cancer
   - multipharmacy prescriptions

- inadequate provision of nutrients in food provided by hospitals or nursing homes
- financial constraints
2. Reduced appetite:
   - raised cytokines
   - inadequate dialysis leading to uraemia
   - suppression of appetite due to peritoneal dialysis; this may be due to glucose absorption, abdominal pressure from the dialysate fluid, or constipation
   - anaemia or other micronutrient deficiencies
   - old age
   - depression.
3. Increased nutritional losses:
   - losses during dialysis: vitamins, minerals, proteins and amino acids
   - persistent proteinuria
   - protein loss during peritonitis.
4. Altered metabolism:
   - inflammatory response as a result of the dialysis process
   - untreated acidosis
   - inadequate dialysis
   - low physical activity
   - intercurrent illness/infections, causing raised requirements
   - hyperparathyroidism.

ASSESSING NUTRITIONAL STATUS

This should be done regularly and systematically for all patients as physical deterioration can occur rapidly and is difficult to reverse. It is important to identify malnutrition to rehabilitate the patient early and to improve clinical outcome. The National Institute for Health and Clinical Excellence (NICE) guidelines (2006) have recommended that 'All hospital in-patients on admission and out-patients at first appointment should be screened for presence or risk of malnutrition'.

The European Society for Clinical Nutrition and Metabolism (ESPEN) guidelines (2002) has described the prerequisites of a useful assessment tool. This tool should have the following features:

- good predictive validity – the individual identified 'at risk' will benefit from intervention
- good content validity – it will include 'all' relevant components of the problem it is meant to solve
- high reliability – small interobserver variation
- practical
- linked to 'specific protocols for action'
- rapid and simple, so that it can be performed by admitting staff or community health care teams.

The authors of the K/DOQI guidelines recommended that further work needed to be done in order to *identify and validate* the optimal panel of measures for screening and assessment of nutritional status in patients with renal diseases (K/DOQI 2000). In the meantime, nutritional assessment should incorporate a number of complementary measures that at least include dietary assessment and body composition measures (Engel et al 1995, Appendix 11.6). The MUST tool (Stratton et al 2003, www.bapen.org.uk/the-must.htm) and Subjective Global Assessment contain both these elements, although so far only SGA has been validated for use with patients with renal diseases.

Methods of dietary assessment

- 24-hour recall: this is quick and assesses recent intake.
- 3-day food diary: this can include a weekend day and one HD day, and gives a better illustration of the variety of foods eaten. It may also reveal the disruption to meal times caused by a dialysis day – for HD patients significant decreases in all nutrients can occur in three days out of seven.
- Urea content of 24-hour urine samples in predialysis patients and urine plus dialysate collection in PD patients can be used to calculate urea nitrogen appearance. This is equivalent to dietary protein intake in nutritionally stable patients (24-hour urine and PD dialysate collection can also be used to estimate protein losses).
- In HD patients, changes in plasma urea measurements, collected for dialysis adequacy tests, can be used to calculate the protein catabolic rate (PCR). This is only equivalent to protein intake in nutritionally stable patients (urinary urea also needs to be included).

Techniques to assess body composition

The best known techniques are listed below.

- Height and weight (BMI).
- Mid upper arm anthropometry: mid-arm circumference (MAC), triceps skinfold thickness and mid-arm muscle circumference (MAMC). MAC is easy to perform, non-invasive and training can reduce observer error repeatable to an acceptable degree. Skinfolds are more prone to observer error; a measure of muscle function may be a better way of assessing muscle mass (e.g. grip strength, sit-to-stand test or walking test; Mercer et al 1998).
- Bioelectrical impedance: quick and non-invasive, but it is an indirect measure and it is influenced by hydration and electrode placement (Lindley et al 2005).
- Dual-energy X-ray absorptiometry (DEXA): measures bone mineral content and density. It relies on assumptions about hydration status which may not be valid in patients with renal diseases, particularly for the measurement of lean body mass. DEXA expensive and not widely available (Mazess et al 1990).

The Dialysis Outcome Quality Initiative (K/DOQI, 2000) guidelines have indicated the need for more information regarding 'the appropriate parameters to be used for assessment of body composition', and also stated that 'patient subgroups needed to be identified: elderly, obese, severely malnourished, physically very inactive who would benefit from specialised combinations of body composition measures'.

Subjective global assessment

Subjective global assessment is an assessment of nutritional status and was first performed on surgical patients (Detsky et al 1987). It is based on patient history and physical examination. A simple questionnaire is usually completed by a trained nurse or dietitian.

History

The history includes weight changes, dietary intake, gastrointestinal symptoms, functional status and can include co-morbid disease.

Physical examination

Physical examination takes into account loss of subcutaneous fat, muscle wasting, oedema and ascites. Each section is rated on a three- or seven-point scale by the interviewer. An overall score is then assigned depending on the severity of symptoms. For the three-point scoring system, subjects are given a score of A, B or C (A for well nourished, B for mild–moderate malnutrition and C for severe malnutrition). The 7-point score subdivides these categories into A, A−, B+, B, B−, C+ and C, or sometimes a numerical score is used: SGA scores of 6–7 (well nourished), 3–5 (mild–moderate undernutrition) and 1–2 (severe undernutrition; Appendix 11.5).

The seven-point SGA was developed for the CANUSA study (Churchill et al 1996) and was found to positively correlate with BMI, percentage body fat and MAMC (Visser et al 1999). A 1 unit lower SGA score was associated with a 25% increase in the relative risk of death and a 1 unit increase in score was associated with reduction in days hospitalised. Reproducibility was good: 81–91% when two observers were compared.

K/DOQI Guidelines (2000) stated that 'SGA is a valid and clinically useful measure of protein-energy nutrition status in maintenance dialysis patients'. The Renal Association (2002) also supports use of the seven-point SGA.

TREATMENT OF PROTEIN ENERGY MALNUTRITION

Intervention should start as soon as malnutrition is identified. A protocol should be in place so that the appropriate intervention is initiated immediately (a good example of this is illustrated by the MUST tool, which describes the actions to be taken for each level of malnutrition). This may require nursing staff to start monitoring the patient with food charts or to start supplements in the first instance, and alert the renal dietitian who will carry out a full dietary review and liaise with the renal team regarding an appropriate plan of nutrition support.

The primary aim of nutrition support is for the patient to meet their nutritional requirements (macronutrients and micronutrients) in the least invasive, most effective way. Protein and energy requirements are calculated using the formula previously shown. The patient's protein and energy intake can be calculated from food intake charts or a 24-hour recall.

Requirements − current intake = nutrient deficit

This deficit has to be met using the following methods of nutrition support.

- Oral − for patients who are able to eat and drink normally: fortified foods or foods with a high nutrient content or sip feeds; support and encouragement with eating, if necessary.
- Nasogastric or gastrostomy feeding for patients who are unable or unwilling to eat or drink normally. Oral and tube feeding can be combined (e.g. tube feeding overnight, while the patient sleeps and encouraging normal eating/drinking during the day).
- Intraperitoneal amino acids (IPAA) with PD.
- Intradialytic parenteral nutrition (IDPN) during HD.
- Total parenteral nutrition (TPN) for patients whose gastrointestinal tract is not functioning sufficiently.

Nutrition support is ineffective without close teamwork and each member of staff agreeing to carry out specific roles. All healthcare workers directly involved in in-patient care should receive training in the following (NICE guidelines 2006):

- the importance of nutrition
- indications for nutrition support and delivery
- when and where to seek advice on nutrition support.

Oral nutritional support

The key stages in providing oral nutritional support (ONS) are:

- identifying any barriers preventing the patients from meeting their requirements and referral to other specialists, if necessary
- involving the patient in deciding which type of supplementation is appropriate.

Barriers to meeting requirements

Gastrointestinal problems should be identified by the nutrition screening tool. If chewing and/or swallowing is a problem, the consistency of food may need to be modified. The catering department will have to be notified and referral to the speech and language therapist may be appropriate. People who lose weight rapidly often find that their dentures no longer fit properly; unfortunately this problem cannot usually be remedied during the patient's stay. Thrush infections are common in undernourished or immunosuppressed patients. This can cause a sore mouth, taste changes and swallowing problems, and can be relatively easily treated with antifungal agents. Constipation and diarrhoea are equally deleterious to the patient's appetite, and need to be identified and treated.

Motivating and encouraging the patient at meal times is often necessary and needs to be supervised by a member of the nursing team. Actively involving older people in their nutritional care and allocating a nurse to oversee their nutritional needs can improve intake by 30% (Pederson 2005). If active depression is an underlying cause, it may be useful to involve the help of a qualified counsellor.

Prior to admission, the patient may have had a long period of deterioration due to the lack of ability or facilities to cook and shop. These problems may be resolved by a social worker and involvement of other family members or friends. If physical weakness is a problem, a physiotherapist or occupational therapist can suggest exercises to strengthen the patient or tools to assist the patient.

In hospital, physical weakness may prevent the patient cutting up their food or removing packaging. Poor vision may also be a problem. Assistance must be provided when these problems are identified. Loss of muscle mass is one of the main consequences of PEM and, in elderly people in particular, this leads to decreased capacity for the activities of daily living, loss of independence and decline in mental status. Physical activity and physiotherapy can improve muscle mass and should be part of nutritional support in the elderly patient (Suetta et al 2004).

Food supplementation

This may involve providing fortified foods, snacks or drinks with high nutritional content. Some of these can be given between meals so that the patient can eat little and often. Examples of these foods include sweet biscuits, cakes, cheese and biscuits, yogurt and mousses.

Supplement drinks, mousses and soups are available as well as protein and energy powders, although the latter are more likely to be added during food preparation. The supplement drinks and desserts should be prescribed as a medicine and their listing on the drug chart may help improve distribution and monitoring of intake. The drinks may be milk shakes, juice drinks and yogurt drinks. The flavours can include various fruits, vanilla, chocolate, neutral and savoury. Mousses and bars are available and may be useful for patients with reduced fluid allowances.

The renal dietitian will be aware of the nutritional content of any supplements as well as potassium and phosphate content. The ratio of protein to energy may vary, which may suit the needs of different patients. A malnourished patient's potassium and phosphate intakes are usually poor and they may even have low plasma levels, but it is always necessary to be aware of the potassium content; powdered drinks that require the addition of milk may be unsuitably high in potassium. The patient will usually need to continue phosphate binders unless they are extremely malnourished.

Nursing and/or catering staff need to ensure that the supplements/fortified foods are given to the patient at the right time, at the correct temperature and that they are actually consumed by the patient.

Nasogastric and gastrostomy feeding

The insertion of a percutaneous enteral gastrostomy (PEG) feeding tube enables long-term tube feeding to be carried out without the discomfort of a nasogastric feeding tube. The NICE guidelines recommend PEG placement if nasogastric tube feeding is not appropriate or if feeding is likely to be required for more than 4 weeks. Renal formulae are available with reduced electrolyte content but high nutrient density to reduce the fluid intake. Surveys have shown that the majority of (non-renal) patients (83%) accepted the PEG well. In comparison with nasogastric feeding, there were fewer complications, greater comfort, better quality of life and better nutritional efficacy (Loser et al 2005). In adult dialysis patients, there have been fewer reports of gastrostomy use. Peritonitis was a frequent complication in PD patients (Fein et al 2001), although PEG feeding in children seems more successful and perhaps some lessons need to be learnt from the techniques used in paediatrics (Coleman et al 1998).

Dialysate containing 1.1% amino-acid solution will provide a net gain of 18 g amino acids from one 2-L exchange. It is important to ensure that energy requirements are being met otherwise positive nitrogen balance will not be achieved. Studies have indicated an improvement in nitrogen balance with increases in albumin, the dialysate seems to be well tolerated (Tjiong et al 2005, Taylor et al 2002, Steele et al 1998).

Nutritional peritoneal dialysis

Parenteral formulas containing 50–70 g amino acids and 1000 kcal from fat and carbohydrate can be safely delivered via the venous return during the HD treatment. Glucose monitoring during treatment is essential to prevent hyperglycaemia and fluid balance can be adjusted accordingly. An oral multivitamin and mineral supplement may be required to ensure efficient use of the protein and calories. The cost of IDPN is ten times that of oral supplementation, therefore the latter method should be encouraged first. A number of small studies have shown that IDPN promotes positive nitrogen balance (Pupim et al 2002, Cherry et al 2002).

Intradialytic parenteral nutrition

This may require daily recording of food intake charts and weighing the patient regularly. Food records are best completed as the meal is being finished in order to observe the patient and note any problems, as well as record the amount and type of food eaten. Patients can often forget what they have eaten within a couple of hours. Monitoring of biochemistry and fluid balance is also crucial for patients with renal disease (very low as well as high levels of potassium and phosphate are possible). Arm anthropometry such as MAC can be repeated monthly.

Monitoring nutritional support

TRANSPLANTATION

Renal transplantation is thought to offer the patient with established renal failure the best chance of rehabilitation and good quality of life. They no longer have to undertake the time-consuming and exhausting process of dialysis, and uraemic waste products are removed much more effectively.

There is a general improvement in well-being; however the metabolic effects of chronic renal failure – anaemia, bone disease, muscle wasting and cardiovascular disease – will be present in many of the newly transplanted patients. The immunosuppressive and antihypertensive therapy can exacerbate these conditions as well as creating additional problems, such as increased risk of diabetes, and susceptibility to infections and certain types of cancer (Cohen & Galbraith 2001).

POSTOPERATIVE TRANSPLANT CARE

Appetite may initially be poor postoperatively and steroids can increase protein catabolism; therefore, both kidney and gastrointestinal function should be monitored. The rate at which biochemistry and urine output return to normal can vary (sometimes within a couple of days post surgery, or it can take several weeks) and needs to be monitored closely. There may be an 'oliguric stage' where fluid and electrolyte restrictions are still required. This can progress to a polyuric stage, where intravenous support may be necessary to prevent fluid and electrolyte levels dropping below normal; dehydration at this stage can damage the new kidney. Nutritional requirements and the need for nutrition support can be assessed as previously described. Uncomplicated surgery increases metabolic rate by 5–20% and this should be included in the protein and energy requirements.

LONG-TERM POST-TRANSPLANT CARE

The advice given to patients should include healthy eating (with some advice on food hygiene), exercise, and avoidance of smoking and exposure to too much sun. One of the positive aspects of transplantation is that the dietary restrictions are relaxed; however, it is necessary to reinforce advice on healthy eating to help reduce the risk of obesity, cardiovascular disease, diabetes and also cancer.

Nutrient requirements are based on recommendations for the general population. The 'Balance of Good Health' is an appropriate model on which to base nutritional advice and meal suggestions (British Nutrition Foundation: *http://www.nutrition.org.uk*).

CARDIOVASCULAR DISEASE

Cardiovascular disease is the cause of 60% of deaths in transplanted patients and the incidence of CVD is five times greater than expected for age and gender. The main risk factors are obesity, hypertension, hyperlipidaemia, diabetes, sedentary lifestyle and smoking. The European Best Practice Guidelines (EBPG 2002) for renal transplantation also list hyperhomocysteinaemia as a risk factor.

Obesity is common with a successful transplant (Heaf et al 2004) and is multifactorial.

- The patient's appetite increases due to the increased feeling of well-being and release from dietary constraints. Relaxation of restrictions post transplant can lead to a more liberal intake of high-calorie foods, such as dairy products, fried potato products and chocolate.
- Steroids stimulate the patient's appetite.
- Activity and exercise levels may be low. Patients are often reluctant to exercise for fear of damaging the new kidney, and also because of lack of confidence and low exercise tolerance owing to previous inactivity.

The combination of an increased calorie intake and low activity levels leads to a rapid gain in body fat. Obesity contributes to hypertension, hyper-lipidaemia and insulin resistance, and these in turn contribute to CVD. Graft survival is also lower in the obese and the patient should be made aware of the risk of obesity at an early stage, pretransplant if appropriate.

Regarding the other CVD risk factors:

- elevated levels of serum triglyceride cholesterol are found in 36% and 63% of transplant patients, respectively
- arterial hypertension is present in 60–85% of patients
- post-transplant diabetes affects 4–18% of patients
- homocysteine is elevated, although not to the same level as on dialysis.

Control of calorie intake, and increasing energy expenditure through activity and exercise are usually necessary. Additionally, poor eating habits may have formed whilst adhering to the dietary restrictions on dialysis: intake of fruit and vegetables and other 'cardioprotective' foods, such as oily fish are often low (very few patients have the recommended five portions of fruit and vegetable per day, or fish twice a week). Regular reinforcement of healthy eating advice can help reduce weight gain (Patel 1998), improve lipid levels (Lawrence et al 1995) and also help control hypertension.

BONE DISEASE

An improved lean body mass (muscle) and bone strength may also result from diet and exercise advice. Alendronate, vitamin D and calcium supplements may be required to improve bone strength.

DIABETES

The development of post-transplant diabetes is exacerbated by immuno-suppressive agents: steroids, tacrolimus and ciclosporin. Elderly, black and Hispanic patients are most at risk. Graft loss is four times greater for patients who have diabetes. Fasting blood glucose should be checked every three months in all non-diabetic transplanted patients. Diet and exercise interventions help reduce the risk of metabolic syndrome and developing diabetes (Engel 2003).

SUMMARY OF DIETARY ADVICE

- Monitor biochemistry and blood pressure control. In particular lipid levels (cholesterol and triglycerides), blood glucose, potassium, bone minerals, PTH and haemoglobin.
- Aim for acceptable body mass index: 'balance of good health' is an appropriate food model to use.
- Emphasise eating a variety of fruit and vegetables: aim for at least five portions per day.
- Encourage high-fibre foods (soluble and insoluble).
- Encourage fish, particularly oily fish, lean meats and pulses.

- Foods high in sugar, saturated fat and salt should be used sparingly.
- Dairy products should be low fat – with attention to meeting calcium requirements.
- Alcohol consumption should be within usual recommendations.
- Be aware of good food hygiene practices.
- Encourage physical activity and regular exercise.
- Avoid smoking and too much sun exposure.

Ideally, a team of specialists should be available to help with the rehabilitation of transplanted patients, including the dietitian, nurse, physiotherapist, social worker and counsellor.

DIETARY MANAGEMENT IN PAEDIATRICS

Chronic renal failure may present after birth or later in life and can proceed to established renal failure during childhood (Watson 1991). The profound effects that chronic renal failure can place upon growth (Kari et al 2000) and development, particularly during infancy, necessitate early nutritional management on a long-term basis. Fluctuating clinical and biochemical disturbances with changes in treatment require constant review and readjustment of the nutritional prescription by an experienced dietitian (Coleman 2001). Infants may present with particular problems, such as anorexia and vomiting, and an understanding of the psychosocial effects often proves to be as important as the dietary advice (Norman et al 1995).

Nutritional assessment should include the regular monitoring of growth (weight, height and head circumference) and dietary analysis by means of food diaries or dietary recall. Biochemical assessment with frequent review of fluid balance and prescribed medication, such as phosphate binders and antireflux agents is recommended. The maintenance of normal serum calcium and phosphate levels is crucial to achieve bone development, and nutritional measures have a large part to play, particularly in controlling phosphate levels (Norman 2004).

The dietary aims in managing children with chronic renal failure are dependent upon age, stage of chronic kidney disease and nutritional assessment. Oral nutritional supplements have an important role, and are frequently used. However, experience has shown that attempting to achieve adequate nutrition this way can be stressful for families due to vomiting, palatability and compliance.

A proactive approach to maintaining good nutrition and growth without the use of growth hormone has resulted in a programme of early instigation of dialysis in combination with nutritional support (Coleman et al 1998, Lederman et al 1999). Although nasogastric tubes are used successfully, supplementary feeding using a gastrostomy button device may be more suitable in the long term (Watson et al 1998). The button also provides a convenient route for the administration of medication, which has undoubted benefits for the child and family.

Dialysis is seen only as a holding measure before transplantation. Most children do very well and resume normal eating and drinking post transplant (Coleman et al 1998). However, even if the transplant is successful with normal renal function, concerns remain that there may be a prolonged transition to exclusive oral nutrition in infants and children who commenced nutritional support via an enteral route early in life. Support should be provided to encourage oral stimulation from the time of commencement of tube feeding (Pugh & Watson 2006). Such children may continue to require a period of nutritional support post transplant. Conversely, the lifting of dietary restrictions and steroid treatment in other children may require energy intake to be reduced to prevent rapid weight gain. A healthy, no-added-salt diet and exercise should be encouraged with ongoing dietetic advice.

Maintaining good nutrition in this group of children requires support from all members of the multidisciplinary team (Watson 1995). An agreed philosophy of nutritional care and dietetic time to attend ward rounds regularly, outpatient clinics and psychosocial meetings are essential. Home and school visits with frequent telephone contact are invaluable support measures.

SUMMARY

This chapter has provided the opportunity for the reader to improve current theoretical and practical knowledge of renal nutrition. However, dietary advice is constantly changing as a result of new research findings and evidence-based guidelines. It is important that a positive effort is made continuously to review practice and always to involve patients in the decision-making process.

ACKNOWLEDGEMENTS

With grateful thanks to Marianne Vennegoor who was the original author of this chapter and to Pearl Pugh who updated the section on paediatric nutrition from Janet Coleman's original script.

References

Aguilera A, Codoceo R, Selgas R et al. Anorexigen (TNF-alpha, cholecystokinin) and orexigen (neuropeptide Y) plasma levels in peritoneal dialysis (PD) patients: their relationship with nutritional parameters. Nephrol Dial Transplant 1998; 13: 1476–1483.

Bansal VK. Potassium metabolism in renal failure: nondietary rationale for hyperkalemia. J Renal Nutr 1992; 2: 8–12.

Berlyne GM. A course in renal disease, 2nd edn. Oxford, Blackwell Scientific Publications, 1968.

Block GA, Hulbert-Shearon TE, Levin NW et al. Association of serum phosphorus and calcium phosphate product with mortality risk in chronic hemodialysis patients: a national study. Am J Kidney Dis 1998; 31: 607–617.

Brenner B. Hemodynamically mediated glomerular injury and the progressive nature of kidney disease. Kidney Int 1983; 23: 647–655.

Canada–USA Peritoneal Dialysis Study Group. Adequacy of dialysis and nutrition in continuous peritoneal dialysis: association with clinical outcomes. J Am Soc Nephrol 1996; 7: 198–207.

Carfray A, Patel K, Whitaker P et al. Albumin as an outcome measure in haemodialysis in-patients: the effect of variation in assay method. Nephrol Dial Transplant 2000; 15: 1819–1822.

CARI guidelines. Caring for Australasians with renal impairment – protein restriction to prevent the progression of diabetic nephropathy, 2006. (www.cari. org.au/index.php).

Cherry N, Shalansky K. Efficacy of intradialytic parenteral nutrition in malnourished hemodialysis patients. Am J Health-Syst Pharm 2002; 59: 1736–1741.

Chung SH, Heimburger O, Stenvinkel P, Wang T, Lindholm B. Influence of peritoneal transport rate, inflammation, and fluid removal on nutritional status and clinical outcome in prevalent peritoneal dialysis patients. Perit Dial Int 2003; 23: 174–183.

Churchill DN. An evidence based approach to earlier initiation of dialysis, Am J Kidney Dis 1997; 30: 899–906.

Churchill DN, Taylor DW, Kesehaviah PR. Adequacy of dialysis and nutrition in continuous peritoneal dialysis: association with clinical outcomes. J Am Soc Nephrol 1996; 7: 198–207.

Cohen D, Galbraith C. General health management and long term care of the renal transplant recipient Am J Kidney Dis 2001; 38(Suppl 6): S10–S24.

Coleman JE. The kidney in clinical paediatric dietetics, 2nd edn. Shaw V, Lawson M,eds. Oxford: Blackwell Scientific Publications, 2001: 158–182.

Coleman JE, Watson AR. Growth post-transplantation in children previously treated with chronic dialysis and gastrostomy feeding. In: Khanna R, ed. Advances in peritoneal dialysis. Toronto: University of Toronto Press, 1998: 271–273.

Coleman JE, Watson AR, Rance CH et al. Gastrostomy buttons for nutritional support on chronic dialysis. Nephrol Dial Transplant 1998; 13: 2041–2046.

Davidson A. Interdialytic weight gain in Indo-Asians on haemodialysis. Br J Renal Med 2000; 5: 23–25.

Davies SJ, Phillips L, Griffiths AM, Russell LH, Naish PF, Russell GI. What really happens to people on long-term peritoneal dialysis? Kidney Int 1998; 54: 2207–2217.

Delahanty LM. Implications of the diabetes control and complications trial for renal outcomes and medical nutrition therapy. J Ren Nutr 1998; 8: 59–63.

Detsky AS, McLaughlin JR, Baker JP et al. What is subjective global assessment of nutritional status? J Parenteral Enteral Nutr 1987; 11: 8–13.

EDTNA/ERCA nutritional guidelines, 2002. Available from: www.edtna-erca.org.

Engel B. Nutritional management of diabetic renal transplant recipients. In: G Frost, Dornhurst A, Moses R, eds. Nutritional management of diabetes. London: John Wiley and Sons, 2003.

Engel B, Kon SP, Raftery MJ. Identification of malnutrition in haemodialysis patients. J Ren Nutr 1995; 5: 62–66.

ESPEN guidelines for nutrition screening 2002. Clin Nutr 2003; 22: 415–421.

European Best Practice Guidelines for Renal Transplantation 2002. Nephrol Dial Transplant 2002; 17(Suppl 4).

Fein PA, Madane SJ, Jorden A, Babu K, Mushnick R, Avram MM, Grosman I. Outcome of percutaneous endoscopic gastrostomy feeding in patients on peritoneal dialysis. Adv Perit Dial 2001; 17: 148–152.

Fine A, Cox D. Modest reduction of serum albumin in continuous peritoneal dialysis patients is common and of no apparent clinical consequence. Am J Kidney Dis 1992; 20: 50–54.

Fissell RB, Bragg-Gresham JL, Gillespie BW et al. International variation in vitamin prescription and association with mortality in the Dialysis Outcomes and Practice Patterns Study (DOPPS). Am J Kidney Dis 2004; 44: 293–9.

Fouque D, Laville M, Boissel JP. Low protein diets for chronic kidney disease in non diabetic adults. Cochrane Review 2006; issue 3.

Fouque D, Wang P, Laville M et al. Low protein diets delay end-stage renal disease in non-diabetic adults with chronic renal failure. Nephrol Dial Transplant 2000; 15: 1986–1992.

Friedman AN. Adiposity in dialysis: good or bad? Semin Dial 2006; 19: 136–140.

Ginn H, Rigalleau V, Aparicio M. Which diet for diabetic patients with chronic renal failure? Nephrol Dial Transplant 1999; 14: 2577–2579.

Goodman WG, Goldin J, Kulzon BD et al. Coronary artery calcification in young adults with end-stage renal disease who are undergoing dialysis. N Engl J Med 2000; 342: 1478–1482.

Grimble RF. Nutritional modulation of cytokine biology. Nutrition 1998; 14: 634–640.

Hadfield C. The nutritional adequacy of a low protein diet. J Ren Nutr 1992; 2(Suppl 1): 37–41.

Hakim RM, Lazarus JM. Initiation of dialysis. J Am Soc Nephrol 1995; 6: 1319–1328.

Halverson NA, Wilkens KG, Worthington-Roberts B. Interdialytic fluid gains in diabetic patients receiving hemodialysis treatment. J Ren Nutr 1993; 3: 23–29.

Hart PD, Wade A, Engel B, Marsh FP, Powell-Tuck J. Low protein diets in chronic renal insufficiency. BMJ 1992; 304: 640.

Heaf J, Jakobsen U, Tvedegaard E, Kanstrup I, Fogh-Andersen N. Dietary habits and nutritional status of renal transplant patients. J Ren Nutr 2004; 14: 20–25.

Heimburger O, Bergstrom J, Lindholm B. Is serum albumin an index of nutritional status in continuous ambulatory peritoneal dialysis patients? Perit Dial Int 1994; 14: 108–114.

Henderson IS, Leung AC, Shenkin A. Vitamin status in CAPD. Perit Dial Bull 1984; 4: 143–145.

Hong SY, Yang DH, Chang SK: Plasma homocysteine, vitamin B6, vitamin B12 and folic acid in end-stage renal disease during low-dose supplementation with folic acid. Am J Nephrol 1998; 18: 367–372.

Ifudu O, Dawood M, Homel P et al. Excess interdialytic weight gain provokes antihypertensive drug therapy in patients on maintenance hemodialysis. Dial Transplant 1997; 26: 541–559.

Ikizler TA, Greene JH, Wingard RL, Parker RA, Hakim RM. Spontaneous dietary protein intake during progression of chronic renal failure. J Am Soc Nephrol 1995; 6: 1386–1391.

Johnson DW Dietary protein restriction as a treatment for slowing chronic kidney disease progression: the case against. Nephrology 2006; 11: 58–62.

Jones CH, Wells L, Stoves J, Farquhar F, Woodrow G. Can a reduction in extracellular fluid volume result in increased serum albumin in peritoneal dialysis patients? Am J Kidney Dis 2002; 39: 872–875.

Kari JA, Gonzalez C, Ledermann SE, Rees L. Outcome and growth of infants with severe chronic renal failure. Kidney Int 2000, 57: 1681–1687.

Kaysen GA. Nutritional management of nephrotic syndrome. J Ren Nutr 1992; 2: 50–58.

Kaysen GA, Kumar V. Inflammation in ESRD: causes and potential consequences. J Ren Nutr 2003; 13: 158–160.

Klahr S, Levey AS, Beck GJ et al. The effects of dietary protein restriction and blood-pressure control on the progression of chronic renal disease. N Engl J Med 1994; 330: 878–884.

Konings CJ, Kooman JP, Schonck M et al. Fluid status, blood pressure, and cardiovascular abnormalities in patients on peritoneal dialysis. Perit Dial Int 2002; 22: 477–487.

Kopple JD, Wolfson M, Chertow GM et al. Clinical practice guidelines for nutrition in chronic renal failure. Am J Kidney Dis/J Ren Nutr 2000; 35: S17–S140.

Lawrence IR, Thomson A, Hartley GH et al. The effect of dietary intervention on the management of hyperlipidaemia in British renal transplant patients. J Ren Nutr 1995; 5: 73–77.

Lederman SE, Shaw V, Trompeter RS. Long-term enteral nutrition in infants and young children with chronic renal failure. Paediatr Nephrol 1999; 13: 870–875.

Lim VS, Flanigan MJ. Protein intake in patients with renal failure: comments on the current NFK–DOQI guidelines for nutrition in chronic renal failure. Semin Dial 2001; 14: 150–152.

Lindley E, Devine Y, Hall L, Cullen M, Cuthbert S, Woodrow G, Lopot F. A ward based procedure for assessment of fluid status in peritoneal dialysis patients using bioimpedance spectroscopy. Perit Dial Int 2005; 25(Suppl 3): S46–S48.

Loser C, Aschl G, Hebuterne X et al. ESPEN guidelines on enteral nutrition – percutaneous endoscopic gastrostomy (PEG). Clin Nutr 2005; 24: 848–861.

Lowrie EG, Lew NL. Death risk in hemodialysis patients: the predictive value of commonly measured variables and an evaluation of death rate differences between dialysis facilities. Am J Kidney Dis 1990; 15: 458–482.

Makoff R. Vitamin replacement therapy in renal failure patients. Mineral Electrolyte Metab 1999; 25: 349–351.

Mandayam S, Mitch WE. Dietary protein restriction benefits patients with chronic kidney disease. Nephrology 2006; 11: 53–57.

Marckmann P. Nutritional status of patients on hemodialysis and peritoneal dialysis. Clin Nephrol 1988; 29: 75–78.

Mazess RB, Barden HS, Bisek JP, Hanson J. Dual-energy x-ray absorptiometry for total-body and regional bone-mineral and soft-tissue composition . Am J Clin Nutr 1990; 51: 1106–1112.

McCann L. Subjective global assessment as it pertains to the nutritional status of dialysis patients. Dial Transplant 1996; 25: 190–202, 225.

McIntyre C, Harper I, Macdougall IC et al. Serum C-reactive protein as a marker of infection and inflammation in regular dialysis patients. Clin Nephrol 1997; 48: 371–374.

McKenzie SI, Henderson IS. The effect of increased dietary fibre intake on regular haemodialysis patients. In: Stevens E, Monkhouse P, eds. Aspects of renal care. London: Baillière Tindall, 1986: 172–178.

Mercer TH, Naish PF, Gleeson NP, Wilcock JE, Crawford C. Development of a walking test for the assessment of functional capacity in non-anaemic maintenance dialysis patients. Nephrol Dial Transplant 1998; 13: 2023–2026.

Millward DJ, Jackson AA. Protein/energy ratios of current diets in developed and developing countries compared with a safe protein/energy ratio: implications for recommended protein and amino acid intakes. Public Health Nutr 2003; 7: 387–405.

Muth I. Implications of hypervitaminosis A in chronic renal failure. J Ren Nutr 1991; 1: 2–8.

National Institutes of Health. Morbidity and mortality of dialysis. NIH consensus statement. Bethesda, MD: National Library of Medicine, Office of Medical Applications of Research, National Institutes of Health, 1993: 1–33.

National Kidney Foundation. K/DOQI Clinical practice guidelines for nutrition in chronic renal failure. K/DOQI paediatric guidelines. Am J Kidney Dis 2000; 35(Suppl 2): S105–S136.

National Kidney Foundation. K/DOQI clinical practice guidelines for managing dyslipidemias in chronic kidney disease. Am J Kidney Dis 2003a; 41(Suppl 3): S1–S92 (www.kidney.org/professionals/kdoqi/guidelines_lipids/index.htm).

NICE guidelines. Nutritional support in adults – oral supplements, enteral tube feeding and parenteral nutrition, 2006. www.nice.org.

Norman LJ, Coleman JE, Watson AR. Nutritional management in a child on chronic peritoneal dialysis; a team approach. J Hum Nutr 1995; 8: 209–213.

Norman LJ, Macdonald IA, Watson AR. Optimising nutrition in chronic renal insufficiency – growth. Paediatr Nephrol 2004; 19: 1245–1252.

Orth SR, Ritz E The nephrotic syndrome. N Engl J Med 1998; 338: 1202–1211.

Pagenkemper JJ, Burke KI, Roderick SL et al. Potassium availability in selected bran products: implications for the renal patient. J Renal Nutr 1994; 4: 27–31.

Patel MG. The effect of dietary intervention on weight gains after renal transplantation. J Ren Nutr 1998; 8: 137–141.

Pederson PU. Nutritional care: the effectiveness of actively involving older patients. J Clin Nurs 2005; 14: 247–255.

Pedrini MT, Levey AS, Lau J et al. The effect of protein restriction on the progression of diabetic and nondiabetic renal disease: a meta-analysis. Ann Intern Med 1996; 124: 629–632.

Pender FT. The effect of increasing the dietary fibre content of diets of patients with chronic renal failure treated by haemodialysis at home. J Hum Nutr Dietet 1989; 2: 423–427.

Pugh P, Watson AR. Transition from gastrostomy to oral feeding following renal transplantation. Adv Perit Dial 2006; 22: 153–157.

Pupim LB, Flakoll PJ, Brouillette JR, Levenhagen DK, Hakim RM, Ikizler TAJ. Intradialytic parenteral nutrition improves protein and energy homeostasis in chronic hemodialysis patients. Clin Invest 2002; 110: 437–439.

Ramirez G, Chen M, Boyce W et al. Longitudinal follow up of chronic haemodialysis patients without vitamin supplementation. Kidney Int 1986; 30: 99–106.

Renal Association and Royal College of Physicians. Treatment of adult patients with renal failure: recommended standards and audit measures. London: Renal Association and Royal College of Physicians of London, Royal College of Physicians Publication Unit, 2002.

Rocco MV, Makoff R. Appropriate vitamin therapy for dialysis patients. Semin Dial 1997; 10: 272–277.

Roubenoff R, Heymsfield SB, Kehayias JJ, Cannon JG, Rosenberg IH. Standardization of nomenclature of body composition in weight loss. Am J Clin Nutr 1997; 66: 192–196.

Sexton J, Vincent M. Remedying calcium and phosphate problems in chronic kidney disease. Pharm J 2004; 274: 561–564 (www.pjonline.com).

Sherman RA, Cody RP, Rogers ME et al. Interdialytic weight gain and nutritional parameters in chronic dialysis patients. Am J Kidney Dis 1995; 25: 579–583.

Spiegel DM, Anderson M, Campbell U et al. Serum albumin: a marker for morbidity in peritoneal dialysis patients. Am J Kidney Dis 1993; 21: 26–30.

Steele M, Yokum D, Armstrong A. Efficacy of intraperitoneal amino acid (IPAA) dialysate in an Asian vegetarian patient with chronic hypoalbuminaemia. EDTNA–ERCA J 1998; 24: 28–32.

Stenvinkel P, Heimburger O, Lindholm B et al. Are there two types of malnutrition in chronic renal failure? Evidence for relationships between malnutrition, inflammation and atherosclerosis. Nephrol Dial Transplant 2000; 15: 953–960.

Stenvinkel P, Heimburger O, Paultre F, Diczfalusy U, Wang T, Berglund L, Jogestrand T. Strong association between malnutrition, inflammation, and atherosclerosis in chronic renal failure. Kidney Int 1999; 55: 1899–1911.

Stenvinkel P. Interactions between inflammation, oxidative stress, and endothelial dysfunction in end-stage renal disease. J Ren Nutr 2003; 13: 144–148.

Stratton RJ, Green CJ, Elia M. Disease related malnutrition an evidence based approach. Oxford: CABI International, 2003.

Suetta C, Magnusson SP, Rosted A et al. Resistance training in the early postoperative phase reduces hospitalization and leads to muscle hypertrophy in elderly hip surgery patients —a controlled, randomized study. J Am Geriatr Soc 2004; 52, 2016–2022.

Tan CC, Harden PN, Rodger RSC et al. Ranatidine reduces phosphate binding in dialysis patients receiving calcium carbonate. Nephrol Dialy Transplant 1996; 11: 851–853.

Taylor GS, Patel V, Spencer S, Fluck RJ, McIntyre CW. Long-term use of 1.1% amino acid dialysis solution in hypoalbuminemic continuous ambulatory peritoneal dialysis patients. Clin Nephrol 2002; 58: 445–450.

Tjiong HL, van den Berg JW, Wattimena JL et al. Dialysate as food: combined amino acid and glucose dialysate improves protein anabolism in renal failure patients on automated peritoneal dialysis. J Am Soc Nephrol 2005; 16: 1486–1493.

Todorovic VE, Micklewright A. A pocket guide to clinical nutrition. Birmingham: British Dietetic Association, 2004.

UK Prospective Diabetes Study (UKPDS). Intensive blood–glucose control with sulphonylureas or insulin compared with conventional treatment and risk of complications in patients with type 2 diabetes (UKPDS 33). Lancet 1998; 352: 837–853.

Vennegoor M, ed. Enjoying food on a renal diet. London: King Edward's Fund for London, 1982.

Vennegoor M, ed. Enjoying food on a renal diet. London: King Edward's Fund for London, 1992.

Vennegoor M, ed. Nutrition for patients with renal failure. Portsmouth: EDTNA–ERCA, 1986.

Visser R, Dekker FW, Boeschoten EW, Stevens P, Krediet RT. Reliability of the 7-point subjective global assessment scale in assessing nutritional status of dialysis patients. Adv Perit Dial 1999; 15: 222–225.

Walters BA, Hays RD, Spritzer KL, Fridman M, Carter WB. Health related quality of life, depressive symptoms and malnutrition at start of hemodialysis initiation. Am J Kidney Dis 2002; 40: 1185–1194.

Watson AR. Disorders of the urinary tract. In: Levine MI, ed. Jolly's diseases of childhood. 6th edn. Oxford: Blackwell Scientific Publication, 1991: 226–268.

Watson AR. Strategies to support families of children with end-stage renal failure. Paediatric Nephrology 1995; 9: 628–631.

Watson AR, Coleman JE, Warady BA. When and how to use nasogastric and gastrostomy feeding for nutritional support. In: Fine RN, Alexander SR, Warady BA, eds. CAPD/CCPD in children, 2nd edn. Boston: Kluwer Academic Publishers, 1998: 281–301.

Waugh NR, Robertson AM. Protein restriction for diabetic renal disease. Cochrane Reviews 1997 (updated 2000).

Wolk R. Micronutrition in dialysis. Nutr Clin Pract 1993; 8: 267–276.

Wood R, Alexander C, Crawford M, Paterson A. The need for vitamin supplements reviewed. Br J Ren Med 1998; 3(2): 17–20.

World Health Organization. Obesity. Preventing and managing the global epidemic. Geneva: WHO, 1998.

Yale JF. Oral antihyperglycaemic agents and renal disease: new agents, new concepts. J Am Soc Nephrol 2005; 16(Suppl 1): S7–S10.

Young GA, Kopple JD, Lindholm B et al. Nutritional assessment of continuous ambulatory peritoneal dialsysis patients: an international study. Am J Kidney Dis 1991; 17: 462–471.

Further reading

Engel B, Vennegoor M, James G, Singh S. Setting standards and achieving optimal nutritional status. British Dietetic Association renal nutrition group standards for adult renal patients over 18 year olds. 1998.

ESPEN guidelines for nutrition screening (2002). Clin Nutr 2003; 22: 415–421.

European Best Practice Guidelines for Renal Transplantation (2002). Neprol Dial Transplant 2002; 17(Suppl 4).

K/DOQI. Clinical practice guidelines for nutrition in chronic renal failure. National Kidney Foundation. Am J Kidney Dis 2000; 35: S1–S140.

National Kidney Foundation. K/DOQI clinical practice guidelines for bone metabolism and disease in chronic kidney disease. Am J Kidney Dis 2003b; 42(Suppl 3): S1–S202 www.kidney.org/professionals/kdoqi/guidelines_bone/index.htm

Useful websites

K/DOQI National Kidney Foundation: www.kidney.org
EDTNA–ERCA: www.edtna-erca.org

Cochrane Renal Group: www.cochrane-renal.org

APPENDIX 11.1   CALCULATION OF BODY MASS INDEX AND IDEAL BODY WEIGHT

Body mass index (BMI) can be calculated by dividing the weight in kilograms by the height in metres squared.

If the patient has oedema, the BMI will be overestimated and is not valid. In estimating oedema-free body weight (BW_{ef}), weight should be measured after HD or after drainage of dialysis fluid in PD.

Example

A person weighs 65 kg and is 1.70 m tall

$$BMI = 65/(1.7 \times 1.7) = 22.5 \, kg \, m^{-2}$$

Normal range: 18.5–24.9
Underweight < 18.5
Pre-obese (overweight): 25–29.9
Obese class I: 30–34.9
Obese class II: 35–39.9 (obese)
Obese class III: > 40 (morbidly obese)

The K/DOQI guidelines recommend the use of adjusted oedema-free body weight (aBW_{ef}) to calculate protein or energy requirements or to assess intake. The following method can be used.

Standard body weight: a BMI between 18.5 and 24.9 $kg \, m^{-2}$ and its corresponding weight in kilograms, is considered within the normal range (WHO 1998). However, given the increased mortality of patients at the lower end of the 'normal' range it may be prudent to calculate the standard weight for a BMI of 23 and this can be used in the equation below. The following equation has been suggested:

Ideal body weight (IBW) = aBW_{ef}
$$= BW_{ef} + ((standard \, body \, weight - BW_{ef}) \times 0.25)$$

These figures should be used to calculate protein and energy requirements for individual patients.

Note: the important point for audit purposes and comparison across renal units is to note clearly how you have calculated IBW. As there is no consensus regarding this issue, a simpler method would be to use the weight corresponding to a BMI of $23\,kg\,m^{-2}$.

APPENDIX 11.2   FOODS WITH A HIGH AND LOW SODIUM (SALT) CONTENT

It may not be possible to eliminate all the listed foods or meals, unless a low-sodium alternative is available. A compromise may be reached by allowing some salty foods for sandwiches or main meals, but preparing the rest of the meals at home without salt. Adding herbs and spices during meal preparation or thereafter compensates for the loss of salt.

APPENDIX 11.3   FOODS WITH HIGH AND LOW PHOSPHORUS CONTENT

All foods with a high protein content also contain a fair amount of phosphorus. However, some of these foods are an essential part of the diet and cannot be eliminated.

APPENDIX 11.4   FOODS WITH HIGH AND LOW POTASSIUM CONTENT

FOODS WITH A HIGH POTASSIUM CONTENT

Snacks
- Bombay mix, curu snacks, peanuts and raisins, potato crisps, potato hoops, tortilla chips, Twiglets, vegetable samosas.

Sweets
- Chocolate-plain, milk or white – and all sweets containing chocolate or cocoa.
- Liquorice Allsorts, toffees, fudge and other sweets containing nuts, chocolate and dried fruit.

Beverages
- Coffee in excess.
- Milk powder and drinks containing milk powder, such as Ovaltine, Horlicks, Complan, Build-up, drinking chocolate, milk shakes, Nutrament, cocoa powder.
- Fruit juices unless exchanged for fruit, tomato juice, carrot juice, vegetable juice, cane sugar juice, pomegranate juice, guava, mango and lychee juice.
- Strong ale, barley wine, vintage cider, red wine, sweet white wines, sweet sherry and port.

Appendix 11.2   Foods with a high and low sodium content

Avoid	Suitable alternative
Dairy products	
Salted butter or margarine	Use unsalted or salt-reduced alternatives instead
Cheese, cheese spreads	
Meat and meat products	
Canned and cured meat products such as bacon, gammon, salt beef, corned beef, ham, tongue, all types of sausages, pâtés	Fresh-cooked meat Fresh-cooked poultry Fresh-cooked fish
Meat pies, quiches and sausage rolls	Home-cooked meals
Processed meals	
Fast food-type meals	
Vegetables	
Canned vegetables, sauerkraut, instant potato powder, salted potato crisps	Fresh or frozen vegetables
Nuts	
Roasted and salted nuts	
Miscellaneous	
Salt, sea salt, salt substitutes such as Lo Salt, Solo, Selora	Herbs, spices
Mayonnaise, salad dressings	Home-made dressings, i.e. French dressing
Bottled sauces, pickles	Vinegar, lemon, lime juice
Canned or packet soups or ready-made soups	Home-made soup
Pasta sauce, curry paste, soya sauce	Home-made sauces
Meat or yeast extracts and bouillon cubes, packet gravy, gravy cubes or powders	Use herbs and spices for curries Use fresh ingredients for pasta dishes
Foods containing monosodium glutamate	
Salted savoury snacks	
Asian foods	
Poppadums, samosas, other savoury snacks, chutneys, pickles, chevra, chana	
Greek foods	
Taramasalata, canned vine leaves, houmus	Home-made houmus
Chinese foods	
Dried fish, salted fish	
Peking duck and similar products	

Appendix 11.3   Foods with high and low phosphorus content

Foods with a high phosphorus content	Foods with a low phosphorus content
Cereals	
Natural Bran, All-Bran, Bran Flakes, Bran Buds, cereals containing nuts	All other breakfast cereals
Rye bread	Porridge
Crispbread containing rye	Wholemeal or white bread, croissant
Oatcakes, scones	Puri, pitta bread, chapatti, nan
Soya flour	Yorkshire pudding
	Flour, barley, sago
	Semolina, tapioca, cornflour, custard powder
	Pasta, noodles, rice, wild rice
Dairy products	
Milk, yoghurt (see allowance allocated by renal dietitian)	Cream, crème fraîche
Evaporated and condensed milk	Fromage frais, quark
Milk powder, Horlicks	Cottage cheese and curd cheese
Most types of hard cheese, e.g. cheddar	Full-fat or reduced-fat cream cheese, such as Boursin, Philadelphia, roulé, mascarpone, riccota
Stilton, cheese spread	
Eggs (no more than one daily); however, these quantities may need to be adapted for vegetarian diets	Egg white, meringue
Meat and meat products	
Liver, kidney, liver pâté and liver sausage, black pudding	Beef, veal, lamb, pork, chicken, turkey, sausages, meat pies (see meal plan suggested by the renal dietitian)
Fish and fish products	
Fish with edible bones, such as anchovies, herring, kippers, pilchards, salmon, sardines, sprats, whitebait, fish roe, fish paste	Fresh or smoked fish, such as cod, haddock, halibut, plaice, mackerel, tuna, fish fingers, fish cakes
	Canned fish, such as tuna, salmon with all bones removed
	Cockles, mussels, squid
	Occasionally use: crab, lobster, prawns, scampi, trout
Vegetables	
Pulses, such as dried peas, dried beans, lentils, baked beans, chick peas	All other vegetables
Savoury snacks	
All types of nuts such as peanuts, peanut butter	Popcorn, corn snacks
Bombay mix, chevra, chana, ganthia	
Poppadoms	
Sweets	
Chocolate, cocoa powder, Ovaltine, Mars bars, Snickers, Bounty, halva, burfi with nuts	Sweets, barley sugars, butterscotch, mint, fruit pastilles, starburst, sherbets, jelly babies, wine gums, marshmallows, Turkish delight, chewing gum, plain toffee and fudge, lollipops, ice lollies
Cakes and pastries	
Chocolate cake, Battenburg cake	All other types of cakes, biscuits, pastries
Any cakes and pastries containing chocolate or nuts	Doughnuts, cream cakes, gingerbread
Biscuits	
Chocolate biscuits, Jaffa cakes	Plain biscuits, such as Digestives

Foods with a high phosphorus content	Foods with a low phosphorus content
All biscuits containing nuts or chocolate	Cream crackers, Rich Tea, shortbread, sponge fingers, cream-filled biscuits
Puddings Milk pudding, custard, bread pudding, Christmas pudding, fruit pies or crumbles, sponge Chocolate mousse, chocolate ice cream, desserts containing nuts and chocolate	Pancakes, pastries, sweet or savoury, fruit jelly, sorbets Plain ice cream, cheesecake
Beverages Milk and milk drinks, such as milk shakes, Build-up, Complan, Nutrament, drinking chocolate, cocoa, Bournevita, Ovaltine, Jamaican punch	Tea, coffee Soft drinks, Lucozade, fruit squash, lemon barley, blackcurrant drink, lime juice cordial, Crusha syrup, rosehip syrup
Condiments and miscellaneous Meat and yeast extracts, such as Marmite, Bovril, Vegemite Marzipan, peanut butter Seeds such as sesame, tahini Chocolate and nut spread	Sugar, jam, marmalade, honey, lemon curd, golden syrup Gelatine, yeast, pickles, chutney, tomato ketchup, tomato purée, lemon juice, vinegar, mustard, mayonnaise, salad cream, salad dressing, tartare sauce, chilli sauce, soya sauce, herbs and spices, apple sauce, cranberry sauce, redcurrant jelly, horseradish, mint sauce, mint jelly

Fruit

- Avocado pear, banana, fresh blackcurrants or redcurrants.
- Dried fruit, such as dried apples, dried apricots, dried banana chips, currants, dates, dried figs, prunes, raisins, sultanas and other dried fruits.

Nuts

- All types of nuts, including peanut butter and marzipan.
- All types of seeds, such as sesame seeds.
- Chocolate and nut spread.

Vegetables

- Ackee, Jerusalem artichokes, beetroot mushrooms, spinach, celeriac, squash, grilled or fried tomatoes, fried onions, potato waffles.
- Plantain and green bananas.
- Sun-dried tomatoes, tomato purée or sauce in excess.
- Dried pulses, such as dried beans, red kidney beans, broad beans, butter beans, black-eyed beans, dried peas, chick peas, lentils.
- Vegetables that can be taken instead of potatoes.
- Yam, sweet potato, plantain or green banana in small quantities, pulse vegetables and parsnips.

Cereals

- All-Bran, Bran Flakes, oatbran flakes, Fruit and Fibre, oat and wheat bran, Raisin Splitz, Shredded Sultana Bran.

Cakes and biscuits

- Fruit cake, mince pies, Christmas cake, ginger nuts.
- Oat cakes, rye crispbread.
- All biscuits and cakes containing dried fruit, nuts or chocolate.

Pudding and desserts	• Bread pudding and Christmas pudding. • Desserts containing chocolate.
Meat substitutes	• Fresh soya bean products, vegetarian meat substitutes, bean milk.
Miscellaneous	• Tomato ketchup, tomato chutney, tomato purée, tomato sauce (can be taken in small quantities). • Meat and yeast extracts (dried or paste). • Salt substitutes containing potassium chloride (i.e. low-salt products).

FOODS WITH A LOW POTASSIUM CONTENT

These can be given as alternatives to high-potassium foods.

Sweets	• Sugar, jam, marmalade, honey, lemon curd, Golden Syrup. • Boiled sweets, barley sugars, peppermints, plain fudge, butterscotch toffee, Turkish delight, fondant sweets, jelly babies, fruit pastilles, fruit gums, sherbets, marshmallows, lollipops, ice lollies, chewing gum.
Drinks	• Tea – black or with a little milk. • Soft drinks: tonic, Seven-Up, lemonade, Lucozade (bottled only), soda water, mineral water, dry ginger ale, ginger beer, American ginger ale, bitter lemon, sparkling orange and other soft drinks with a low juice content. • Fruit squash or barley water with a low natural juice content. • Whisky, gin, vodka, brandy, rum and liqueurs in small quantities. These can be mixed with water, soda, lemonade, tonic and any of the above soft drinks.
Fruit	• Crystallised or glacé fruit.
Cereal	• Rice, wild rice, noodles, pasta. • Bread, pitta bread, croissant, puri, chapati. • Cream crackers, water biscuits. • Cornflakes, Rice Krispies. • Plain cake, pastry and biscuits. • Flour, barley, sago, semolina, tapioca.
Fat (see dietitian's advice on the use of these products)	• Slightly or unsalted margarine, butter, low-fat spreads, oil, olive oil. • French dressing, mayonnaise, salad cream. • Double cream, crème fraîche, cream cheese.
Condiments	• Spices, such as allspice, cinnamon, ginger powder, mustard powder, nutmeg, pepper. • Vinegar, Worcester sauce, mustard, chilli sauce.

- Basil, bayleaf, caraway seeds, chilli powder, cloves, coriander, curry powder, dill, mint, oregano, paprika, parsley, sage, tarragon, thyme, tumeric, etc.
- Garlic, lemon juice, Tabasco.
- Piccalilli, horseradish, chutney and sweet pickles.

Dried herbs or spices in moderation

- Basil, bayleaf, coriander, dill, oregano, mint, tarragon, thyme, etc.

Fresh herbs in moderation

POTASSIUM PORTIONS

Potassium portions or exchanges can be used to encourage variety. Most fruits and vegetables contain potassium in varying quantities. Each portion contains approximately 5 mmol (200 mg) potassium. Quantities are based on fresh or boiled vegetables or on fresh, stewed or canned fruit.

Note: one portion contains 10 mmol potassium. 150 g boiled potatoes may be replaced by:

Potatoes, tubers and pulses

- 150 g new potatoes, peeled
- 75 g baked potato in skin
- 75 g new potatoes, boiled in skin
- 75 g roast potato
- 50 g chips (2 tablespoons) or 6 oven chips
- 25 g = 1 small packet potato crisps (no salt)
- 2 potato croquettes
- 150 g boiled parsnips
- 150 g ravioli or spaghetti in tomato sauce
- 150 g yam, sweet potato, dasheen, eddoes, coco, boiled bread fruit
- 150 g rice and peas (without coconut)
- 75 g boiled green banana or plantain.
- 150 g soaked and boiled butter beans, haricot beans, black-eyed beans, baked beans in tomato sauce, dried peas, split peas, chick peas
- 150 g lentils, boiled
- 100 g red kidney beans, boiled.

VEGETABLES

(Note: one portion is approximately 5 mmol (200 mg) potassium)

The following vegetables are low in potassium. As a guide, one portion is about 3–4 heaped tablespoons.
Boiled and drained vegetables such as:

Low potassium content

- asparagus (6 medium spears)
- runner beans
- beansprouts
- bamboo shoots
- cauliflower
- carrots
- globe artichoke

- red, white or Savoy cabbage
- Chinese leaves
- marrow
- pumpkin
- peas (processed, canned, frozen, mushy peas)
- onions boiled, pickled or silverskin
- spring greens.

Medium–high potassium content

The following vegetables have a medium–high potassium content. As a guide, one portion is 2–3 heaped tablespoons of boiled, drained vegetables such as:

- aubergine
- french beans
- broccoli
- celery
- courgettes
- curly kale
- mangetout
- leeks
- capsicum (red or green)
- turnip
- sweetcorn kernels, on the cob or baby sweetcorn, fresh or canned
- turnip.

High potassium content

The following vegetables have a fairly high potassium content. As a guide, one unit is 75 g of boiled, drained vegetables such as:

- brussel sprouts (6)
- fennel okra (6 pods)
- spinach
- kohlrabi
- mushrooms (boiled in water first)
- tomatoes (canned).

Raw vegetables

A small portion – use a mixture of the following:
- beetroot
- red cabbage
- carrots
- celery
- chicory
- coleslaw
- corn kernels
- cucumber
- lettuce
- mustard and cress
- peppers (red, green, yellow or orange)
- radish

- spring onions
- tomato (no more than half a tomato)
- watercress.

Fruit

Canned, bottled, stewed or baked fruit in water contains less potassium than raw fruit. Drain fruit before measuring a portion, as the juice also contains potassium and should be discarded.

Low potassium content

The following fruits have a low potassium content. As a guide, one unit of fruit is 6 tablespoons of most canned fruits (except those mentioned in lists of fruits with medium or high potassium content), or 150 g of fresh fruit, for example:

- 1 apple
- 1 clementine
- ½ grapefruit
- mango
- a thin slice of melon – cantaloupe, galia, honeydew, watermelon
- 1 small orange
- 2 passion fruits
- 1 medium-sized pear
- 1 satsuma
- 1 tangerine.

Medium–high potassium content

The following fruits have a medium–high potassium content. As a guide, one portion is 100 g (canned, 4 tablespoons or fresh):

- apricots (canned in syrup or juice)
- blackberries (fresh or stewed)
- blackcurrants
- 12 cherries
- gooseberries (fresh or stewed)
- 6–8 kumquats
- 1 lemon or lime
- loganberries (fresh)
- 6 lychees (fresh)
- 1 nectarine
- paw paw (papaya)
- 1 medium peach (fresh or in natural juice)
- pineapple (1 medium thick slice)
- 2 pomegranates
- plums: depending on size, 1 large or 3–4 small
- raspberries (fresh)
- rhubarb (stewed or canned)
- 1 sharon fruit
- 8 strawberries.

Fairly high potassium content

The following fruits have a fairly high potassium content. As a guide, one unit is 75 g of canned or fresh:

- damsons
- 5 dates (fresh or dried)
- 1 figs (fresh)
- 4 greengages (fresh)
- 1 kiwi fruit
- 6 prunes (dried or canned)
- ½ banana.

APPENDIX 11.5   SUBJECTIVE GLOBAL ASSESSMENT

SUBJECTIVE GLOBAL ASSESSMENT RATING FORM	
Patient Name: ID#: Date:	
HISTORY	

WEIGHT/WEIGHT CHANGE: *(Included in K/DOQI SGA)*
1. **Baseline Wt:**   _____(Dry weight from 6 months ago)
   Current Wt: _____(Dry weight today)
   Actual Wt loss/past 6 ms: _____ % loss:_____(actual loss from baseline or last SGA)
2. **Weight change over past two weeks:**_____No change_____ Increase _____Decrease
	Rate 1-7

DIETARY INTAKE No Change_____(Adequate) No Change_____(Inadequate) 1. Change: Sub optimal Intake: _____Protein_____Kcal_____ Duration_____ Full Liquid: _____ Hypocaloric Liquid _____ Starvation _____	

GASTROINTESTINAL SYMPTOMS *(Included in K/DOQI SGA-anorexia or causes of anorexia)*
    Symptom: **Frequency:***   **Duration:**+
    _____ None   _____   _____
    _____ Anorexia   _____   _____
    _____ Nausea   _____   _____
    _____ Vomiting   _____   _____
    _____ Diarrhea   _____   _____
            Never, daily, 2-3 times/wk, 1-2 times/wk > 2 weeks, < 2 weeks	

FUNCTIONAL CAPACITY
    Description   **Duration:**
    _____ No Dysfunction   _____
    _____ Change in function   _____
    _____ Difficulty with ambulation   _____
    _____ Difficulty with activity (Patient specific "normal") _____
    _____ Light activity   _____
    _____ Bed/chair ridden with little or no activity _____
    _____ Improvement in function _____	

DISEASE STATE/COMORBIDITIES AS RELATED TO NUTRITIONAL NEEDS Primary Diagnosis_____Comorbidities_____ Normal requirements _____Increased requirements_____ Decreased requirements_____ Acute Metabolic Stress:_____ None _____Low _____Moderate _____ High	
PHYSICAL EXAM	

_____ Loss of subcutaneous fat (Below eye, triceps,   _____Some areas_____All areas
              biceps, chest) *(Included in K/DOQI SGA)*
_____ Muscle wasting (Temple, clavicle, scapula, ribs,   _____Some areas_____ All areas
              quadriceps, calf, knee, interosseous *(Included in K/DOQI SGA)*
_____ Ederma (Related to undernutrition/use to evaluate weight change)	

OVERALL SGA RATING	
Very mild risk to well-nourished = 6 or 7 most categories or significant, continued improvement. Mild-moderate = 3, 4, or 5 ratings. No clear sign of normal status or severe malnutrition. Severely Malnourished = 1 or 2 ratings in most categories/significant physical signs of malnutrition.	

HAEMODIALYSIS REVIEW PROFORMA

Name:.. **Date of review**:...

1. Blood results

	Date	Date	Trend	Comments
Hb (also Check MCV, B12, folate, ferritin)				
Sodium				
Potassium				
Urea				
Creatinine				
Adj Calcium				
Phosphate				
Albumin				
PTH				

2. Hours on dialysis per week / dialysis adequacy (kt/v)...

Comment / Action...

3. Dry weight (kg):.. ht (m)............ BMI (kg/m^2)................................

Weight change since last review? Is this significant, desirable,

undesirable?.. ideal weight[1] (kg)....................

Comment/ Action:...

4. Urine output (ml)...................................... Fluid allowance (ml).......................................

5. Weight gain between dialysis (subject to local standards)

Good (<1.5kg) ❏   OK occasionally (1.5 – 2.5kg) ❏   Poor (> 2.5kg) ❏

Comment/ Action (check sodium intake)...

6. Potassium: mmol/l (subject to local standards)

Low ❏   Good ❏   Acceptable occasionally ❏   Poor ❏
(<3.5)   (3.5 – 6.0)   (6.1 – 6.5)   (>6.5)

Comment / Action:...

---

[1] This weight can be used to calculate protein and energy intake: g/kg or kcal/kg (Q 10)

7. **Phosphate: mmol/l** (subject to local standards)[2]

Low ❑   Good ❑   Acceptable occasionally ❑   Poor ❑
(<1.1)   (1.1 – 1.6)   (1.7 – 1.8)   (>1.8)

Phosphate binders used (check timing and amount taken) :

....
....

Comment / Action:..
....

8. **Other medication:**

9. **Meal Plan:** check protein, energy, sodium, potassium, phosphate as well as balance of good health

Breakfast

Lunch

Evening Meal

Snacks / Drinks

10. **Daily energy & protein intake** (assess from diet history or diet diary)

Average DPI (g/day)...

Average energy intake (kcal/kg/day)[3]...

DPI (g/kg/day)[3] (subject to local standards)

Low ❑   Acceptable ❑   Good ❑   High ❑
(<0.9)   (0.9 – 1.0)   (1.0 – 1.2)   (>1.2)

Comment / Action:...
....

---

[2] (Calcium × Phosphate product = 4.8 mmol^2/l^2)
[3] Ideal weight can be used

Chapter 12

Renal transplantation

Raymond Trevitt

CHAPTER CONTENTS

**LEARNING OUTCOMES
FOR THIS CHAPTER**

- To analyse the risks and benefits of renal transplantation
- To identify the contraindications to transplantation
- To understand the importance of pretransplant assessment
  and the nursing role in the pretransplant clinical care pathway
- To explore donor and recipient matching, and its relevance to graft
  survival
- To understand cadaveric and living donation
- To evaluate critically the possible options to increase cadaveric
  donor supply
- To outline the nursing care for the renal transplant recipient
  in the pre-, peri- and postrenal transplant phase
- To explain the use of immunosuppressive regimens in individual
  recipient situations

INTRODUCTION

Renal transplantation is now widely acknowledged as the treatment of choice for those with established renal failure (ERF). Since the time of the first transplants in the 1950s, advances in antirejection therapies, surgical techniques and tissue matching have enabled kidney transplantation to evolve from an experimental procedure to the treatment that can offer the best quality of life and the most cost-effective care for kidney patients.

Many patients view a kidney transplant as the gateway to 'personal liberation' and as the opportunity to restore 'control over one's life' (Galpin 1992). A successful transplant offers freedom from the practical and psychological difficulties and restrictions of long-term dialysis; freedom from dependence upon a machine, fluid bag or partner; freedom from fluid and dietary restrictions; a return of sexual functioning and fertility with the possibility of parenthood; and a return to an almost normal lifestyle.

A study from the University of Maryland reported similar findings, noting that 'Older age was associated with smaller, but still significant, improvement in quality of life' (Connerney & Bartlett 2001). Thus, older patients may wish to spend more time evaluating the risks and benefits associated with transplantation before joining the transplant waiting list.

Most research studies clearly show that, for the majority, kidney transplantation has the greater rehabilitation potential and that the quality of life for patients with functioning grafts is superior to that which is usually achieved on dialysis (Evans et al 1985, Jofre et al 1998, Morris & Jones 1988). However, research into quality of life has received much criticism, and individual perception and assessment of quality of life is known to be affected by a wide range of independent and personal variables. But, for many of those with renal failure, transplantation offers an improved quality of life, and may be the most significant factor for patients when considering transplantation.

COST-EFFECTIVE CARE

Transplantation is the most cost-effective treatment option for end-stage renal disease. The cost of 1 year of haemodialysis or peritoneal dialysis is similar to that of a renal transplant in the first year. However, thereafter the cost of continuing care for the transplant patient is one-fifth of the cost of dialysis per year.

NATIONAL WAITING-LIST FIGURES FOR KIDNEY TRANSPLANT

The improvement in quality of life and cost-effectiveness of this treatment support the suggestion that renal transplantation is the treatment of choice for the majority of patients. Unfortunately, such a goal is not possible at present because of the limited supply of cadaveric organs. The current UK waiting list for kidney transplantation stands at more than

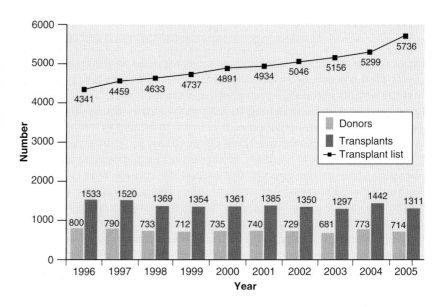

5000 patients (Fig. 12.1). About 1700 renal transplants are performed in the UK each year. We therefore need to explore ways of increasing donor numbers in order to offer all suitable patients the chance of a transplant.

CONTRAINDICATIONS TO RENAL TRANSPLANTATION

Although the majority of patients may request a transplant, transplantation may not be suitable for all those with ERF because of possible medical complications.

MALIGNANCY

Malignant disease must be excluded prior to transplantation as the immunosuppressive regime may cause accelerated growth of the tumour and may encourage secondary spread. If the patient is known to have had a tumour removed in the past, it is important to ascertain the type of tumour, the stage of tumour development and the treatment received. In selected cases, transplantation may still be possible provided that curative treatment has been given and sufficiently long follow-up has occurred to exclude recurrence. The importance of time to transplant following treatment of a malignancy is shown by Penn's (1997) paper using data from the USA. In 1137 recipients who had been treated for a malignancy prior to transplantation, the recurrence rate was:

- treatment < 2 years pretransplant – 54%
- treatment 2–5 years pretransplant – 33%
- treatment > 5 years pretransplant – 13%.

RECURRENT DISEASE

It is also important to consider the patient's primary renal disease as in some cases the disease may recur and destroy the new kidney (Table 12.1). Renal disorders with a very high recurrence rate include focal segmental glomerulosclerosis (FSGS) (causing massive proteinuria and scarring of the glomeruli) and mesangiocapillary glomerulonephritis (an immunological disorder of the glomeruli). However, transplantation may still be considered but only after counselling and explanation of the risks to the patient. Most centres would advise against living related donation in this situation.

Other conditions, such as Goodpasture's syndrome and the other vasculitic illnesses, need to have been fully treated before going ahead with transplantation because of the risk of damage in the new kidney in the presence of active disease. Twelve months is normally considered the earliest that transplantation would be considered, to allow antibody levels to fall. Several other diseases, such as diabetes, can cause microscopic changes in the kidney after many years but rarely lead to graft loss.

HEPATITIS VIRUS AND HUMAN IMMUNODEFICIENCY VIRUS

Patients who are hepatitis B or hepatitis C positive may be at risk of progressive liver disease after transplantation owing to the impact of the immunosuppressive therapy. Similarly, the immunosuppression would have an adverse effect in the presence of human immunodeficiency virus (HIV), reducing life expectancy. In most centres, infection with HIV is classed as an absolute contraindication to transplantation. Opinions differ with regard to transplantation in the presence of hepatitis B and hepatitis C. Decisions are taken on an individual basis with regard to level, type of infection and the extent of liver damage. However, many patients with hepatitis B and C have no or quiescent disease. Lamivudine inhibits hepatitis B viral replication and has been used with some success post-transplant (Lee et al 2001).

Type of glomerulonephritis	Recurrence (%)
Focal segmental glomerulosclerosis	30
Membranous nephropathy	10
Mesangiocapillary type I	20–30
Mesangiocapillary type II	95
Immunoglobulin A nephropathy	50
Henoch–Schönlein purpura	80
Antiglomerular basement membrane nephritis	5
Idiopathic crescentic glomerulonephritis	?

Data from Mathew (1988) with permission.

Table 12.1
Recurrence of glomerulonephritis in renal transplants.

DIABETES MELLITUS AND CARDIOVASCULAR DISEASE

Many people with diabetes can receive a renal transplant, but they are at risk from other complications of their diabetes. Cardiovascular disease is seen primarily in those with type 2 diabetes, and may contribute to higher levels of morbidity and death. Also, it is important to assess vessel patency prior to transplantation, as severe atherosclerosis of the iliac vessels may at worst preclude transplantation and at best complicate the transplant surgery.

EVALUATION FOR TRANSPLANTATION

AGE

Morbidity and mortality after kidney transplantation tend to increase with age and therefore the age of the recipient must be classed as a risk factor. Age must also be considered within the context of other risk factors, such as advanced cardiovascular disease. Most centres do not have age barriers for transplantation. Health is assessed on an individual basis, and physiological rather than chronological age and the existence of other risk factors are seen as the important assessment issues. Many units have patients of 70 years and over who have progressed well following a kidney transplant. With demand far exceeding supply and studies reporting smaller changes in improvements in quality of life for the older age groups, some may question the use of such a precious and scarce resource in older people. This debate continues, with some centres now attempting to match kidneys from older cadaveric donors with the older recipients, although tissue match is the major deciding factor (Box 12.1).

POLYCYSTIC KIDNEY DISEASE

This inherited kidney disease can result in several members of a family receiving ERF treatments. The native cystic kidneys may be very large, thus leaving little space for the transplant, and there may also be an increased risk of bleeding and infection. Occasionally, it may be necessary to perform a unilateral, or in severe cases a bilateral, nephrectomy prior to transplantation.

Box 12.1   Ethical discussion point on shortage of donor organs

- Renal transplants: demand far exceeds supply
- Younger patients are shown to gain greater life satisfaction after a transplant
- Older patients are at greater risk of complications

Discussion
Should younger patients be given priority over the older group?

URINARY TRACT

It is important to assess that there are no problems with the bladder and urethra, and that there will be no difficulties following transplantation; if it is felt that the bladder capacity is unacceptably low, surgical enlargement may be possible. In the presence of a history of repeated urinary tract infections with bilateral reflux, it may be necessary to undertake a bilateral nephrectomy prior to transplantation to reduce the risk of post-transplant infection.

CARDIAC DISEASE

Routine investigations, such as an electrocardiogram (ECG) and cardiac history, are essential for all patients. Those patients who are in the high-risk groups for cardiovascular disease (e.g., older patients, those with diabetes or ischaemic heart disease) should be reviewed by a cardiologist and should undergo further investigation. Patients who have a history of myocardial infarction should be symptom-free for 1 year prior to transplant.

GASTRIC ULCERATION

A history of indigestion and/or gastric ulceration must be noted and endoscopy undertaken if active ulceration is a possibility, as those with active ulceration risk bleeding after transplantation due to the action of the steroid therapy. Treatment with H_2 receptor blocking agents (such as ranitidine) should be given prior to transplantation if active disease is present. Many centres also use ranitidine prophylaxis in all recipients during the first 6 postoperative months.

RESPIRATORY DISEASE

Routine chest X-ray is essential for all patients, and any infection must be treated. Pulmonary tuberculosis will require treatment before transplantation. Patients with a history of tuberculosis, and those who have visited or lived in high-risk areas will require prophylactic treatment with isoniazid and pyridoxine for at least 1 year following transplantation.

Patients should also be strongly advised to stop smoking and should be offered information regarding smoking cessation strategies and support systems.

OBESITY

Obesity may make the transplant surgery difficult and increase the risk of postoperative complications. Nutritional advice should be given pre- and post-transplantation (see Ch. 11).

ORAL HYGIENE

Dental hygiene and assessment of dental state are essential. Any gum infection or dental problems should be dealt with prior to transplantation. Ciclosporin can cause gum hypertrophy, which is made much worse in the presence of poor hygiene.

PRETRANSPLANTATION PREPARATION

Patients may be referred for transplantation during different phases of the disease process; some may be in the predialysis stage, others may already be established on dialysis therapy. UK guidelines allow a patient to be listed on the cadaveric list when he or she is within about 6 months of requiring dialysis. A pre-emptive cadaveric transplant gives a better outcome compared to having to spend time on dialysis, and the longer the wait, the worse the survival (Meier-Kriesche et al 2000). A planned pre-emptive transplant from a living donor gives the best outcome in terms of graft success and recipient health. Early transplantation before the need for dialysis therapy is welcomed from a clinical perspective, but may prove difficult psychologically if emotional adjustments have not been successfully negotiated, and the patient and family are still reeling from the impact of the disease. A structured approach to predialysis education and counselling should include discussion of suitability for transplantation, and the likelihood of any potential living donors being found. Appropriate patients can then be seen for pretransplant education and assessment, and friends or relatives who are interested in living donation can be contacted at this early stage. An overview of the psychological support required for those pretransplantation is outlined in Ch. 3.

An important part of this support is the pretransplantation information group for patients and families, and details are provided in Ch. 3. Boxes 12.2–2.5 show useful checklists for the pretransplant stage. A systematic approach to assessing patients for suitability for transplantation should include those approaching established renal failure as well as those on dialysis. This is of particular importance when a suitable living donor may be found, thus allowing pre-emptive transplantation.

SPECIFIC PRETRANSPLANT ANXIETIES AND FEARS

Specific issues concerning body image are discussed in Ch. 3; other anxieties include acceptance of the transplant as part of the 'self' and guilt over benefiting from traumatic death. There are also very specific challenges relating to patients' education and understanding of their immunosuppressive therapy.

It is vital that patients understand the need to continue with their antirejection therapy for as long as they have their transplant. Many patients believe that it will only be necessary to take the drugs until the kidney settles into the body. There are great challenges for the transplant team to ensure that patients are well informed about their medication.

One prospective study (Vlaminck et al 2004) found that non-compliance in renal transplant patients more than 1-year post-transplantation is associated with an increased risk of late rejection and a higher increase in serum creatinine during the following 5 years.

> **Box 12.2** Prabramsplant information and assessment proforma: checklist used by the transplant nurse specialist in stage 1–information and discussion.
>
> 1. Desire to receive a transplant
> 2. Benefits of a renal transplant:
>   - Improved quality of life
>   - Freedom from dialysis
>   - Normal healthy diet
>   - Freedom from fluid restrictions
>   - Travel freely (may require special vaccinations)
>   - Employment
>   - Improved fertility (majority) – contraception
> 3. Risks/disadvantages of a renal transplant:
>   - Immunosuppression
>   - Adherence with medication and healthcare advice
>   - Drug side-effects:
>   - Ciclosporin:
>   hirsutism (electrolysis available)
>   gum hyperplasia (dental care)
>   tremor
>   nephrotoxic/hepatoxic
>   - Steroids:
>   body image changes
>   weight gain/hunger
>   mood swings
>   bone problems
>   changes in control of diabetes
>   Azathioprine
>   some hair loss
>
> susceptible to infections
> - Tacrolimus:
>   increased blood glucose levels
> - Mycophenolate mofetil:
>   diarrhoea
>   nausea
>   leukopenia
> - Sirolimus:
>   delayed healing
>   increased lipid levels
>   acne
> - Susceptible to infections and viruses
> - Lymphoma and cytomegalovirus infection
>   – risks and treatment
> - Risk of rejection/biopsies
> - May lose financial benefits – annual prescription
> 4. Clinical:
>   - Blood pressure
>   - Pulse
>   - Dental check: date of last check
>   - Last cervical smear: date of last smear
>   - Breast self-examination
>   - Weight
>   - Height
>   - Body mass index > 25 < 35

Butler et al (2004) carried out a meta-analysis of 36 studies on adherence and concluded that the risk of graft loss was increased sevenfold in non-adherent patients.

A variety of explanations have been given for these difficulties. They include the effects of immunosuppression on physical appearance, inability to accept the lifestyle limitations, misinformation given by one patient to another, poor education given by staff and fear of long-term side-effects. Sometimes, those who have had difficulty in accepting dialysis are exemplary transplant recipients because the post-transplant lifestyle is especially precious.

It is inappropriate to refuse transplantation to patients who are perceived as high risk for non-compliance (Case study 12.1). It is important to offer extensive pretransplant counselling to explore the reasons for not taking healthcare advice and, if necessary, offer additional post-transplant support in order to help facilitate adherence to medication therapies. This may necessitate changing to an immunosuppression regime with a different side-effect profile.

Box 12.3 Pretransplant information and assessment proforma: checklist used by the physician to evaluate clinical assessment and information

Clinical history
1. Renal disease and disease progression: dialysis status
2. Previous medical history, noting previous blood transfusions, pregnancies and previous transplants
3. Previous surgery
4. Current clinical status
5. Social history, family status
6. Smoking, alcohol, recreational drugs
7. Current medications, allergies
8. Immunological status, blood group

Clinical assessment
1. Cardiac assessment
2. Respiratory assessment, tuberculosis risks/contacts
3. Urological assessment
4. Gastrointestinal assessment – previous gastric ulceration, treatment and outcome
5. Abdominal assessment – previous surgery, Tenckhoff site

6. Vascular assessment – assess pulses
7. Dentition
8. Gynaecological status

Information: discussion
1. Risks:
   - Surgical, anaesthetic, death rates, patient survival rates
   - Graft survival rates – cadaveric and living donor
   - Lymphoma
   - Cytomegalovirus
   - Cardiovascular
   - Skin cancer
2. Further investigations required
3. Live donor possibility or cadaveric list
4. Immunosuppression regimen required
5. Decision
   - On cadaveric transplant waiting list
   - For live donor programme
   - Await further investigations
   - Patient undecided – does not want a transplant
   - Unsuitable for transplant due to ....

Box 12.4 Pretransplant assessment proforma used by the transplant nurse specialist in stage 3: routine investigations

1. Blood group
2. Tissue typing
3. Biochemistry
4. Haematology
5. Liver function tests
6. Lipid levels
7. Virology:
   - Hepatitis B and C
   - Cytomegalovirus
   - Human immunodeficiency virus
   - Epstein–Barr virus
   - Varicella zoster virus
8. Chest X-ray
9. Electrocardiogram–cardiac referral if required
10. Midstream urine
11. Further specific investigations required

Box 12.5   Pretransplant assessment proforma used by the transplant nurse specialist in stage 4

1. Orientation: tour of the unit
2. Waiting list: how it works, how to manage waiting time
3. Planning for the transplant call: arrange child/pet/others care
4. Transplant call: what to expect, transport
5. Contact numbers: holiday arrangements
6. Inpatient care: ward environment and policies – information
7. Final cross-match: booklet
8. Pre- and postoperative care
9. Transplant nurse specialist: contact card – further contact

---

Case study 12.1

Claire, a 16-year-old, received a cadaveric transplant and her initial recovery was excellent. But, at 3 months post-transplant, she missed several appointments and refused to discuss her feelings with her parents or staff. At this time, Claire moved in with a friend and did not attend clinic for 3 weeks. Frequent contact by family and transplant personnel was ignored. Finally, she was admitted with acute rejection, which resulted in graft loss. She returned to dialysis.

One year later, she asked to go back on the transplant list for a second graft. Some medical and nursing staff were reluctant to offer a second chance owing to the shortage of kidneys, and difficulties with taking medication. Discussions with Claire highlighted the difficult issues for her with the previous graft, which included changes in body image and a desire to be a 'normal teenager' experiencing life without parental control.

If she received a second transplant, Claire agreed to work closely with the transplant nurse specialist in the post-transplant phase to explore future difficulties. The medical staff agreed to plan a specific immunosuppressive regimen that would minimise the particular side-effects that she had found distressing.

Claire received a second transplant and made an excellent recovery.

TRANSPLANT WAITING LIST

Once the pretransplant assessment has been completed satisfactorily and the tissue-typing and blood-grouping details are finalised, the name of the patient will be added to the national waiting list. Waiting time is impossible to predict.

It is important to explain to patients that the transplant waiting list is very different from other hospital waiting lists in that they do not simply have to wait until their name reaches the top to receive a graft. The transplant list is essentially a pool of recipients, and each transplant is allocated on the basis of the closest match, irrespective of time waiting. Therefore, their name will join the recipient pool and they must wait for the best match for them. This is a difficult concept to understand

and some patients become distressed if another patient, who has waited less time, is transplanted before them.

It is also important that patients do not sit by the phone all day waiting for 'the call', thus greatly restricting their lifestyle. Patients are encouraged to keep as active and as healthy as possible whilst waiting and to continue as normal a lifestyle as possible. Some patients may still feel ambivalent about a transplant at this time. Specific fears and anxieties may need to be explored and support given within the context that patients must be allowed the time to decide the best treatment for themselves. Ongoing contact with the transplant nurse specialist is vital during the waiting time and it is recommended that those who are waiting are contacted every 12 months and offered support and reassurance. Support is especially important at times of additional stress, such as when a fellow dialysis patient receives or rejects a kidney.

DONOR AND RECIPIENT MATCHING

IMMUNE SYSTEM: OVERVIEW

The human body has a complex system of defences that can provide protection against infection and disease. This system has the ability to target, isolate and destroy potentially harmful invaders. This destruction is achieved in three stages: first, by the recognition of structures on the invader (antigens), which are not present in the host. Antibodies and T cells that can recognise the antigens as 'foreign' are then produced. These antibodies and T cells then attach to the invader and destroy it both directly and by recruiting other mechanisms of destruction. Exactly the same happens to a transplant unless it is from an identical twin. The 'foreign' antigens on the transplant induce antibodies and T cells. These target the transplanted organ and do their very best to destroy it. The term 'transplant antigens' is used to describe those antigens that are most important in this regard. Only two are really important: the human leukocyte antigen (HLA) system and the ABO system (see below). In order to prevent rejection, it is necessary to circumvent the immune system (by matching and cross-matching) and to suppress the immunological response.

COMPONENTS OF THE IMMUNE SYSTEM

Leukocytes (white blood cells)

These comprise the cells which produce the antibody (B lymphocytes), recognise the foreign antigens (T lymphocytes), directly destroy invaders (activated T lymphocytes), or can be called in to help with the destruction process (monocytes, polymorphs and eosinophils). Thus, it can be seen that the lymphocytes play several roles and therefore have the major influence on graft acceptance.

These comprise 20% of the total white blood cell count and are made up of several groups of cells with specialised functions. The term 'orchestra' is often used to describe the mode of operation. Each section of the orchestra is made up of individuals with similar but not identical characteristics. The overall result of the orchestra playing is a result of each section performing in concert with the others.

There are two types of lymphocyte:

- T cells, which have antigen recognition structures fixed to their surface
- B cells, which have antigen recognition structures that can be secreted (antibodies).

T cells and B cells can be naive or activated. T cells can be activated to various functions, namely, helper, killer or tolerant status. B cells can be activated to produce antibody or memory.

Each naive lymphocyte has an antigen recognition structure that is unique, for example, different from other members of its section and thus capable of seeing a different antigen. In this way, literally millions of 'foreign' antigens can be recognised. Each time a recognition event occurs, a naive cell becomes activated and divides. Thus, even if a single cell recognises an antigen as foreign, it keeps dividing until it forms a significant number of identical cells (a clone), all capable of recognising the antigen.

Depending on influences from other sections, T cells can help B cells produce antibody (helper T cells), kill targets bearing the antigen directlyh (killer T cells), or become tolerant (i.e., capable of recognising the antigen but not producing a damaging response to it). B cells can produce antibody in around 8–10 days if they see it for the first time (naive B cells) or within 24h if they have seen it before (memory B cells). B cells produce much more antibody if they get help from the T cells, which can themselves see the same antigen.

One point about antibody production relevant to transplantation is that the process which produces it is long-lived. This is very positive for vaccination programmes, where having antibody around for years and years is very beneficial, although negative of course for transplantation.

Lymphocytes

ABO BLOOD GROUPS

The ABO system of human blood groups was described by Landsteiner in 1902. Blood group is determined by A and B antigens on the surface of the red blood cells. Each individual has one of the four basic blood group types: O, A, B or AB.

Each individual has antibodies to the blood group antigens that they do not express (Table 12.2). Antibodies against the blood group antigens can cause hyperacute rejection and, therefore, matching of blood group between donor and recipient is vital. Blood group O organs can be transplanted into all groups; O is classified as the universal donor. Blood group

Table 12.2 The ABO blood group system

Blood group	Percentage of population	Antigens expressed	Antibodies expressed	Acceptable donor blood group
O	47%	None	Anti-A, Anti-B	O
A	42%	A	Anti-B	O, A
B	8%	B		Anti-A O, B
AB	3%	AB	None	O, A, B, AB

AB recipients can receive organs from all groups; AB is classified as the universal recipient. A small proportion of people with group A belong to a subgroup defined as A2, and have reduced expression of A antigen. These kidneys may be transplanted into O or B, or A2B into AB recipients with low anti-A titres (Nelson et al 1998).

HISTOCOMPATIBILITY ANTIGENS

A further set of proteins that can trigger the B and T cell response are the transplantation antigens or the histocompatibility antigens. The histocompatibility antigens can be divided into two groups – major and minor.

Major histocompatibility complex (MHC)

This system, first discovered in the mouse by Peter Gorer at Guy's Hospital in the late 1930s is, as the name suggests, the most important system in transplantation and indeed in immunity to infection. The human system is termed HLA (for human leukocyte antigen) and was identified by Dausset, van Rood and Payne in the 1960s (Klein 1986). The sera from pregnant women were found to have antibodies that recognised lymphocytes from their partners and from some random blood donors. The reason for this is that pregnancy is in some ways like a transplant. Passage of blood from partner or child to mother results in T cells and antibody being produced to the foreign antigens on the blood cells. Since the most potent foreign antigens are those of the HLA system, most of the mother's response is directed against them and the long-lived antibody-producing cells remain in her blood. These antibodies can persist for over 40 years.

The HLA system is complex. There are four main series important for transplantation: A, B, C and DR (donor-related). There are over 30 antigens in each series. Each person can have two from each series (one from each parent). The permutation on 2/30 from A, 2/30 from B, 2/30 from C and 2/30 from DR means that, outside of a family, it is very rare for individuals to have identical HLA types. Luckily for matching in renal transplantation, DR is dominant. However, most of the antibody and T-cell response is produced to A, B and C.

The rules for HLA and matching are not nearly as clear-cut as the rules for ABO, but there are several strong guidelines.

- Transplantation of a kidney into someone who has antibodies directed to a foreign (mismatched) HLA antigen on that kidney will result in hyperacute rejection.
- Transplantation of a kidney into someone who has strong memory to a foreign (mismatched) HLA antigen on that kidney will result in very rapid rejection.
- Transplantation of a kidney with two mismatches at DR will have more rejection than one with one mismatch at DR, and both will have more rejection than a kidney with no DR mismatches. However, rejection episodes can be treated or mismatched patients given additional immunosuppression. The total number of mismatches has a bearing on long-term outcome (Fig. 12.2, Collaborative Transplant Study 2006).

DONOR AND RECIPIENT MATCHING

The majority of organs for transplant come from cadaveric donors. It is essential to match for blood group and to achieve the best DR match possible. Since antibodies can be induced to pregnancies or transfusions or previous transplants, and can be boosted by infection, regular screening of patients on the waiting list is necessary to maintain knowledge of their current antibody status. Donors are avoided if they contain any mismatch to which the recipient has antibodies in current or recent serum.

DONOR AND RECIPIENT CROSS-MATCHING

As a final check for current antibody and for the accuracy of past screening, a recent sample and selected past samples from the recipient are always checked against donor cells before transplantation.

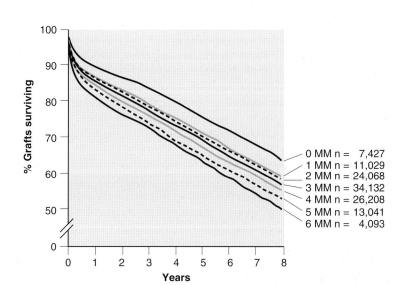

Figure 12.2
Influence of HLA matching on survival (first cadaveric renal transplant) 1985–2004. Statistics prepared by Collaborative Transplant Study. MM, mismatch.

0 MM n =   7,427
1 MM n = 11,029
2 MM n = 24,068
3 MM n = 34,132
4 MM n = 26,208
5 MM n = 13,041
6 MM n =   4,093

UK MATCHING SYSTEM

Within the UK, each transplant centre has a local list of recipients awaiting transplant. There is also a national list held at UK Transplant in Bristol. Each cadaveric donor is tissue-typed at the local transplant centre and the details sent to Bristol, where the closest tissue match is found from the central computer. The kidneys are then sent to the recipient centre for transplant.

A new scheme for the national allocation of kidneys was adopted in the UK in July 1998, replacing the previous beneficial matching scheme (Gilks et al 1987). The new scheme was the result of work by Task Forces of the UK Transplant Kidney and Pancreas Advisory Group and is based on rigorous analyses of the National Transplant Databases to determine factors that influence renal transplant outcome in the age of modern immunosuppression (Morris et al 1999). The scheme is based on HLA matching, gives priority to paediatric patients, some priority for highly sensitised patients (i.e., patients with high levels of HLA antibodies) and uses a point score to differentiate between equally matched patients. Local patients have priority over national patients.

The scheme has three tiers. Tier 1 kidneys are offered to patients with no mismatched HLA antigens at HLA-A, -B and -DR (termed a 000 mismatched transplant). If there are no such patients in tier 1, then kidneys are offered in tier 2 to favourably matched patients (i.e. no mismatch at HLA-DR and a maximum of one mismatched antigen at both the HLA-A and HLA-B locus; 100, 010, 110 mismatch grades). If there are no patients in either tier 1 or 2 and the kidneys cannot be used locally, then the kidneys are offered in tier 3 to the transplant unit with the highest balance of exchange. Monitoring the scheme has shown an increase in the proportion of well-matched transplants and of the number of highly sensitised patients transplanted in the UK (Fuggle et al 1998). However, there are still geographic variations in access to transplantation, both nationally and regionally, related to factors such as donation rates and distribution of kidney disease (Rudge et al 2003).

PRETRANSPLANT CROSS-MATCH

Prior to transplant, a cross-match test is performed in the tissue-typing laboratory. A blood sample from the recipient is mixed with lymphocytes from the donor. If the donor cells react (die), the result is termed a positive cross-match; the recipient is adversely reacting to the donor antigens. In the presence of a positive cross-match, transplantation cannot proceed, as the transplant would be rejected.

SENSITISATION

When there is a positive cross-match, the recipient is sensitised to that donor. The higher the level of sensitisation, the greater will be the difficulty in finding a transplant that will not reject.

Sensitisation can occur during pregnancy (to partner's antigens), during blood transfusion and after transplantation. In order to reduce the risk of sensitisation, it is important to minimise the giving of blood transfusions.

Some recipients may have a high level of sensitisation. The patient's serum is tested periodically against a representative panel of cells from many donors. If the patient does not react with the various donors tested, then they are classified as unsensitised. If the blood reacts with 50% of donors (50% of the panel or 50% panel reactive antibody; PRA), they are 50% sensitised, and if blood reacts with 100% of donors, they are highly sensitised. Unfortunately, some highly sensitised candidates wait many years for a compatible transplant, although the antibodies responsible for sensitisation can decrease with time.

Antibodies can be removed by administration of intravenous immunoglobulin. This is most useful with a planned living donor, and may be combined with combinations of plasma exchange or immunoadsorption, where it may allow a negative cross-match to be obtained followed by transplantation (Glotz et al 2002, Schweitzer et al 2000).

CADAVERIC (HEART–BEATING) DONATION

The majority of renal transplants in the UK result from cadaveric donation. Cadaveric donors are patients who have suffered irreversible brain stem damage (brain stem death) and are maintained on a ventilator within a critical care unit.

CAUSES OF BRAIN STEM DEATH

The most common causes of brain stem death are listed in Box 12.6.

Cerebral swelling resultant from trauma or anoxia and intracerebral bleeding can cause raised intracranial pressure, which forces the cerebral hemispheres through the tentorial hiatus, thus compressing the brain stem and interrupting its blood supply. Such herniation of the cerebral tissue is usually described as 'coning' and results in irreversible damage to the brain stem.

Box 12.6   Common causes of brain stem death

- Intracerebral bleed or infarction
- Head trauma
- Cerebral hypoxia due to:
  - respiratory arrest
  - cardiac arrest
  - smoke inhalation/carbon monoxide poisoning
- Cerebral tumour
- Drug overdose
- Intracranial infection

BRAIN STEM FUNCTIONS

The brain stem is responsible for the capacity to breathe spontaneously and the capacity for consciousness. If the brain stem is irreversibly damaged, then there is loss of function and it is argued that the 'irreversible loss of the capacity for consciousness and the irreversible loss of the capacity to breathe' constitutes brain stem death, which constitutes death of the person (Pallis 1994).

Brain stem death diagnosed by signs of irreversible damage to the brain stem is an accepted concept in most countries of the world.

BRAIN STEM DEATH DIAGNOSIS

Tests to diagnose brain stem death originated from the Harvard Medical School criteria (Harvard Medical School 1968), which were published in the USA in 1968. A UK Code of Practice for the diagnosis of brain stem death was agreed by the Conference of Medical Royal Colleges in 1976, 1979, 1991 and 1998 (UK Code of Practice 1998). The application of the Code and the criteria for diagnosis of death remain under discussion (Bell et al 2004, Park 2004).

The clinical diagnosis of brain stem death involves three steps. The first step is to ascertain that the following preconditions have been met.

- The patient is deeply comatosed and on a ventilator.
- The patient has been maintained on the ventilator for sufficient time to ascertain that the brain damage is irreversible.
- There is a positive diagnosis of the cause of the coma.

The second step is to exclude other possible causes of coma, which are:

- primary hypothermia ($< 35°C$)
- drug intoxication or alcohol intoxication
- metabolic and endocrine disturbances.

The third step is to perform testing to ascertain:

- absent brain stem reflexes
- apnoea (loss of capacity for spontaneous breathing).

Tests for brain stem death (absent brain stem reflexes) are as follows.

- The pupils are fixed and dilated: there is no response to light.
- The corneal reflex is absent; the patient does not blink when the cornea is stimulated.
- Vestibulo-ocular reflexes are absent; there are no eye movements during or after slow injection of 20 mL of ice-cold water into each external auditory meatus.
- Cranial nerve response to pain is absent: there is no response to stimulation of any somatic area.
- Gag reflex is absent: there is no response to tracheal and bronchial stimulation by a suction catheter.
- No respiratory movements occur when the respiratory centre is stimulated (apnoea testing).

The UK Code of Practice recommends that brain stem death testing should be carried out by two medical practitioners 'who have expertise in this field'. One should be a consultant and the other a consultant or senior registrar. Neither of the doctors should be a member of the transplant team or associated with potential transplant recipients.

Declaration of brain stem death

The Code of Practice also recommends that testing should be performed twice to ensure that there has been no observer error. The interval between the tests is normally at the discretion of the critical care staff who will also consider the needs and circumstances of the family.

Repetition of testing

The time of completion of the first set of tests is legally the time of death, and this should be recorded as such on the death certificate.

Time of death

CRITERIA FOR MULTIPLE ORGAN DONATION

- The patient is aged 0–80 years.
- The patient has suffered severe and irreversible brain damage resulting in brain stem death.
- The patient is maintained on a ventilator.
- The patient has no major untreated sepsis (discuss with transplant team).
- The patient has no malignancy – except primary brain tumour (discuss with transplant team).
- The patient is HIV- and hepatitis B- and C-negative (discuss with transplant team).

Patients with some degree of sepsis that have been treated may be considered, as may hepatitis B- or C-positive cases, in certain instances. Conversely, other diseases may preclude donation of specific organs. Therefore, it is recommended that critical care staff consider organ donation in all those with brain stem death and refer to the local transplant coordinator for a decision regarding medical suitability.

Patients from high-risk groups (as defined by the Department of Health 2000) should also be excluded. In order to keep transplants safe, the Department of Health guidelines state that 'certain medical and social information' must be given. Therefore, donor families are given an information sheet (Box 12.7) and asked to read these questions and answer 'to the best of their knowledge'.

REQUESTING DONATION

In the UK, the legal requirements for organ donation are laid down in the Human Tissue Act 2004. This Act established the Human Tissue Authority (HTA) as the regulatory body for all matters concerning the removal, storage, use and disposal of human tissues (except gametes and embryos) for scheduled purposes, and includes responsibility for

Box 12.7   Keeping transplants safe: information sheet given to proposed kidney donor families

In order to proceed with organ and tissue donation, the Department of Health[a] guidelines state that we need to ask for certain medical and social information.

Therefore to the best of your knowledge:

Is there a history of behaviour that might increase the risk of HIV, syphilis, hepatitis A, hepatitis B and hepatitis C?

Has your relative ever:

- had any acupuncture, tattoos, ear and/or body piercing within the last 6 months?
- been tested for or known to have HIV, hepatitis B and/or hepatitis C?
- had sex with another man (if a man)?
- received money or drugs as payment for sex?
- injected or snorted drugs?
- been sexually active in Africa (excluding Morocco, Algeria, Tunisia, Libya and Egypt)?
- had sex with anyone in the above list during the last 12 months?

Does your relative have a risk of having an infection of unknown origin? Has he or she ever had:

- a past medical history of jaundice?
- a family history of CJD or confusion?
- an occular tissue transplant (cornea, sclera or occular stem cells)?
- human pituitary-derived growth hormone or gonadotrophin before 1989?
- neurosurgery or operations on tumours or cysts on the spine or implantation of dura mater before August 1992?

Has your relative:

- had a history of neurodegenerative disease of unknown aetiology?
- had a history of disease of unknown aetiology (i.e. multiple sclerosis, Alzheimer's disease, Parkinson's disease or Crohn's disease)?
- had a history of encephalitis?
- had a history of animal bites received overseas in the last 6–12 months?
- had a history of rabies, herpes simplex or unknown virus?
- travelled outside western Europe and had an infection whilst abroad?
- travelled overseas in the last few months? Has he or she contracted malaria or lived for more than 3 months in a malaria risk area (Africa, Asia, South and Central America, Mexico, Mississippi Valley, West Indies, California, Texas, Japan and the Caribbean)?
- had Lyme disease, tuberculosis or brucellosis?
- been tested for toxoplasmosis?
- been tested for cytomegalovirus?
- had a recent viral infection or rash, such as chickenpox, shingles, measles or Epstein–Barr virus?

Thank you for taking the time to read this sheet. If it would be more appropriate, please feel free to discuss the above with the transplant coordinator in private before the donation. All information is treated with the strictest of confidence.

[a] Department of Health Committee on Microbiological Safety of Blood and Tissue Transplantation (2000, revised). Crown copyright material is reproduced with the permission of the Controller of HMSO and the Queen's Printer for Scotland.
CJD, Creutzfeldt–Jakob disease; HIV, human immunodeficiency virus.

living donor transplantation. The HTA's code of practice (2006) on consent sets out guidance on how the law should be applied, encompassing issues of consent.

In practice, it is the next of kin or the patient's executor who is usually approached to give permission for donation. If the patient has signed a donor card, there is no statutory requirement to approach the family, but in practice the views of the family are always sought and, if objections are raised, donation does not occur.

If the next of kin cannot be notified, the body remains in the possession of the hospital. In such cases, the hospital manager can give permission for donation as long as reasonable enquiries have been made and that there is no reason to believe that the deceased had expressed objections.

Religious beliefs

As far as it is known, no major religious groups in the UK object to the principles of organ donation and transplantation. Some groups feel that it is only permissible if donors themselves had requested donation. These groups include, in particular, Orthodox Jews, Christian Scientists and some Hindu groups. Jehovah's Witnesses have religious objections to blood transfusions, but feel that donating or receiving organs is a matter for all Jehovah's Witnesses to decide for themselves.

It is often thought that the Muslim faith does not support donation, and anecdotal evidence suggests that British Muslims are, in general, reluctant to donate organs. However, recent legislation has approved donation and transplantation in Muslim countries such as Saudi Arabia. Also, a fatwa issued by the Muslim Law Council has stated that Muslims may donate organs. They may carry donor cards and their next of kin may give permission for donating (Carlisle 1995). Previous reluctance to donate may have been cultural rather than religious and, therefore, information and liaison with Muslims will be vital in order to encourage donation.

Several centres within the UK have appointed a renal recipient transplant coordinator for Asian or Afro-Caribbean communities. The aim of these roles is to provide 'continuous direct rapport and liaison with the community by developing specific educational material relevant and appropriate to the patient population' (Jain 1999).

Jain (1999) states that there is a documented 2–4-fold increased prevalence of ERF in the Asian patient group. The major causes are the higher incidence of hypertension and diabetes combined with other reasons, which are, as yet, unknown. In some regions, they represent one-third of the transplant waiting list (Jeffrey et al 2002). There are fewer cadaver organ donations from this community; the reasons for this are complex and multifactorial (AlKhawar et al 2006). Although the three major Asian religions, Hinduism, Sikhism and Islam, encourage organ donation, there is a fear and mistrust coupled with a lack of awareness about brain stem death, the scope and value of organ donation and transplantation. Language and cultural barriers seem to have inhibited the uptake of public health messages pertinent to organ donation and transplantation.

Awareness campaigns have been initiated and living donation has been seen as a possible interim solution as dialogue develops. Culturally sensitive education and support have been introduced coupled with a significant drive to increase public awareness in the Asian, and to a lesser extent Afro-Caribbean communities in the UK. It is too early to assess the impact of these initiatives but a more positive perception of organ donation and transplantation is now reported from within this community.

Other issues inherent to the UK may also be adversely affecting the cadaveric donor rate from within all groups, particularly aspects relating to gaining consent from the bereaved.

Fear of increasing the distress of the family

Critical care staff have expressed fears that offering donation may increase the distress of the bereaved (Wakeford & Stepney 1989); however, experience suggests that offering the choice to donate, if performed with empathy, does not increase distress. Indeed, donor families report that the act of donation brings comfort and something positive in an otherwise negative situation (Buckley 1989). American and UK studies have noted that a fundamental need for relatives during a 'crisis time' is 'to feel there is hope' (Coulter 1989, Molter 1979, Wilkinson 1995). In the presence of a diagnosis of brain stem death, there can be no hope for the patient but donation can be an option of hope with life for others.

Acceptance that death has occurred

It is crucial that the bereaved family have accepted the fact that death has occurred before donation is requested. In the case of brain stem death, the acceptance of death is more difficult for the family as they are asked to accept a 'new concept of death'. The accepted concept and image of death involves a cold, lifeless body without a heartbeat; however, in the case of brain stem death, the family are presented with an image of a warm patient with a heartbeat who appears (due to the ventilator) to be breathing. Therefore, the visual message is one of life but the verbal message is one of death. In such cases, denial is often enhanced and relatives must struggle to understand and accept the situation. Denial may be particularly acute in the case of an intracerebral bleed where there is no outward sign of injury or trauma.

Clear communications must ensue, the core message being that there is no hope of recovery. Irreparable damage has occurred and the brain has died – death of the brain stem is death of the person.

When to offer donation

It is damaging to approach the family too early, as trust may be lost. One study examined the reasons for relatives' refusal (Mori/UKTCA/BACCN Marketing & Opinion Research International Ltd/United Kingdom Transplant Coordinators' Association/British Association of Critical Care Nurses 1995) and noted that a refusal may have been because the family were 'approached too early by inexperienced staff'. This study also reports that 'Consent for donation rates are higher in cases where the request is made after the second set of brain stem tests'. Furthermore, a study from the USA noted that relatives were more likely to agree to donation if the explanation of brain stem death and the request for organ donation were clearly separated in time (Garrison et al 1991). Thus it is important for the family to have accepted that death has occurred before donation is offered, also to inform the family of the death and to request donation at separate meetings. In Spain, organ donation increased by 100% over 10 years following a comprehensive public education programme supported by increased resources in hospitals (Miranda et al 2003).

All studies report that the person who has established a trusting relationship with the family is the most appropriate person to offer donation. It is important that the requestee has a positive view of donation and can offer it in a positive way.

Who should offer donation?

There are no 'right' words; each situation is unique and families will have their own individual responses. The family should be asked if they have any objection to donation rather than for permission to proceed. Some families will require time to consider their decision. Many relatives will have additional questions concerning the process of donation and its implications at this time. It may be helpful for the family to meet with the transplant coordinator, who can answer specific questions. The family may require reassurance on the following issues.

How to offer donation

- The donor will feel no pain.
- There will be dignity and respect throughout the donor surgery.
- The body will not be grossly mutilated or disfigured.
- The surgical wound will be sutured.
- They can view the body after surgery and the funeral will not be delayed.

The transplant coordinator will work closely with other healthcare professionals to answer further questions and to facilitate the wishes of the family. The coordinator can also reassure the family that he or she will be present throughout the surgery and at the end to oversee and continue care. The coordinator will ensure that the bereaved can see the deceased after surgery in the chapel of rest if this is their wish.

It is important to stress that organ donation is a voluntary 'unconditional gift'. One case, much publicised, reported that the bereaved had stated that the organs 'must only be given to white recipients'. Such a condition is totally unacceptable and there is now legislation that prohibits the placing of any conditions when agreeing to organ donations (see Case study 12.2).

Unconditional gift

Case study 12.2

A 58-year-old female who had been investigated as a living donor for her son suddenly collapses from a subarachnoid haemorrhage 1 month before the planned transplant and is declared brain stem dead.

The family agree to cadaveric donation but stipulate that one kidney *must* be given to her son.

It is illegal to place this condition upon the donation.

Discussion question:
- Should the son receive one of the kidneys donated?

Continuing care after donation

Letters of thanks containing brief anonymous information concerning the transplant recipients are given or sent to the donor family after the donation. Further help and support are also offered. Many families state that the news of the successful transplants is a source of comfort. More recently, transplant coordinators have arranged meetings between donor families and recipients. Such meetings have been requested by both parties and have followed careful counselling and preparation to ensure the willingness of all individuals involved.

Refusal to donate

A Mori/UKTCA/BACCN (1995) study reported a 38% refusal rate. The five most common reasons given for refusal were as follows.

- The relatives did not want surgery to the body (24%).
- The patient had stated in the past that donation was not to take place (21%).
- The relatives felt that the patient had suffered enough (21%).
- The relatives were divided over the decision (19%).
- The relatives were not sure whether the patient would have agreed to organ donation (18%).

As part of recent measures to improve organ donation rates in the UK, a potential donor audit has been established by UK Transplant. Results from the first full year of the audit show that the overall relative refusal rate for heart-beating solid organ donation is 41.5%. Age and gender of the potential heart-beating donor has little impact on the relative refusal rate, but relatives of ethnic minority groups are more than twice as likely to deny consent than those of white potential heart-beating donors (Barber et al 2005).

Refusal rates at this level represent a desperate lost potential. Therefore, it is vital that information programmes to allay fears and to present the successes of transplantation continue. It is also helpful to implement education for healthcare staff to examine the issue of requesting donation so that personnel will feel comfortable when offering this option of hope to the family.

Transplant coordinator groups have introduced workshops on breaking bad news and the approach for donation for nursing and medical colleagues working in intensive care and emergency departments. Such workshops utilise informed actors and provide a forum and a safe environment for staff to examine sudden traumatic death, the reactions of relatives and responses that will facilitate the approach for donation.

If the family agree to donation, the ventilation continues and the preparations for the donor surgery are made, but if the family refuse donation, then ventilation will cease.

It is always helpful for the family if the deceased carried a donor card, was registered as a donor on the National Register or had discussed the issue with them. Most families want to fulfil the wishes of their loved one and, if they know the thoughts of the deceased with regard to donation, then the question and decision are no longer difficult for them.

CLINICAL CARE OF A POTENTIAL ORGAN DONOR

Brain stem death results in changes to normal homeostatic mechanisms; such changes will ultimately result in cardiac arrest. Once permission has been given for donation, it is important to stabilise the condition of the donor to ensure optimal condition of the organs for transplantation. The care can be very complex and is outside the scope of this book; but further reading can be found in Novitzky (1998).

THE ROLE OF THE TRANSPLANT COORDINATOR

All renal transplant centres depend on regional transplant coordinators. They are senior practitioners (usually with a nursing background) who offer a 24-h service to intensive care units with regard to organ donation. The role of the transplant coordinator at the time of donation is to offer:

- advice regarding suitability of a potential organ donor
- advice regarding donor clinical care
- advice and/or help with the approach to relatives
- organisation of the organ donation procedure and surgery
- support of the family and staff.

The transplant coordinator will usually attend at the donor hospital to offer advice and support to the donor family and critical care staff. Organisation of the organ donation is complex and the transplant coordinator will attempt to make all arrangements with a minimum of distress to the donor family and the critical care staff. The majority of organ donations today are multiple donations, and it is the transplant coordinator who organises the necessary blood and clinical tests, liaises with the heart, liver, renal and ophthalmic teams and arranges the donor surgery (Box 12.8).

Organisation of the organ donation procedure and surgery

PERMISSION FROM THE CORONER

If the case comes under the jurisdiction of the coroner (or procurator fiscal in Scotland), then permission must be obtained to proceed to organ donation. Cases usually requiring the coroner's permission include:

- road traffic accident
- suspicious deaths/suicide
- deaths less than 12 h after surgery
- traumatic deaths.

It is unusual for permission to be withheld except in the case of suspected murder.

REMOVAL OF KIDNEYS FROM A MULTIORGAN DONOR

It is most common now for kidneys to be taken out as part of an operation from a multiorgan donor. This requires careful coordination between

---

Box 12.8   Organ donation: role of the transplant coordinator

- Arrival at donor hospital
- Meet with critical care staff
- Assess potential donor suitability
- Advice regarding donor clinical care (if requested)
- Meet with donor family; offer advice and support (if requested)
- Permission from the coroner or coroner's officer
- Organise clinical tests and blood tests:

Clinical tests	Blood tests
12-lead ECG	ABO blood group
Chest X-ray	Biochemistry:
Approx. size and weight of donor	– urea and electrolytes
Arterial blood gases	– liver function tests
– full blood count	
– virology screen	

  – HIV
  – hepatitis B and C
  – cytomegalovirus
  – toxoplasmosis
  – syphilis
- Contact UK Transplant re super-urgent cases
- Liaise with heart, liver, renal and ophthalmic teams
- Liaise with theatre staff and obtain theatre time:
    – accompany donor to theatre
    – assist surgical teams
    – support theatre personnel
- Final care of donor
- Contact with donor family offering information and/or support
- Information and thanks to donor hospital personnel

ECG, electrocardiogram; HIV, human immunodeficiency virus.

---

the liver, renal and thoracic teams involved to make sure that there is no compromise to viability in any of the transplanted organs (Plates 2–4).

The exact details of the operation vary from centre to centre, but the principles include a generous incision giving good exposure to the organs of interest with the heart still beating, and placement of cannulae for *in situ* perfusion and cooling.

- A bilateral subcostal incision with a midline sternotomy is a common approach to the chest. The heart and lungs are inspected and mobilised first to allow rapid removal at a later stage.
- A careful laparotomy is carried out before dissection of the major blood supply to the liver. The common bile duct is transected and the gallbladder incised and flushed to prevent biliary autolysis.
- Cannulae are placed into the aorta and portal vein via the mesenteric vein for perfusion. The distal inferior vena cava is cannulated and used for vascular drainage. Ventilation ceases when the aorta is cross-clamped. Perfusion starts simultaneously to minimise warm ischaemia.
- The organs are removed; first, heart and lungs, followed by the liver and then the kidneys. Careful cooperation between teams is required to minimise damage to the various organs. The pancreas is used for transplantation with increasing success; concurrent retrieval with the above organs has not been associated with adverse outcome.

Before closure of the abdominal incisions, specimens of donor lymph nodes and spleen are removed for histocompatibility and tissue typing.

SURGICAL TECHNIQUE FOR CADAVERIC DONOR NEPHRECTOMY

If the kidneys are to be removed alone, bilateral nephrectomy is accomplished through a long midline incision or a bilateral subcostal incision. The kidneys are either taken out en bloc or individually on patches of inferior vena cava and aorta. The technique preferred in this centre entails the removal of an individual kidney on a patch of aorta and inferior vena cava. The technique is as follows.

- Abdominal incision and laparotomy are performed as for multiorgan retrieval.
- The aorta is dissected up to the superior mesenteric artery and the inferior vena cava dissected above the renal veins.
- Slings are placed around the aorta and the inferior vena cava above the bifurcation ready for tying at a later stage.
- A catheter is passed into the aorta through an incision just above the bifurcation. The balloon of the catheter is distended with fluid and ties placed around the aorta distal to the balloon to hold it in place. Care must be taken not to overdistend catheter balloons as this can obstruct the lumen of the catheter.
- A similar procedure is carried out with the inferior vena cava just above the confluence of the right and left common iliac veins, and the aorta and inferior vena cava below the catheters are tied off.
- The aorta is tied off in the upper abdomen and perfusion is started through the Foley catheter (Fig. 12.3). As perfusion starts, ventilation is discontinued.

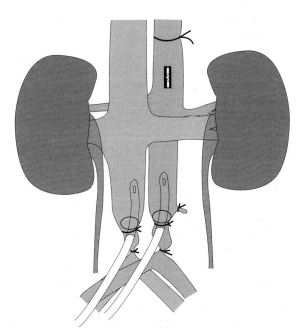

Figure 12.3
Perfusion catheters in situ for cadaveric donor nephrectomy.

- The kidneys begin to get cold at this stage and, while the perfusion fluid is running through into the kidneys and out through the renal veins, the kidneys should be surrounded by ice to assist cooling and prevent rewarming from the adjacent tissues.
- The inferior vena cava above the renal veins is ligated and the blood from the kidneys drains out through the catheter in the inferior vena cava.
- After 2 L of perfusion fluid has flushed through the kidneys and the kidneys are cold, they can be mobilised and the cannulae removed.
- The inferior vena cava is split up the middle and along the back, taking care not to divide the right renal artery. The aorta is also divided anteriorly and posteriorly, taking care to avoid damaging the left renal vein, which crosses in front of the aorta. Having done this, each kidney is taken out with a section of aorta, inferior vena cava and long length of ureter and placed in iced saline, where it is reflushed with preservation fluid.
- Normally, no further dissection is done at this stage, but the kidney is placed in sterile bags and sent at 4°C to the receiving centre. Further dissection of the kidney is performed immediately before subsequent transplantation into the recipient.

Following removal, each kidney is examined for any surgical injury and unusual anatomy and is placed in a sterile bag with a small amount of perfusion fluid. This bag is then placed inside two further polythene bags to ensure sterility. The kidney is finally packed into a transport container with ice.

ORGAN PRESERVATION

The aim of preservation is to maintain the organ in an optimal condition until transplantation can occur. All living cells require oxygen to survive. Once the blood supply to the organ ceases, the lack of oxygen will result in cellular ischaemia. Cooling the organ will reduce the cellular metabolism and thus help to minimise subsequent damage. Ischaemia that occurs before the organ is cooled is termed warm ischaemia.

Warm ischaemia

If the blood supply to the kidneys is interrupted without cooling, the tubular cells suffer warm ischaemia, resulting in acute tubular necrosis (ATN). ATN may be reversible if the warm ischaemia time is limited (approx. 45 min). However, should the warm ischaemia extend longer than 1 h the glomeruli are likely to suffer irreversible damage and the kidney may not regain function. During cadaveric donation (heart-beating donation) the ventilation and blood supply continue until the perfusion system is in place. As perfusion with cooled fluid commences, the ventilation ceases. Thus, the kidney is immediately cooled and the warm ischaemia is limited to approximately 1–2 min only.

The ice should maintain the kidney at approximately 4°C, thus minimising ischaemic damage and enabling transport to the transplant centre. The time from the beginning of cooling to reperfusion and rewarming at the time of transplantation is termed the cold ischaemia time. Most kidneys can be stored for 24–48h if necessary. However, recent studies suggest that prolonged cold ischaemia does reduce the function of the transplant, particularly if the kidney is from an elderly donor. Therefore, most transplant centres transplant kidneys within 24h of removal when possible.

Cold ischaemia

LIVING DONATION

In the early days of transplantation, live related transplants were the only possible option but, with the advent of cadaveric donation from brain-dead donors and improved immunosuppression regimes, most centres concentrated, in the main, on cadaveric donation with fewer live donor transplants. This was due, in part, to the fact that some clinicians struggled with the ethical issue of subjecting a healthy and fit person to the risks of major surgery that had no personal benefit for them, albeit there would be benefit to their family member.

ETHICAL ISSUES

The core factors of the living donation debate involve the critical issue of a balance between 'doing good without doing harm' and the concept of altruism.

The donation will most certainly 'do good' in benefiting the recipient but may also 'do harm' to the donor, as the surgical procedure exposes the living donor to major clinical risks. Mortality from living donor surgery is low; however, donor deaths have been reported. A figure of 1 in 3000 is suggested in UK guidelines on living kidney donation (British Transplant Society/Renal Association 2005). Early postoperative complications may also occur and may include chest infection, deep vein thrombosis, wound infection and postsurgical depression amongst others. Long-term complications have not been demonstrated, with follow-up studies of living related donors, for as long as 20 years, finding no functional abnormalities.

A major study undertaken by Najarian et al (1992) at the University of Minnesota followed living kidney donors for 20 years after donation by comparing renal function, blood pressure and proteinuria in donors with siblings ($n = 57$). The study conclusions found that the donor group had had no progressive rise in serum creatinine; the frequency of hypertension was not higher than in the general population or in sibling controls; and finally, that although 23% of these donors had proteinuria, so did 22% of their siblings. Such proteinuria was mild in most and not associated with hypertension or renal dysfunction. The study postulated

Physical well–being – doing good without doing harm

that renal transplant donors were not at an increased risk of developing renal failure. Data from Sweden on long-term survival showed that kidney donors died of similar causes than did the general population, but that donors live longer than the general population (Fehrman-Ekholm et al 1997).

Psychological well-being – doing good without doing harm

Undoubtedly, many living donors gain psychologically from the act of giving. Studies suggest that donors describe the act 'as one of the most meaningful experiences in their lives' (Fellner & Marshall 1968) and 'view themselves as more worthwhile because of donation' (Simmons et al 1971). The satisfaction of helping a 'loved one' return to a normal lifestyle is very rewarding for many. Indeed, it has been suggested that there may be psychological harm if a donor is prevented from giving (Simmons et al 1977). Thus, living donation presents physical risks but psychological gain for most donors (Thiel et al 2005).

Altruism

Altruism – the act of unselfishness – means giving freely without thought of reward. Much debate has surrounded this concept, with writers in the 1960s and 1970s questioning the fundamental reasons for giving. Kemph (1966) reported that, although donors were 'consciously altruistic' there was 'considerable unconscious resentment' towards the recipient and towards hospital personnel who requested or encouraged the donation. Other studies suggested the presence of a degree of coercion or subtle familial pressure. There were also reports of financial incentives or other 'material rewards' offered by recipients to donors to encourage donation. Although many of these early studies involved small numbers of donors and recipients, the negative findings led many centres to pursue cadaveric options.

Later studies in the 1970s and the 1980s reported more positive psychological findings. Smith et al (1986) found that 97% of donors reaffirmed their decisions and fewer than 15% said that they felt pressurised to donate.

Such positive reports encouraged some centres to increase live donor programmes but many continued with a strong stance against it, mainly because of the physical risks to the donor. However, a study by Levey et al (1986) noted that the physical risks to the donor were 'minimal' and that the benefits to the donor were 'considerable' with regard to self-esteem and self-worth. Surman (1989) stated that 'kidney donation has a favourable outcome for both donor and recipient and that the participation of living related donors in kidney transplantation was now widely accepted'.

Studies in the 1990s have been supportive of live donation but have also noted psychological issues that may need to be addressed. Russell & Jacob (1994) reported that 'psychological side effects, namely donor depression and family conflict were noted but these risks were generally under-emphasised'. More recent studies have also reported positive findings. Jacobs et al (1998) investigated follow-up of 529 living donors who had donated between 1985 and 1996. Study conclusions noted that 'donors scored higher than the general population with regard to quality of life issues'. If given the opportunity, only 4% of the donors said that they would not donate again and 9% were unsure.

BENEFITS FOR THE TRANSPLANT RECIPIENT

Although the ethical issues have been recognised and much debated, the decision to continue with living donation has usually been based upon the very real benefits that ensue for the recipient. Living donation has always demonstrated higher graft survival rates than cadaveric donation. Although recent advances in immunosuppression have narrowed the gap between the two groups (Fig. 12.4), in most cases the living donor grafts still have a 10% better survival rate at 1 year and a significantly higher probability of function in the long term. The closer tissue match achieved with related donation usually results in fewer rejection episodes and a reduced amount of immunosuppression, and the reduced ischaemia time for all living donor kidneys contribute to the better outcome.

The living donation can be planned to take place at the most suitable time (medically and socially) for the recipient and donor. As renal function deteriorates, transplantation can be planned for the predialysis phase, thus avoiding the physical and psychological stress of dialysis adjustments. Studies have shown an improved outcome for recipients transplanted in the predialysis phase. Such benefits have encouraged the expansion of living donor programmes.

TRANSPLANT RATES

Living related donation programmes vary throughout the world but most European countries have a substantial live donor programme. In the countries covered by Eurotransplant, in 2005, 22% of kidney transplants were from living donors; 43% of these were from non-relatives (Eurotransplant 2006, see Fig 12.5). In Europe, Norway has the

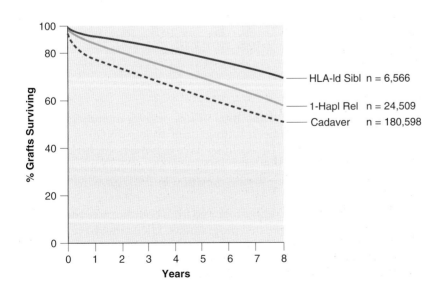

Figure 12.4
Graft survival in living related and cadaveric renal transplants 1985–2004. Statistics prepared by Collaborative Transplant Study, 2006. HLA, identical sibling; 1 haplotype, relative.

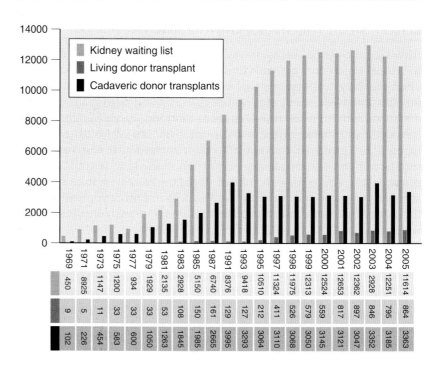

Figure 12.5
Dynamics of the Eurotransplant kidney waiting list and kidney transplants between 1969–2005. Statistics prepared by Eurotransplant.

	1969	1971	1973	1975	1977	1979	1981	1983	1985	1987	1991	1993	1995	1997	1998	1999	2000	2001	2002	2003	2004	2005
Kidney waiting list	450	8925	1147	1200	934	1929	2135	2928	5150	6740	8376	9418	10510	11324	11975	12313	12524	12653	12362	2928	12251	11614
Living donor transplant	9	5	11	33	33	33	53	108	150	161	129	127	212	411	526	579	559	817	897	846	795	864
Cadaveric donor transplants	102	226	454	583	600	1050	1263	1845	1985	2665	3995	3293	3064	3110	3068	3050	3145	3121	3047	3352	3185	3363

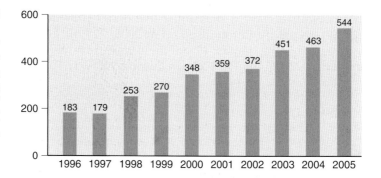

Figure 12.6
Living kidney donors in UK, 1 January 1996 to 31 December 2005. Statistics prepared by UK transplants, fom the National Transplant Database maintained on behalf of transplant services in the UK and Republic of Ireland.

highest rate, with 38% of the total adult, or 69% including paediatric, transplant programme resulting from living donation. Sweden, the USA, Denmark and Greece also have relatively high rates. Until recently, the UK had a low rate with only 5% of the total transplant programme resulting from living donation in 1981, growing to 32% in 2004 (Fig. 12.6).

Following the positive results reported from both Norway and the USA in live related and live unrelated programmes, UK centres have increased live donation. Indeed, transplant clinicians and the Department of Health are now actively promoting live donation.

LIVING UNRELATED DONATION (GENETICALLY UNRELATED–EMOTIONALLY RELATED)

In Norway, parents, siblings, adult children, uncles, aunts, grandparents and spouses were accepted as donors. Spouses are, of course, genetically unrelated but were recognised as 'emotionally related'. The Norwegian experience showed that transplantation between spouses (partners) can achieve graft survival rates equal to the best achieved with cadaveric organs. Similar results for transplantation between partners have been reported in the USA (Terasaki et al 1995). UK centres are now utilising spousal/partner donors and also other donors, who have a demonstrable long-term relationship with the recipient, such as close friends. However, all centres stress that the donor must be well motivated and well informed, and that the offer must be 'altruistic' and come from within a 'stable relationship'.

DONOR EXCHANGE AND ALTRUISTIC NON-DIRECTED DONATION

The Human Tissue Act (2004) expanded the criteria for living donation. Ross et al (1997) proposed to increase the number of living kidney donations by using kidneys from living ABO or cross-match incompatible donors through an exchange arrangement between two living kidney donor-recipient pairs. Only a small proportion of potential living donor pairs would be eligible for an exchange on the basis of blood group or cross-match incompatibility. There are two variations to this concept: (1) altruistically unbalanced, when only one pair is incompatible; and (2) an indirect exchange between a live donor-recipient pair with a cadaveric donor–recipient pair on the basis of incompatibility between the living donor-recipient pair. Ross et al (1997) acknowledged that all exchanges increase the potential for coercion and rejected altruistically unbalanced exchanges because of this.

The indirect ABO-incompatible exchange, however, may also disadvantage group O recipients and the concept remains controversial (Ross & Woodle 2000).

Non-directed altruistic donation, whereby a donor gives a kidney to be anonymously allocated by UK Transplant, is clearly permissible within the Act, although numbers are expected to be very small.

BUYING AND SELLING OF ORGANS

Living related and living unrelated transplantation in the UK is controlled by strict laws to prevent the possibility of illegal practices, such as financial payments and coercion. The unrelated group have been monitored by a government committee entitled ULTRA (Unrelated Live Transplant Regulatory Authority). The aim of this body was to ensure that there is no reward or coercion and that a 'long-standing relationship' is evident between donor and recipient. Prior to 2006, legislation precluded the use of altruistic donors who wish to give anonymously to the donor pool. Such donors have been utilised in the USA and New Zealand.

In the UK, the Human Tissue Act 2004 came into place in 2006. This new Act places the principle of consent at the centre of living donation, and indeed to all issues relating to donation and the taking of, storage and use of human tissues and organs. It covers England, Wales, Northern Ireland with the Human Tissue (Scotland) Act 2006 covering Scotland. The Human Tissue Authority, established in 2005, will implement the provisions of the Act and the EU Tissue and Cells Directive, which also came into force in 2006. Prior to the Human Tissue Act, living related transplants were approved through genetic blood testing using an approved tester, whilst living-unrelated or living-related donors, where a genetic relationship cannot be proven, were approved through ULTRA. Under the new Act, the approval process will be the same for directed genetically or emotionally related organ donation. Local independent assessors, trained and accredited by the Human Tissue Authority, assess all donor/recipient pairs and, where the requirements are met, give approval to proceed. The new Act also allowed the development of national paired organ donation and non-directed organ donation programmes, with an HTA panel deciding on whether approval is given or not.

The buying and selling of organs does occur in some of the developing countries and is an accepted practice. Indeed, some clinicians have suggested that a similar system, strictly controlled by legislation, could be introduced in the UK to increase transplant rates. The ethical and moral ramifications would be immense and at present such a concept is illegal and totally unacceptable to most.

DONOR AND RECIPIENT MATCHING

Individual tissue type is inherited as half from each parent. Therefore, matching within a nuclear family unit will usually result in a potential donor who is HLA-identical, a one-haplotype match or a mismatch.

Immunological aspects (example as for donor–related (DR) matching)

Matching for the MHC will take place, however. Figure 12.7 demonstrates tissue-type inheritance using the DR locus.

Therefore, potential donors may be:

- HLA-identical, as with DR1:3 (siblings)
- a one-haplotype match, as with DR1:3 and DR1:8 (siblings)
- DR1:4 and DR1:3 (parent–child)
- unmatched, as with DR1:3 and DR4:8 (siblings).

The long-term graft survival rates are better with better matching, but a mismatched living donor kidney transplant gives better results overall than well-matched deceased donor transplants (Gjertson 2003). Parents are usually very willing to donate, but siblings may be ambivalent and experience a crisis of loyalties between the family of birth and the family of marriage.

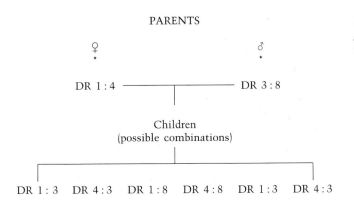

PARENTS

Figure 12.7
An example of tissue-type
inheritance.

PSYCHOLOGICAL ISSUES

The question of the possibility of living related donation may bring unity to a family group but it may also bring conflict. Parents will often offer early in the disease process and are extremely well motivated, but problems can arise if one parent is 'more suitable' due to tissue matching or physical constraints. The 'less suitable' parent may feel rejected and excluded from the donation and transplant process.

Siblings may be willing or ambivalent, and it may be difficult to express ambivalent feelings because of societal concepts of family loyalty and love. A sibling of a patient has expressed the wish that 'the request had never been made, as once verbalised it was impossible to refuse without feeling enormous guilt'. Married siblings may wish to donate but may encounter hostility from their partner who feels that the risks are too great and that responsibilities to the family of marriage are more important than loyalty to the family of birth.

Ongoing psychological support is a necessary part of a living donor programme. Donor and recipient must be well informed concerning the risks and benefits, and also the psychological difficulties that may develop. Separate meetings, both for the donor and the recipient, with medical staff and nurse/counsellor should be planned so that feelings, fears and anxieties can be discussed with honesty. The motivation to donate should be explored and, if appropriate, the donor offered the opportunity to withdraw without guilt or family conflict.

Similarly, the decision to receive should be explored and the recipient offered the opportunity to refuse. Some patients have refused living donation, preferring to wait for cadaveric grafts so as not to 'inflict my disease on my family'. The dynamics of the donor and recipient relationship must be well understood so that help and advice may be offered if difficulties arise.

ASSESSMENT AND PREPARATION OF DONORS

The living donor must be:

- well motivated
- in excellent health with two normal kidneys and normal renal function

- compatible for blood group and cross-match with the recipient, although a small number of transplants are being carried out across this barrier after removal/suppression of antibodies, and it remains to be seen how the donor exchange programme in the UK develops after 2006.

The assessment and preparation for living donation are extensive and normally carried out in stages over several weeks or months. Different centres will conduct tests at different stages but most units complete the same catalogue of tests in order to ensure that the criteria are fulfilled. The British Transplant Society and Renal Association (2005) have produced guidelines on this. Usually the assessment involves three stages. At each stage, the donor meets with medical staff and the nurse counsellor. Various tests are grouped together for each visit, thus minimising the disruption to the donor's working and personal life. Prior to stage 1, the donor will have received written information regarding the risks and benefits and the preoperative and postoperative experiences. Preliminary blood grouping and tissue typing may have occurred before the stage 1 visit (if not, they will be completed during this visit).

Stage 1

The donor and recipient and other family members are invited to the transplant centre to meet with the transplant surgeon and the nurse counsellor. At this meeting, the risks and benefits are explored, as are the forthcoming tests and the pre-, peri- and postsurgery experiences.

The donor and recipient have the opportunity to meet separately with the nurse counsellor alone, so that individual thoughts and anxieties can be explored in privacy. This is also an opportunity to explore the donor–recipient relationship. Such meetings help to initiate a trusting relationship with the nurse counsellor so that support can be available throughout the experience.

Assessment at stage 1

- Age: the donor must be above the age of consent. The assessment criteria are for physical health rather than chronological age, although renal function and physical fitness decline with age.
- Informed consent: the donor must be able to understand the risks that may ensue.
- Preliminary medical history: hypertension, if severe or of long-standing, untreated diabetes and other problems that would suggest anaesthetic risk to the donor may prevent donation.
- Renal disease: familial renal disease may exclude from donation.
- Smoking: smokers should be advised to stop prior to donation because of increased anaesthetic risks. They may also be referred for lung function tests and exercise ECG if smoking has been heavy over a prolonged period of time.
- Drug or alcohol abuse: this is investigated fully and may preclude from donation.
- Obesity: donors who have an unacceptable body mass index (BMI) will be asked to reduce weight prior to surgery.
- Blood and clinical tests: taken at visit 1 stage 1 (Box 12.9).

Box 12.9   Stage 1 donor blood and clinical tests

- Blood group
- Tissue typing: T- and B-cell cross-match
- Urea, electrolytes, creatinine, thyroid function
- Liver function tests: fasting glucose
- Haemoglobin and clotting screen,
- Viral screen
- Urine tests (midstream urine, urinalysis, albumin/creatinine ratio)
- Blood pressure, pulse, weight and height

Box 12.10   Investigations at stage 2 prior to medical assessment

Blood tests
- Repeat tissue typing
- Urea and electrolytes two readings of these tests are preferable at stages 1 and 2
- Liver function test
- Haematology

Clinical tests
- Chest X-ray
- Electrocardiogram
- Ultrasound scan of renal system

Urine tests
- Midstream urine, urinalysis, 24-h urine (× 2) for creatinine clearance and protein

---

If the initial assessments are satisfactory and the donor still wishes to donate, further tests are completed prior to a medical assessment, which should be performed by a nephrologist who is not responsible for the recipient (Boxes 12.10 and 12.11).

If the results of the tests and the medical evaluation are satisfactory, the donor assessment will proceed to stage 4. Stage 4 includes glomerular filtration rate (GFR) estimation, renal angiography and dimercaptosuccinic acid (DMSA).

Throughout the assessment programme the donor is assured that it is possible to retract the offer to donate at any time. Such a decision will be strictly confidential, and support and advice will be available. If the donor wishes, a medical reason not to donate can be provided. This medical reason is seen within the context of a 'benevolent decision' to enable the donor to retract without family conflict or distress, thus promoting full altruism. This technique has been successfully used in living donor programmes (Hilton & Starzomski 1994).

Once the tests are completed, the donor and partner will meet with the nurse counsellor and the surgical team that will be performing the

Box 12.11   Stage 3: medical assessment

The nephrologist in this centre will meet with the donor and ascertain that the donor is well informed, able to consent, really motivated and altruistic. He/she will tell the donor that he/she is 'their doctor and their advocate'. He/she will then proceed to answer three critical questions:

1. Is the donation safe for the recipient?
2. Is the donor fit for a nephrectomy?
3. Can the donor afford the gift?

Is the donation safe for the recipient?
Assessment of:

- Donor infection
- Donor age, blood pressure
- Donor – exclude history of cancer
- Donor kidney function: glomerular filtration rate (GFR)
- Anatomically safe: renal angiogram – how many arteries, can the kidney be transplanted with minimal technical risk?

Is the donor fit for a nephrectomy?
To establish donor health, an in-depth medical history

will be taken and a physical examination completed, paying specific attention to the following issues:

- General health and past medical history, especially cardiac and respiratory
- Anaesthetic and bleeding history
- Thrombosis history/oral contraceptive (the donor will be asked to stop contraceptive 3 months before surgery)
- Drugs, alcohol and smoking
- Allergies
- Specific evaluation for undeclared cancer, hypertension, cardiac disease, respiratory disease, risk of deep vein thrombosis
- GFR and renal angiogram results

Can the donor afford the gift?
- Is the blood pressure acceptable? (Any hypertensive damage should exclude the donor)
- Is renal function normal for age and gender?
- Is the 24-h urine protein < 300 mg?
- Is the fasting glucose normal?
- Is there a risk of renal disease in later life?

nephrectomy. The nurse counsellor can further explore any fears and anxieties, and can fully outline the preoperative and postoperative procedures. The surgeon can give details of the kidney to be removed and size and placing of surgical scar.

Two separate surgical teams are usually involved with a living related donation. The donor team assume responsibility for donor care and the transplant team take responsibility for recipient care. The donor and recipient are usually both nursed within the transplant centre in separate rooms. However, they may be nursed together if they so wish, if there are language or other difficulties.

The recipient will also be offered the opportunity to meet the nurse counsellor and the transplant surgeon to discuss preoperative and postoperative care, and any specific fears and anxieties. The recipient clinical preparation will be completed as outlined above. Providing all the assessment tests are satisfactory, the preoperative assessment for both donor and recipient will occur in the week before surgery (Box 12.12).

The donor and recipient are usually admitted on the day before transplant and, at this stage, a further medical history and physical examination will be performed, along with an anaesthetic and physiotherapist assessment.

Box 12.12   Stage 4: preoperative assessmentof donor and recipient

Investigations
- Glomerular filtration rate and dimercaptosuccinic acid
- Renal angiography

Other tests
- Final cross-match
- Methicillin-resistant swabs (throat, nose, axilla, groin) Staphylococcus aureus
- Midstream urine, urinalysis

- Biochemistry
- Liver function tests
- Haematology and clotting screen
- Electrocardiogram, blood pressure, pulse, temperature
- Chest X-ray

A preoperative dialysis plan for the recipient will be agreed, if required

---

PREOPERATIVE CARE FOR THE DONOR

The immediate preoperative care for the living donor will be similar to that given to patients undergoing conventional nephrectomy. However, particular attention is paid to informed consent, preoperative hygienic care and premedication.

SURGICAL TECHNIQUE OF NEPHRECTOMY

Living donor nephrectomy is always emotionally taxing surgery and can be technically difficult. The estimated mortality from living donor nephrectomy is 1 in 3000 (British Transplant Society/Renal Association 2005). Thus, while very rare, the risks are certainly not negligible, and major morbidity or death is very traumatic not only for the relatives but for the members of the surgical team themselves.

The traditional approaches (and those still most-used in the UK) for removing a kidney from a live donor are either transabdominal, intraperitoneal, or via the loin over the 11th or 12th rib, either spreading or removing the 11th or 12th rib. The intra-abdominal approach is usually through a transverse incision in the right or left upper quadrant. Laparoscopic nephrectomy is available at a few centres, using an anterior transperitoneal or loin approach, and this procedure is discussed in more detail in a later section.

The kidney may be approached via the abdominal cavity (transperitoneal) or from the loin (extraperitoneal). The kidney is carefully exposed and meticulous dissection is carried out with careful handling of the kidney and careful exposure of the renal vein and artery. The gonadal and adrenal tributaries of the renal vein are ligated and divided, and often a posterior lumbar vein needs ligating and dividing as well.

The renal artery is cleaned and exposed at its junction with the aorta, and the ureter is identified and dissected down to the pelvic brim or just below, where it is ligated and divided. It is very important to avoid too much dissection in the hilum of the kidney and it is also essential to avoid stripping the ureter of its adventitia. The blood supply to the ureter normally comes from the renal artery, branches from the gonadal vessels and the external iliac artery and branches of the superior vesicle artery. In a transplant kidney, the blood supply to the ureter is entirely dependent on the renal artery and it is essential to keep a good amount of adventitia around the ureter to allow the blood to reach the distal ureter. One of the major complications after transplantation is ischaemia of the lower end of the ureter, and this is normally due to stripping of the ureter or loss of a lower pole artery at the time of the donor surgery.

When the kidney is free and attached just by the artery and the vein, the artery is ligated and divided first, followed by the vein. The kidney is removed and placed in iced saline where perfusion is started immediately and, after careful inspection, any further dissection is carried out and a renal biopsy is taken.

POSTOPERATIVE MANAGEMENT: LIVING DONOR

The postoperative care for the living donor is similar to the care given for a conventional nephrectomy. Nephrectomy is recognised as painful surgery requiring frequent analgesia in the early postoperative phase. In most centres, patient-controlled analgesia using an opiate is utilised.

Hydration: fluid and electrolyte balance

Paralytic ileus may occur as a result of the retroperitoneal dissection and the handling of the bowel. Therefore, the intake of oral fluids must commence slowly and only increase as ileus resolves and bowel sounds are evident. In practice, hydration is maintained by intravenous infusion for the first 24–48 h until oral intake is sufficient. Close monitoring of fluid and electrolyte balance is necessary until dietary intake is adequate.

The passing of urine may prove difficult due to the pain of movement and anxiety, so often a urinary catheter is inserted under anaesthetic so that urinary output can be closely monitored and pain minimised. The catheter is usually removed on the second postoperative day. Regular midstream urine specimens should be obtained for microscopy, culture and sensitivity during hospitalisation. Monitoring of urine output is important to determine the function of the remaining kidney.

Wound management

Wound management should include regular inspection to exclude complications of bleeding and infection.

Emotional support

During the early postoperative period, emotional support should be offered, as should frequent information regarding the progress of the recipient. Donor and recipient should be reunited at the earliest opportunity and encouraged to spend time together. The donor may experience a feeling of anticlimax after the surgery due to a release of the preoperative tension and anticipation. Such anticlimax may combine with postanaesthetic 'blues' to form a mild depression with emotional lability. Staff should recognise the altruism of the act and offer understanding and reassurance.

The majority of living donors will be discharged between the fourth and fifth postoperative day. It is recommended that they continue their postoperative recovery at home for approximately 6 weeks to 2 months. Return to work will be variable depending on type of employment, and its physical and psychological demands. Physical monitoring may include one or two further assessments by the surgical team.

Most centres now monitor donors annually, although this may be done by the General Practitioner. Annual follow-up is recommended in the British Transplant Society/Renal Association (2005), and UK Transplant gathers data from these annual follow-ups. Emotional support should continue as appropriate, with help available if difficulties arise.

Loss of earnings and travel can be reimbursed by the recipient's local Primary Care Trust if authorised by the Specialist Health Care Commissioners. Donors should be made aware of this at an early stage in the work-up process. Reimbursement is not obligatory and depends on circumstances and locally agreed guidelines.

Discharge

LAPAROSCOPIC DONOR NEPHRECTOMY

Transplant centres in the USA started this type of donor surgery in 1995 and, by 2005, over 60% of centres in the USA offered it (Giessing et al 2005). A recent survey found that five centres in the UK offer laparoscopic donor nephrectomy (Brook & Nicholson 2004). Donors can expect to be discharged in about 3 days rather than five. Less postoperative analgesia is required and time taken to return to normal activities is reduced by at least half (Waller et al 2002, Wilson et al 2005).

The technique requires a high degree of training of surgeons. The donor is placed in the flank position and the abdomen insufflated with carbon dioxide gas. Entry ports are made into the abdomen for the camera and instruments. After isolating the kidney, it is enclosed by a bag to aid removal through another incision. The hand-assisted laparoscopic technique entails an incision large enough to allow insertion of the surgeon's hand to assist with the laparoscopic procedure.

Laparoscopic donor nephrectomy is thought to increase the number of potential living donors; Kuo & Johnson (2000) reported that 47% of donors did so only because this technique was offered to them.

Li Ming et al (2004), from the Johns Hopkins University Hospital, Maryland, USA, report 381 laparoscopic donor procedures without mortality. They observed a significant decline in both donor and recipient morbidity with experience.

Donor mortality and morbidity rates

Further reports from another centre compared their first 70 laparoscopic donors with a historic open nephrectomy group and found comparable morbidity rates (Flowers et al 1997). These two groups conclude that 'in centres with a large experience and expertise in advanced laparoscopic techniques, the donor operation can be performed safely and without excess morbidity'. However, most UK surgeons remain ambivalent and believe that the transperitoneal approach for the open operation has less morbidity than has been previously reported. Further larger studies are necessary before true comparisons can be drawn between the two techniques.

Laparoscopic donor studies have found that the advantages to the donor include reduction in operative blood loss, postoperative pain, wound-related problems, length of hospitalisation and a speedier recovery to normal activities and work (Flowers et al 1997, Troppman et al 2003).

Risks to the kidney transplant

There have been some reported problems with the kidneys retrieved via laparoscopic techniques. However, after several refinements to the surgical technique, donor early recovery of graft function, longer term renal function, and 3-year patient and allograft survival are similar for live donor kidneys obtained by either a laparoscopic or an open surgical technique (Derweesh et al 2005).

For further reading and explicit diagrams showing the laparoscopic surgical technique, refer to Morris (2001).

INCREASING DONOR ORGAN SUPPLY

As stated earlier, cadaveric organ donor rates and kidney transplant rates in the UK have remained fairly constant during the last 10 years. Such rates are insufficient to meet demand and the renal transplant waiting list continues to rise. If the renal transplant rate continues at the same level, many hopeful dialysis patients will be denied their 'treatment of choice' (Fig. 12.1). Extending the living related and unrelated programmes will increase the supply of kidneys, livers and, in some cases, lungs for transplantation, but it is crucial that the UK continues to explore and introduce initiatives to increase the cadaveric organ supply. UK Transplant, since 2001, has increased the number of living donor co-ordinators, supported the development of non-heart-beating programmes and provided additional donor co-ordinators to support existing teams and provide in-house expertise within hospitals.

A document released in June 2000 by the British Medical Association highlights the inability of the current system of organ donation to meet the increasing demand and outlines various ways of overcoming the difficulties by increasing the availability of organs for transplantation. This report believes that a multifaceted approach is needed. One way is to have more direct appeals for people to register as potential donors by:

- addressing common concerns and misconceptions
- facilitating registration on the National Health Service organ donor register.

The British Medical Association also suggests improvements to the UK transplant coordination system and infrastructure by:

- placing 'key donation' personnel in every hospital (these personnel will work with the regional coordinators)
- adopting required referral, whereby all staff routinely refer any suitable patient who has died to the transplant coordination service
- developing the national transplant coordination service, with an increase in the number of transplant coordinators
- establishing additional critical care beds
- making the list of criteria for exclusion of patients as potential organ donors less restrictive.

These suggested changes are, in part, based upon the very successful Spanish organ donation system (Table 12.3). As can be seen from this table, Spain has an increasing number of cadaveric donors, rising to 35.1 per million population in 2005, compared to only 13.5 cadaveric donors per million in the UK and Ireland.

In 1989 the official agency for transplantation in Spain, the National Transplant Organisation, created a national network of specially trained, dedicated and strongly motivated hospital physicians to take charge of the whole process of organ donation in 139 hospitals. The aim of these appointments was to improve:

Country	Cadaveric donors pmp in 2004
Greece	6
Slovakia	10.2
Switzerland	12.6
Germany	13
Sweden	13.7
United Kingdom	13.8
Poland	14.7
Holland	15.5
Norway	19.6
Czech Republic	20.5
Finland	20.9
France	21
Italy	21.1
Portugal	21.2
Belgium	21.8
Republic of Ireland	22.1
Austria	22.6
Spain	34.6

Table 12.3
Cadaveric organ donation across Europe in 2004. Statistics prepared by the Council of Europe (2005).

- detection of potential organ donors
- management of the donors
- approach to the family
- the support of the mass media, and to reimburse hospitals adequately for the expenses that result from donor care and donor surgery.

Results of the Spanish initiatives show that cadaveric organ donors rose from 550 in 1989 to 1334 in 1999 – a 42% increase. This increase was sustained in 2000. The rates of cadaveric organ donation per million inhabitants (31.5) are the highest in the world, and patients on the Spanish waiting list have the best chance of receiving an organ (Fig. 12.8).

The British Medical Association report also lists the following initiatives to increase the numbers of donors:

- increasing the pool of living donation (related and unrelated donors)
- increasing the numbers of non-heart-beating donors, i.e. patients who die of cardiac arrest, in general wards, accident and emergency or intensive care, who may donate liver and kidneys a short period after death
- introducing presumed consent (opt-out).

ASYSTOLIC DONATION (NON-HEART-BEATING)

An initiative at the Leicester General Hospital in 1992 showed that asystolic (non-heart-beating) donation could become an increasingly important source of renal organs. Leicester identified asystolic donors in the medical wards, and the accident and emergency department of the local hospital. At the time of asystole and following certification of death (providing that there were no medical contraindications to donation), an intra-aortic catheter was inserted and ice-cold perfusion of the kidneys commenced. Such perfusion reduces the warm ischaemic damage and allows time for medical/nursing colleagues to approach the family and the coroner for

Figure 12.8
Cadaveric organ donors in Spain, per million population 1989–2005. Statistics prepared by the Spanish National Transplantation Organisation (ONT).

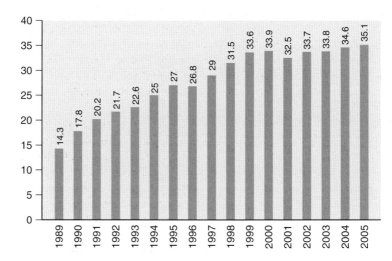

permission to proceed to donation. If permission was granted, the kidneys must be removed within 40–45 min of asystole in order to avoid irreversible renal damage.

Ethical concerns about the insertion of the catheter before consent has been given by the family were widely discussed during the planning of this programme and health personnel, the coroner and the general public groups that were consulted gave consent to this initiative. However, following the widely reported problems with organ retention after post-mortem without family consent that occurred at Alder Hey and other hospitals, it was decided by the Leicester group that they must obtain consent before insertion of the intra-aortic catheter. This decision undoubtedly affected the length of time between asystole and cold perfusion of the kidneys. However, the Human Tissue Act 2004 made the wishes of the potential donor central to any decision to proceed.

Interestingly, results suggest a marginally higher rate of relative consent in asystolic donation than is usually achieved in brain stem death donation. This may be due to the skill of the staff requesting and also the fact that with asystole the patient appears 'dead' in the conventional sense (cold, pale and cyanosed), thus there may be less psychological denial for the family.

Several other centres have introduced asystolic donation programmes and they are providing a useful additional supply of kidneys. However, the limiting factors will be the need for a rapid response time from the retrieval teams and the need for catheter insertion expertise. Such factors may preclude donation from hospitals that are some distance away from the transplant centre.

OPTING IN/OPTING OUT

Within the UK the general public are encouraged to 'opt in' by making the voluntary decision to donate organs. This decision is supported by carrying a donor card or registering with UKT and informing relatives of this wish. Thus, donation is a voluntary gift.

Research suggests that approximately 75% of the general public support donation and about 22% had joined the NHS Organ Donor register by 2006 – over 13 million people. More people who have not registered will carry an organ donor card; however, problems with this system are that, in practice, the donor card may not be available at the time of death, or relatives may either be unaware of the donor's wishes or may choose to ignore them. Several patient groups, and the British Medical Association, have pressed for the introduction of an 'opting-out' system, whereby everyone is deemed to wish to donate unless they have registered an objection. The opting-out system has been introduced in Europe (namely Austria and Belgium), and appears to be successful. However, with a true opting-out system, the wishes of the family are not considered. At present, it is felt by the major health groups in the UK that the denial of the family's wishes is unacceptable practice. Therefore, the government has decided to continue to support opting-in with the introduction of the national registry, whereby those wishing to donate can register their wishes on to the national computer. The computer can be accessed by critical care staff should death occur. However, relatives will still be asked for consent.

The British Medical Association suggests that by adopting a presumed consent (softer opt-out option), close relatives would not be asked to give permission but rather informed that the individual had not registered an objection. Unless the family object, the donation will proceed and this donation becomes a default position.

Additional areas that the British Medical Association suggests require further consideration include:

- elective ventilation
- living kidney exchange.

ELECTIVE VENTILATION

A protocol for increasing organ donation after cerebrovascular death was implemented in the early 1990s (Feest et al 1990), and this protocol stated that 'patients fulfilling the criteria as potential organ donors could be identified on the medical wards; once identified, the relatives could be approached with regard to donation and if permission was given, the patient moved to intensive care for ventilation to facilitate donation'. (This practice became widely known as 'elective ventilation'.) The programme proved successful and, in 19 months, the hospital reported eight such donations. It was suggested that these results, if replicated throughout the UK, would greatly increase the numbers of donor organs.

However, a legal ruling in 1993 described the act of elective ventilation as 'unlawful' as 'the ventilation was deemed not to have been initiated for the benefit of the patient' (New et al 1994). With the advent of this ruling the elective ventilation programmes were discontinued, but discussions regarding the ethical and legal issues continue in the hope that solutions may be found.

PAIRED LIVING KIDNEY EXCHANGE

Paired living kidney exchange is an exchange system whereby a donor who is incompatible with the intended recipient could donate a kidney to another person whose own donor would provide a kidney in return. Such exchanges have taken place in the USA, Europe and South America, but the necessary reforms in the UK only took place in 2006.

CONCLUSIONS

The British Medical Association recommendations were welcomed by all transplant groups. It is hoped that these innovations will indeed increase donation rates, but it is feared that with growing waiting lists the demand may always outstrip supply. (For further reading and to view the British Medical Association Organ Donation Review 2000, visit www.bma.org.co.uk). The solution in the long term may be the introduction of xenotransplantation.

XENOTRANSPLANTATION (TRANSPLANT OF ANIMAL ORGANS INTO HUMANS)

The United Kingdom Xenotransplantation Interim Regulatory Authority was formed in 1997 to advise the government. To debate all the ethical, moral and practical issues regarding the use of other species for transplantation is beyond the scope of this book. However, from a biological viewpoint, closely related non-human primates, such as chimpanzees, would be the most preferable for transplantation, since there is no hyperacute rejection problem. However, it has been universally agreed that such species would be ethically unacceptable and impractical since they are endangered species, and dangerous to use because of the possibility of viral transfer or similar disasters. For practicality, the acceptable species would be those in current large-scale usage for food production, such as the pig.

The most obvious and immediate problem confronting the use of xenografts is the problem of hyperacute rejection. Connection of a suitably prepared pig kidney to the blood circulation of a dialysis patient initially results in normal perfusion of the kidney, which becomes pulsatile and pink and may even briefly produce urine. However, within minutes, the pulsatility of the kidney lessens, and then ceases, the kidney becoming initially blue and finally almost black as the circulation ceases due to thrombosis. This typical pattern of rapid graft failure was initially described in human kidney allografts and was termed hyperacute rejection. The cause was subsequently shown to be the presence in the recipient of high-titre antibody against the donor tissue, binding the antibody causing complement activation and subsequent activation of the clotting cascade. Blood group ABO incompatibility was a potent source of antidonor antibody that was easily avoided, but some cases of hyperacute rejection still occurred, even after blood group matching. In the case of human allografts, it was possible to avoid this fairly rare occurrence by testing for the presence of antidonor antibody and avoiding transplantation when antibody was detected. However, in the case of xenotransplantation between distantly related species, antibody is always detectable despite matching for blood groups, and this antibody came to be known as heterophile or natural antibody.

Two fundamental recent discoveries are the basis for a number of new approaches to prevent xenograft hyperacute rejection, for example, by blocking or removing the natural antibody or infusing human complement regulatory proteins. The recent advent of transgenic manipulation has also allowed the concept of developing herds of animals that express high levels of human complement regulatory proteins on their cells. Research is moving so rapidly that already herds of transgenic pigs have been produced and organs from these pigs are undergoing preclinical experimental studies with partially encouraging results.

It now seems likely that combinations of the above approaches will eventually allow transplantation of organs between species such as pigs and humans, avoiding destruction of the graft by hyperacute rejection. However, this is likely to be only the first of several barriers to successful xenograft usage. Other barriers include the processes of cellular rejection that may well be entirely different to those seen in allograft rejection, the problem of species compatibility for crucial molecular and biochemical pathways, the risk of disease transmission and, of course, the animal rights movement, which promotes heated debate on the moral acceptability of xenotransplantation.

For further information regarding xenotransplantation, refer to Soin & Friend (2001).

PREOPERATIVE MANAGEMENT FOR A RENAL TRANSPLANT RECIPIENT

THE TRANSPLANT CALL

Transplant recipients report mixed reactions of relief, excitement, anxiety and sadness when they receive the transplant phone call: relief that the waiting time may be over; excitement for the new life ahead; anxiety that the surgery may be difficult or that the transplant may fail; and sadness that a family elsewhere has experienced tragedy in order for the kidney to become available (Dubovsky & Penn 1980).

During the telephone conversation, the recipient is informed that a transplant may be possible and to travel to the transplant centre and have nothing further to eat or drink. Brief questions are also asked to clarify current health status and to exclude any infections or other problems that may prevent transplantation.

Some centres contact two recipients for each transplant so that should a positive cross-match occur for one, a second recipient is already prepared, thus minimising the cold ischaemia time. It has been found that contacting two recipients can lead to repeated disappointments, anger and depression; therefore it is preferable to only call one recipient to the transplant centre in the first instance.

NURSING ADMISSION

Upon arrival, the recipient and family are welcomed by the nursing team and helped to familiarise themselves with the unit. Brief information is given regarding the forthcoming blood and clinical tests; questions are answered and anxieties explored during the nursing admission procedure (Box 12.13).

MEDICAL ASSESSMENT

Immediate medical assessment and blood tests are required to assess fluid and electrolyte status (as dialysis may be needed prior to surgery), also to complete the final tissue typing cross-match test, and therefore the medical assessment immediately follows the nursing admission procedure (Box 12.14).

Box 12.13   Nursing admission procedure

- Blood pressure, pulse, temperature, respirations
- Current weight: dry weight
- Past medical history – renal disease
- Dialysis history – current practice, and date and time of last dialysis
- Current health status – recent relevant health events (i.e. blood transfusion/infections)
- Normal urine output, if any
- Social information
- Allergies
- Name band applied

Box 12.14   Medical assessment procedure

- Medical history
- Renal disease history
- Dialysis history
- Current health status – recent relevant events
- Allergies
- Medical examination
- Blood tests:
  - urea and electrolytes
  - liver function tests
  - tissue typing cross-match
  - viral screen (as in pretransplant assessment)
  - cross-match for 2–4 units of blood available for transplant surgery
- Clinical tests:
  - chest X-ray
  - electrocardiogram
  - midstream specimen of urine, urinalysis

PREOPERATIVE DIALYSIS

The results of the medical assessment and blood tests will determine the need for dialysis. Fluid overload and electrolyte imbalance (particularly hyperkalaemia) must be corrected, as they represent an anaesthetic risk and may enhance post-transplantation difficulties. Haemodialysis with minimal or no heparinisation is often necessary to ensure optimal weight and to reduce fluid overload and serum potassium levels.

Peritoneal dialysis patients may require rapid exchanges to achieve optimal fluid and electrolyte status. The peritoneal catheter exit site should be examined for any signs of infection and a swab taken for culture and sensitivity. Also, following the necessary exchanges, the catheter should be drained and a fluid specimen sent for microscopy culture and sensitivity, then the catheter capped, leaving the patient empty of fluid.

INFORMATION AND EMOTIONAL SUPPORT

During the dialysis time, it is often possible to explore individual fears and anxieties, and offer emotional support and information regarding postoperative medications and procedures. Recipients are often emotionally labile at this time ('tears and laughter') and require much emotional understanding and support.

IMMEDIATE PREOPERATIVE CARE

It is usual for the physiotherapist to visit to commence chest physiotherapy and advise regarding postoperative mobility, and for the anaesthetist to perform an assessment. Once the tissue typing cross-match has proved negative, the final preoperative preparation begins (Box 12.15).

SURGICAL TECHNIQUE FOR RENAL TRANSPLANTATION

Before transplantation begins, a catheter is placed into the bladder. This allows drainage of the bladder during the transplant operation. It also allows the bladder to be filled with solution containing antibiotics to facilitate later identification of the bladder for reimplantation of the ureter. The right or left iliac fossa is the normal site for the transplant (Fig. 12.9).

- An incision is made curving from just above the pubic symphysis to just above the iliac crest.
- The inferior epigastric vessels are ligated and divided, and an extraperitoneal approach is made down on to the iliac vessels.
- The external iliac artery and vein are freed, and small branches or overlying lymphatics are ligated and divided.
- Clamps are applied to the external iliac vein and the renal vein is anastomosed to the external iliac vein with continuous 5.0 Prolene sutures.
- Clamps are then applied to the external iliac artery and the renal artery on its patch (known as the Carrell patch) is anastomosed with continuous 5.0 Prolene to the external iliac artery (Fig. 12.10). Sometimes the internal iliac artery is used and an end-to-end anastomosis is performed.
- Once the anastomoses are complete, the clamps are released, taking the venous clamps off first. The kidney normally perfuses quickly and one is often able to see immediate urine production.

Box 12.15   Preoperative preparation

Skin swabs/nose, throat, axilla and groin swabs – for viral, bacterial and methicillin-resistant *Staphylococcus aureus* screening

Swabs and dressings to other dialysis lines (i.e. permanent central venous catheters)

Suppositories (if required)

Bath/shower/hair wash

Operation gown

Marking and dressing (to protect) arteriovenous fistula from inadvertent use of invasive monitoring (e.g., intravenous lines, blood pressure cuffs) and to maintain warmth, thus avoiding clotting

Antithrombosis stockings

Preoperative medications, such as immunosuppressive drugs[a] and aspirin

Medications given immediately preoperatively
 – premedication
 – diabetes mellitus: sliding-scale insulin as appropriate

[a] Note: transplant centres may use differing combinations of immunosuppressive medications.

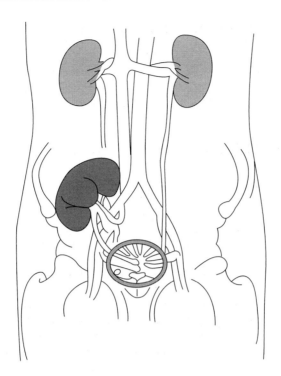

Figure 12.9
Position for the transplant kidney.

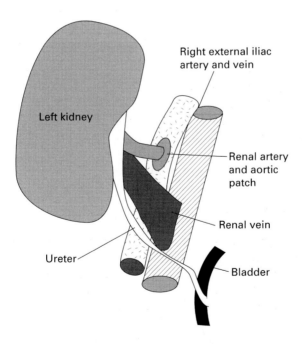

Figure 12.10
The surgical technique for renal transplantation.

- The bladder is then filled through the catheter, and the ureter put into the bladder and then tunnelled submucosally to prevent urinary ureteric reflux (the Leadbetter–Politano technique). Most centres may use an extra vesicle technique, which involves splitting the muscle, laying the ureter just above the bladder mucosa and so into the bladder, and closing the muscle over the top. If the bladder has been opened, it is closed with two layers of Vicryl. Many units are now using ureteric stents, which are left *in situ* for 6 weeks. This practice has reduced the incidence of ureteric complications.

- The wound is closed in the usual fashion and the bladder washed out at the end of the procedure.

RENAL TRANSPLANT REJECTION

There are three types of renal transplant rejection:

- hyperacute rejection
- acute rejection
- chronic rejection or chronic allograft nephropathy (CAN).

HYPERACUTE REJECTION

Hyperacute rejection (Fig. 12.11) occurs rapidly, within minutes or hours of revascularisation of the transplant. It is caused by:

- the presence of preformed cytotoxic antibodies in the recipient's blood (resulting from previous failed transplants, blood transfusions or pregnancies) reacting against the donor's histocompatibility antigens
- ABO incompatibility between the donor and the recipient.

The final lymphocytotoxic cross-match prior to transplant should demonstrate that cytotoxic antibodies are present and transplantation should not take place, thus a hyperacute rejection is a very rare phenomenon today.

Hyperacute rejection may be observed during the transplant surgery. Instead of the kidney becoming distended and pink as the arterial and venous clamps are released, as is usual, with hyperacute rejection the kidney will remain flaccid and become blue. Damage is almost always irreversible and the graft is lost.

ACUTE REJECTION

Acute rejection (Fig. 12.12) is usually a combination of cellular and antibody-mediated rejection, which commonly occurs between 4 days and 2 months after transplantation. The clinical signs of acute rejection may include:

- pyrexia
- renal dysfunction
- weight gain
- fall in urine output
- swelling and tenderness of the transplant
- ankle oedema
- flu-like symptoms.

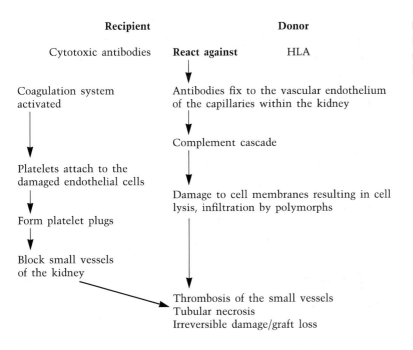

Figure 12.11
Histopathology of hyperacute rejection. HLA, human leukocyte antigen.

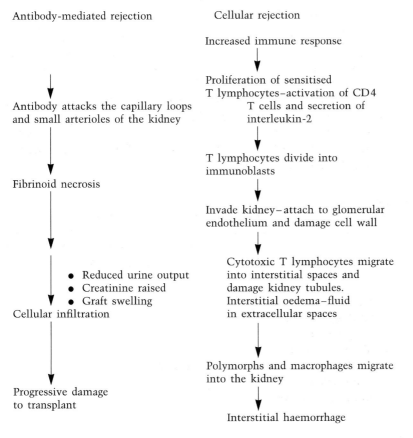

Figure 12.12
Histopathology of acute rejection.

Acute rejection can usually be controlled by increased immunosuppression; however, a severe rejection may result in some loss of overall graft function.

CHRONIC REJECTION OR CHRONIC ALLOGRAFT NEPHROPATHY

Chronic rejection usually occurs over months or years, but may occur much earlier. It is difficult to separate out the contribution of rejection from other factors detrimental to the kidney. The term CAN encompasses all of these; meaning that permanent damage is seen on biopsy (Halloran 2002). There is a gradual occlusion of the lumen of the arteries of the kidney with interstitial fibrosis which destroys the graft. The exact mechanisms involved in chronic rejection are still unclear, and may be immunological or non-immunological. Other factors include donor history and delayed graft function, acute rejection episodes, hypertension, calcinerium inhibitor (CNI) toxicity and infection. The first signs of chronic rejection are usually a gradual worsening of renal function with proteinuria.

IMMUNOSUPPRESSION REGIMES

Until 1997, the most commonly used immunosuppression was a 'triple-therapy' regime involving ciclosporin, azathioprine and prednisolone medications. The advent of newer drugs, such as tacrolimus, mycophenolate mofetil, rapamycin, basiliximab and daclizumab, has allowed centres to use differing combinations of immunosuppressives to match the level of risk relating to potential rejection problems. Other drugs are being developed continuously for use in transplantation; Rituximab and intravenous immunoglobulin (IVIg) are used in high-immunological risk recipients. A consensus has yet to emerge on which particular regime is best for which patients (Vincenti 2003). An example of different protocols according to immunological risk is shown in Box 12.16.

National Institute for Health and Clinical Excellence

The National Institute for Health and Clinical Excellence (NICE 2004) has issued guidance to the NHS in England and Wales on the use of immunosuppressive therapy for renal transplantation in adults. The guidance recommends:

- Basiliximab or daclizumab for induction treatment (immediately after the kidney transplant). These drugs should be used with a combination of other drugs, including a calcineurin inhibitor, such as ciclosporin. The cheapest one of the two (basiliximab or daclizumab) should be used.
- Tacrolimus (a calcineurin inhibitor) can be used instead of ciclosporin when a person needs a calcineurin inhibitor as part of their initial or maintenance immunosuppressive treatment after a kidney transplant. The drug (tacrolimus or ciclosporin) that is least likely to have serious side effects in that particular person should be used.
- Mycophenolate mofetil as part of immunosuppressive treatment after kidney transplant only when a person has to stop taking a calcineurin

Box 12.16   An example of an immunosuppression protocol (Royal London Hospital, 2005)

Low risk renal transplant
Definition
If both recipient *and* donor factors present
Immunological factors (recipient)
- First cadaveric transplant with favourable match (i.e. complete match, 1 mismatch at A or B loci or 1 mismatch at A and B
  and
- Peak PRA of < 10%, on current or historical sera

Nonimmunological factors (donor)
- Donor age < 60 years and no history of ischaemic heart disease (IHD), hypertension (HT), diabetes mellitus (DM), peripheral vascular disease (PVD) or atheroma in the renal artery
  and
- Cold ischaemic time of < 24 h

Immunosupression
- No induction
- Neoral, Cellcept (MMF), prednisolone
[If no rejection at 3rd month *and:*
  – serum creatinine < 130, then withdraw steroid
  – serum creatinine > 130, then consider switch from Neoral to sirolimus]

Medium risk renal transplant
Definition
If any recipient *or* donor factors present
Immunological factors (recipient)
- First cadaveric transplant with no favourable matching
  or
- Peak PRA 10–50%, cross-match negative with DTT
  or
- Cross-match negative on current serum (all sera within 1 year) but borderline positive on historical sera (sera collected > 1 year)
  or
- Live renal transplants
  or
- Afro-Caribbean recipients
  or

- Second graft, with or without favourable matching, following first graft loss due to nonimmunological cause (including CAN diagnosed after 1 year).
  or
- CDC negative but positive flow cytometric cross match on serum collected on the day of transplantation (give IL-2 blocker as soon as possible).

Nonimmunological factors (donor)
- Donor age > 60 years or history of IHD, HT, DM, PVD or atheroma in the renal artery
  or
- Cold ischaemic time of > 24 h

Immunosuppression
- Induction with IL-2 blocker
- Neoral, Cellcept (MMF), prednisolone

High risk renal transplant (1)
Definition
Immunological factors (recipient)
(a) Second transplant following first graft loss due to immunological cause
  or
(b) PRA > 50%

Immunosuppression
- Induction ATG
- Neoral, Cellcept (MMF), prednisolone

High risk renal transplant (2)
Definition
Nonimmunological factors (donor)
- Donor age > 60 years or history of IHD, HT, DM, PVD or atheroma in the renal artery
  and
- Cold ischaemic time of > 24 h

Immunosuppression
- Induction with IL-2 blocker
- Neoral, Cellcept (MMF), prednisolone
Nonimmunological medium and high-risk patients will commence ciclosporin (Neoral) at lower dose of 7.5 mg kg^{-1} day^{-1}

ATG, antithymocyte globulin; CAN, chronic allograft nephropathy; DTT, dithiothreitol; IL-2, interleukin 2; MMF, mycophenolate mofetil; PRA, panel reactive antibody; CDC, complement dependent cytoxicity.

inhibitor, or has to take a lower dose. This could be needed because the calcineurin inhibitor has already damaged the transplanted kidney.

- Sirolimus (rapamycin) as one of a combination of immunosuppressive drugs, but only for people who cannot use calcineurin inhibitors because of their side-effects.

This guidance represents the views of the Institute, and health professionals are expected to take it into account when exercising clinical judgement. However, it does not override the individual responsibility of health professionals to make appropriate decisions for patients. It is not clear how many centres will comply with this guidance, which is itself due for review in 2007.

Ciclosporin (Neoral, Sandimmune)

Ciclosporin is a natural peptide found in two strains of fungi. It was first introduced into clinical immunosuppression in 1983 and is a calcineurin inhibitor. Neoral ciclosporin is in a microemulsion and is more reliably absorbed.

Action

Ciclosporin inhibits interleukin 2 (IL-2) and interferes with the growth and activation of T lymphocytes (Fig. 12.12).

Usually side-effects are dose-dependent and responsive to dose reduction. The commonest side-effects include:

Side-effects

- nephrotoxicity – decreased GFR
- hypertension
- hepatic dysfunction
- hirsutism
- hyperlipidaemia
- hyperkalaemia
- hyperuricaemia
- gum hypertrophy
- hypomagnesaemia
- hypertrichosis.

Other less common side-effects include:

- muscle weakness
- thrombocytopenia.

Ciclosporin may be started immediately before transplant but, because of its known nephrotoxicity, it may be withdrawn for the preliminary phase in the presence of primary non-function due to active tubular necrosis.

Absorption

Ciclosporin is absorbed with variable efficiency by different individuals; therefore, regular monitoring of whole blood levels is necessary. The usual therapeutic range is 150–300 μg mol L^{-1} during the first 3 months of transplantation, with maintenance doses aimed at levels of 90–150 μg mol L^{-1}. Generally, patients who reject due to inadequate ciclosporin levels usually have levels less than 100 μg mol L^{-1}, while patients with ciclosporin nephrotoxicity usually have levels towards the top or above the therapeutic range, but it is an individual response. Some units are now performing C2 monitoring, i.e. measuring blood concentrations 2-h post dose. C2 is thought to predict more accurately individual patient absorptions than traditional trough monitoring, and results in a reduced incidence of acute rejection episodes and acute renal dysfunction.

Tacrolimus (FK506, Prograf)

Tacrolimus is another calcineurin inhibitor, which, like ciclosporin, works early in T-cell activations. Its action inhibits IL-2 and other cytokines that cause early T-cell activation (Fig. 12.12).

Absorption

As with ciclosporin, regular monitoring of whole blood levels is necessary, with maintenance doses aimed at achieving a 12-h trough level of $7–15\,\text{ng}\,\text{mL}^{-1}$ during the first few months, then $5–10\,\text{ng}\,\text{mL}^{-1}$ thereafter.

Side-effects

The commonest side-effects include:

- visual and neurological disturbances
- hypertension
- tremor, headache, insomnia
- raised blood sugar level
- leukopenia
- nephrotoxicity.

Sirolimus (Rapamycin, Rapamune)

Sirolimus acts later in the T-cell activation than ciclosporin and tacrolimus. It inhibits IL-2-mediated signal transduction pathways (Fig. 12.12). Sirolimus is not nephrotoxic, which gives it an advantage over ciclosporin and tacrolimus. It was licensed for use in the UK in 2001.

Side-effects

These include:

- delayed healing (lymphocoele)
- enhanced ciclosporin toxicity, when used together
- hypercholesterolaemia
- hypertriglyceridemia
- thrombocytopenia
- increased levels of MMF (active metabolite mycophenolic acid).

Basiliximab (Simulect), Daclizumab (Zenepax)

These monoclonal antibodies are known as IL-2 blockers. The first infusion is given at induction and subsequent dose(s) according to which type is used.

Action

Basiliximab and Daclizimab work by binding specifically to part of the IL-2 receptor that is only expressed on activated T lymphocytes. Therefore, they help to prevent proliferation of antigen-stimulated T cells. They are used in combination with other immunosuppressives to form a baseline therapy (Box 12.16).

Side-effects   None have been reported.

Azathioprine

Azathioprine is a derivative of the anticancer drug 6-mercaptopurine and was introduced into clinical practice in 1962.

Action   Azathioprine inhibits both DNA and RNA synthesis and prevents growth of lymphocytes (Fig. 12.11).

Side-effects   The main side-effect is neutropenia. If the white blood cell count (WBC) drops to below $3.5 \times 10^9 \, L^{-1}$, the dose should be reduced. If the WBC drops below $3.0 \times 10^9 \, L^{-1}$, the drug should be stopped temporarily.
Other side-effects include:

- alopecia
- general malaise
- muscular pains
- malignancy
- pancreatitis (rare)
- altered liver function
- cholestatic jaundice (rare).

Because of the risk of neutropenia, blood counts must be checked at intervals of not longer than 3 months.

Mycophenolate mofetil

Mycophenolate mofetil was licensed in 1995 and, like azathiaprine, inhibits proliferation of lymphocytes.

Action   Mycophenolate mofetil acts by preventing activated lymphocytes from differentiating and proliferating, and thereby limiting clonal expansion. In the UK, this drug has been used in preference to azathioprine in selected patients who were considered to be at a higher risk of rejection than average (Box 12.16).

Side-effects   Mycophenolate mofetil has significant gastrointestinal adverse effects:

- diarrhoea
- vomiting
- leukopenia
- anaemia.

Prednisolone (corticosteroids)

Action   The action of corticosteroid preparations is complex and involves anti-inflammatory responses with blocking of T cells and interleukin-1 (Fig. 12.12).

These include:

- cushingoid appearance
- fluid retention
- glaucoma
- increased appetite
- hypertension
- psychosis
- peptic ulceration
- increase in blood sugar levels.

Side-effects with long-term treatment are:

- subcapsular cataract
- pancreatitis
- skin thinning
- osteoporosis.

Many centres start steroid reduction at 2 months post-transplant and aim to remove steroid therapy at 1 year post-transplant because of the long-term side-effects.

For further information regarding immunosuppression, see Lee & Devaney (2001).

ACUTE REJECTION

Rejection treatment consists of an increase in the dose of corticosteroids. Usual practice is to administer daily bolus doses of 500 mg intravenous methylprednisolone over a 3-day period (one bolus each day).

Action It is an antibody that reacts with CD3 molecules on the lymphocytes and depletes them.

Muromab-CD3 (Orthoclone; OKT3) monoclonal antibody

Side-effects

These include:

- chest pain
- pulmonary oedema
- gastrointestinal disturbances
- fever
- chills
- dyspnoea
- infections.

This drug can cause rapid pulmonary oedema and therefore it is essential that the patient is evaluated for volume overload and given treatment if necessary prior to administration of the drug.

Action Antilymphocyte globulin (ALG) and antithymocyte globulin (ATG) inhibit and destroy circulatory lymphocytes through antibody action.

Antilymphocyte globulin, antithymocyte globulin – polyclonal antibodies

Side-effects These include:

- rash
- fever/chills
- anaphylaxis
- thrombocytopenia/leukopenia
- myalgia.

POSTOPERATIVE CARE AND COMPLICATIONS FOR THE RENAL TRANSPLANT RECIPIENT

In most cases, the anaesthetist will insert a triple-lumen central venous line via the internal jugular vein immediately prior to surgery. This line facilitates monitoring of fluid status and central venous pressure (CVP), and allows infusion of fluids and medications during surgery and the early postoperative phase.

AIMS OF CARE

The aim of postoperative management is to provide the appropriate care to support primary transplant function and to aid optimal recovery. Initial care involves close monitoring of physical and psychological health, with frequent assessments and adjustments in response to changes in health status.

IMMEDIATE POSTOPERATIVE CARE

Cardiorespiratory status Immediate baseline observations should be recorded, including blood pressure, pulse, respirations and temperature. Such observations should continue every 30 min until stable and thereafter hourly or as appropriate. Twenty-four-hour ECG monitoring may be routine; however, in some centres, such monitoring may only be used for patients in high-risk categories. Close monitoring of respiratory status is essential, as anaesthetic drugs and analgesia may be poorly excreted owing to the reduced transplant function, thus depressing respiratory effort and increasing the risk of pulmonary complication. Early chest physiotherapy is essential.

Pain management The experience of pain is unique to each individual and therefore the use of patient-controlled analgesia is a suitable therapy, as it will provide satisfactory pain management, reduce recipient anxiety, and facilitate deep breathing and movement. An opiate derivative, such as morphine, is commonly used. Pethidine is avoided because of the possible accumulation of metabolites in the presence of reduced renal function. Recipients often report that the presence of the urinary catheter causes the greatest discomfort. Severe pain in the graft in the early postoperative period may be indicative of swelling of the kidney as a result of venous thrombosis.

Inadequate hydration may adversely affect transplant function; therefore, the maintenance of an acceptable venous pressure without the complication of fluid overload is an integral element of care. Fluid intake is usually administered through the central venous line. CVP measurements, recorded hourly, and urinary output measurements, recorded hourly, are used as a guide to appropriate fluid intake.

Fluid intake protocol usually involves fluids being administered through an infusion pump with hourly intake equal to the previous hour's output plus 50 mL, with the aim of achieving a CVP level of approximately 10–15 cmH$_2$O.

Peripheral line perfusion must also be included in the intake total. Infusion of dopamine may be introduced to help maintain pressure and improve transplant perfusion by reducing vasoconstriction of the smaller renal vessels. Monitoring of serum biochemistry and haemoglobin levels is ongoing and the results will determine the type of intravenous fluid given. Often 5% dextrose is alternated with normal saline. Blood transfusion is rarely required.

Oral fluids are usually introduced within the early postoperative phase (as paralytic ileus is rare) and are gradually increased as appropriate. In uncomplicated cases, the CVP line is removed after 48 h and nutrition introduced.

Hydration: fluid and electrolyte balance

A urinary catheter will be *in situ* following the transplant surgery, and the urine may be blood-stained due to the surgical procedures to the bladder and ureter. Clot formation may occur, resulting in pain and anuria. Gentle sterile bladder washouts should be performed to alleviate the problem and re-establish urine flow.

Twenty-four-hour urine output should be recorded and it is, of course, important to note the volume of urine passed from the native kidneys pretransplantation when assessing urinary totals. Daily urine analysis and biochemistry should be noted, and daily catheter specimens obtained for microscopy, culture and sensitivity. The catheter is usually removed on the fifth postoperative day. Some recipients may experience difficulty with voiding and also may have very limited bladder capacity owing to pretransplant bladder atrophy. Reassurance and bladder retraining strategies usually help to solve these problems.

Urine output: catheter care

A wound drain may be present and drainage should be monitored. Observation and aseptic dressing of the wound will be given as appropriate and the sutures removed when healing has occurred. The immunosuppression regime and other contributory factors, such as diabetes or malnutrition, may impede the healing process.

Wound management

Recipients are immunocompromised and, therefore, infection control procedures should be strictly followed. Hand-washing should take place before and after each nursing and medical procedure, and visitors should be monitored for infections. Medications should include prophylaxis against infection and additional treatments should be commenced if infection is suspected.

Infection control

The recipient should be helped to achieve personal and oral hygiene of a high standard and aseptic techniques utilised with regard to wound, peritoneal catheter site, urinary catheter and CVP line care. Catheter tips should be cultured for microscopy and sensitivity when removed.

Postoperative medications

- Ciclosporin, tacrolimus or sirolimus: immunosuppression to prevent rejection.
- Azathioprine or mycophenolate mofetil: immunosuppression to prevent rejection.
- Prednisolone: immunosuppression to prevent rejection.
- Co-trimoxazole (septrin): antibiotic to prevent infection/chest infection, particularly *Pneumocystis carinii*.
- Ranitidine: reduces gastric irritation caused by steroids and prevents gastric bleeding.
- Nystatin pastilles: prevent oral infection (*candida*).
- Aspirin: may be used in some centres to reduce the risk of thrombosis.
- Calcium supplements may be used, particularly in combination with pamidronate, to reduce steroid-induced osteoporosis.

CONTINUING CARE

Recipients usually recover quickly from the anaesthetic and begin early mobilisation to prevent complications. Diet is introduced on day 1. Constipation may be a problem due to anaesthetic, immobility and analgesia, and gentle laxatives or suppositories may be needed. Self-care is usually achieved by the fifth postoperative day.

Sadness may be linked to thoughts of the donor family, and grief and zedy'. It is often helpful to give recipients anonymous details, such as age, sex and cause of death of the donor, and to offer them the opportunity to write a letter of thanks to the donor family. The expression of thanks usually enables recipients to accept the gift of the organ and to move forward to their new lifestyle.

Anxiety is usually linked to the fear of complications, such as rejection, infection and graft loss. Recipients and their families require considerable support, understanding and in-depth information during the early postoperative phase, particularly if difficulties occur.

COMPLICATIONS OF RENAL TRANSPLANTATION

Renal dysfunction – acute tubular necrosis

The most common cause of delayed graft function after renal transplantation is acute tubular necrosis, which may be due to prolonged hypotension in the donor or prolonged ischaemia during the donor or recipient surgery. Dialysis support may be required until adequate transplant function is achieved. Haemodialysis, with reduced heparinisation, can be undertaken as necessary (a frequent clotting screen will be required), and peritoneal dialysis recommended as long as the peritoneum has not been breached by surgery.

CNIs are known to be nephrotoxic and may therefore prolong ATN. Some units may reduce the ciclosporin dosage or withdraw ciclosporin therapy until the ATN is starting to recover. Rapamycin may also prolong ATN as healing is impaired. OKT3 or antithymocyte globulin may be utilised instead of ciclosporin if ATN is thought to be a potential problem.

Acute rejection

Many transplant recipients will experience at least one episode of acute rejection. Acute rejection is usually a combination of cellular and antibody-mediated rejection, which most usually occurs between 4 days and 2 months following transplantation.

The clinical signs of acute rejection may include:

- pyrexia
- fall in urine output
- rise in serum creatinine
- swelling and tenderness of the transplant
- weight gain
- flu-like symptoms
- ankle oedema.

The diagnosis of acute rejection is usually confirmed by a needle biopsy (see Ch. 6), and treatment is commenced immediately with a daily intravenous bolus of methylprednisolone for 3 days. In severe cases, ALG (from horse)/ATG (from rabbit) or OKT3 may be commenced. The rejection is usually controlled by the increased immunosuppression; however, a severe rejection episode may result in some loss of overall graft function.

Vascular complications

Transplant renal artery and renal vein thrombosis   Thrombosis of the renal artery or renal vein is a rare complication. Clinical signs of graft thrombosis usually include pain in the graft, renal dysfunction, anuria and hypotension. Diagnosis may be confirmed by ultrasound scanning (see Ch. 6). Immediate surgical exploration should be undertaken. In the majority of cases the transplant will be lost.

Transplant renal artery stenosis

Renal artery stenosis usually occurs between 6 and 12 months after transplantation. Signs include graft dysfunction and severe hypertension with a bruit on auscultation over the transplant. Diagnosis is confirmed by angiography. In severe cases, intervention may be required either by percutaneous transluminal angioplasty or surgery.

Urological complications

A major urological complication that may occur is avascular necrosis of the distal end of the transplant ureter, resulting in leakage of urine. Surgical reimplantation of the ureter will be required in most cases. This complication has become less common recently owing to the use of a ureteric stent.

INFECTIONS

Bacterial infections

The clinical signs of infection are similar to those of rejection (pyrexia, tachycardia, flu-like illness), therefore it is important that both possibilities are considered and investigations undertaken to exclude either cause.

Chest infections may result from *Pneumococcus, Haemophilus influenzae, Klebsiella* and *Pneumocystis* (Septrin is often given as prophylaxis for *Pneumocystis* during the first 3–6 months post-transplant). Infection may develop rapidly, resulting in the need for ventilation. Early treatment with appropriate antibiotic therapies is essential.

Fungal infections

Oral *Candida* is common and many centres use nystatin as prophylaxis for a short time following transplantation. Oral hygiene of a high standard should be encouraged.

Vaginal *Candida* may also occur and recipients may be reluctant to report this problem, particularly to a male clinician in an outpatient setting. Recipients should be informed that *Candida* is a potential problem and that treatment will be required.

Viral infections

Cytomegalovirus   Cytomegalovirus (CMV) infection is usually acquired during childhood and early adulthood, and is a minor flu-like illness. However, this minor illness can cause major complications in the immunosuppressed transplant recipient. CMV disease, after transplantation, may occur as a result of the following.

- Reactivation of latent disease in a CMV-positive recipient; such reactivation is generally classed as 'secondary CMV'.
- Transmission of CMV from a CMV-positive donor to a CMV-negative recipient through the transplanted organ, or community acquired infection after the transplant. This is classed as 'primary CMV'.

CMV may also be transmitted through whole blood transfusions; hence many centres require that all renal patients receive CMV-negative blood.

CMV vaccinations for all transplant recipients in the pretransplant phase would be an ideal solution to this problem but, as yet, no clinically acceptable vaccines have been formulated. Also matching so that CMV-negative recipients receive CMV-negative grafts would help to minimise the difficulties experienced, but such matching is not always possible in practice. Therefore, primary CMV disease does occur and can cause morbidity and mortality.

The usual time for manifestation of CMV disease is 4–8 weeks post-transplantation. Clinical signs include swinging pyrexia, rigors, malaise and, in extreme cases, pneumonitis, retinitis, gastroenteritis and encephalitis.

Valganciclovir or valaciclovir are widely used as prophylaxis in high-risk recipients (such as CMV-negative recipients receiving CMV-positive grafts, or CMV-positive recipients receiving ATG). Recipients are monitored for serological evidence of CMV activity and treated according to local guidelines. Oral valganciclovir has been used for treatment, although it is licensed only for prophylaxis; however, when the patient is

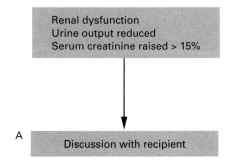

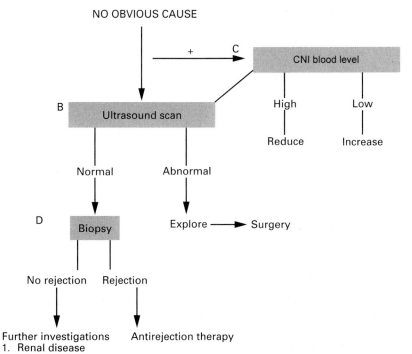

Figure 12.13
Assessment and tests completed in the presence of renal dysfunction during continuing care.

unwell, admission to hospital and treatment with intravenous ganciclovir is necessary.

Herpes simplex (type I and type II) commonly causes problems in the first months following transplantation. Oral and anogenital lesions may occur. Recipients may be reluctant to report such problems owing to anxiety and embarrassment. Therefore, recipients should be aware that these lesions may arise and that they occur because of reduced immunity, not because of other social issues. Sympathetic and understanding care should be offered and treatment with aciclovir may be required.

Herpes simplex and varicella zoster virus

Reactivation of the latent varicella zoster virus may also occur and present as classical 'shingle' lesions. Treatment with aciclovir is necessary to prevent systemic complications. Disseminated varicella zoster (chickenpox) is dangerous in immunosuppressed patients, resulting in some cases of life-threatening illness with encephalitis, pneumonitis and meningitis. The recipients must be aware of the problems associated with such viral infections and should be encouraged to report signs and symptoms or contact with infected others.

BK (Polyoma) virus Most BK virus infections are asymptomatic but it is implicated in ureteric stenoses, late haemorrhagic cystitis and deteriorating graft function. Two factors may account for the increase in BK nephropathy: improvements in biopsy interpretation and the newer immunosuppressants now widely used. Infection is associated with deteriorating renal function but can often be controlled by reducing immunosuppression.

RECIPIENT DISCHARGE FROM HOSPITAL AND CONTINUING CARE

If recovery has been uncomplicated, the transplant recipient may be discharged home on about the seventh to tenth postoperative day.

The educative and developmental intervention is very important for transplant recipients. They must have sufficient knowledge to monitor their health status, be understanding of medication regimes and report problems if they arise. Assessment of learning difficulties should be completed soon after transplant so that relevant interventions may be implemented to aid learning, knowledge and eventual independence. Physical barriers, such as impaired sight and hearing can be aided by electronic blood pressure monitoring equipment. Language and literacy difficulties can be resolved with diagrammatic information, translations and medication presented in daily dosette boxes, all promoting personal independence, although family members may be included in teaching sessions as appropriate.

The 'named nurse' may assess learning abilities (with an informal, non-threatening discussion) post-transplant and plan a teaching information programme, implement this programme and evaluate progress. Written information is given as appropriate both verbally and in the form of a written information booklet. At the time of discharge, the recipient should have the knowledge outlined in Box 12.17.

Drug charts and monitoring booklets should be utilised as part of a self-medication programme introduced as recovery allows or on the second postoperative day.

Immediately after discharge, recipients will be seen very frequently in the outpatient clinic. It is important that nursing intervention identifies developmental needs so that the recipient's knowledge base continues to expand and psychosocial care is offered. Reports suggest that some recipients feel that only the renal function and transplant progress is monitored, not the rehabilitation of the 'whole person'. Therefore, holistic care is essential, addressing psychosocial needs with physical needs; such care may be most appropriately offered by a transplant nurse practitioner who can offer continuity of care as well as understanding and support.

The aim of ongoing care is to empower the recipient to achieve optimal individual rehabilitation. It is essential to help the recipient achieve a balance between monitoring health and gaining normality. One of the most important post-transplant psychosocial tasks that the recipient needs to accomplish is the gradual relinquishing of the sick role and the eventual return to non-patient status (Christopherson 1987). Medical and nursing staff can give a confusing message by referring to recipients as patients and demanding strict adherence to rigid health protocols, whilst at the same time insisting that transplantation offers a return to 'normality'.

Flexibility of care, understanding and encouragement are required to enable recipients to take control of their lives and achieve the highest quality of life possible. Ongoing health monitoring will continue and problems may occur, but advice and support should be available throughout the complete transplant experience.

ONGOING CARE: INFORMATION AND SUPPORT FOR TRANSPLANT RECIPIENTS

- *Peritoneal dialysis catheter*: if transplant function is satisfactory, the peritoneal dialysis catheter is removed at 3 months post-transplant, although there is evidence that removal at time of transplant is advantageous. The ureteric stent is usually removed at 6 weeks after transplant.

Box 12.17   Recipient predischarge knowledge

- Record and report changes in the following and understand the relevance of such changes:
  - pulse
  - temperature
  - respirations
  - weight
  - blood pressure
- Measure and record 24-h urine output
- Understand the action, dosage and side-effects of medication and the need for compliance
- Recognise the signs of rejection
- Recognise the signs of infection
- Have telephone numbers of the transplant centre and know how to contact staff
- Recognise the need to alert transplant personnel in the light of any of these changes

- *Diet:* follow a normal diet, but taking care with weight gain due to increased appetite and freedom from the renal diet. If cholesterol or lipid levels are raised, dietary restrictions may be necessary. Phosphate levels may be low on MMF for a week or so post-transplant.
- *Vaccinations and travel:* transplant recipients should not receive live vaccines. Therefore, it is important to consult the transplant centre before travel immunisations are given. Foreign travel is encouraged but recognition of possible infection sources is necessary so that suitable precautions may be taken.
- *Skin care:* immunosuppression predisposes recipients to skin damage from trauma and sun and increases the risk of skin malignancies. Therefore, dermatological monitoring and advice should be given and recipients should use factor 25–30 sun block during sun exposure and report any skin lesions. Many centres send their patients for a baseline dermatological assessment after transplantation.
- *Fertility:* female patients should be aware of fertility issues and be given advice with regard to birth control measures. Intrauterine devices are not recommended because of the risk of infection. Condoms or the mini-pill are the most appropriate therapies. Recipients of both sexes should, ideally, wait at least 1 year before considering pregnancy. Advice should be available with regard to pregnancy risks in individual cases. Patients of both sexes must be told that they should inform the clinic if they have any plans for pregnancy, so that any medical issues or drug changes can be discussed. Recipients cannot breast feed after delivery as the immunosuppression may transfer to the baby.
- *Employment:* recipients may return to work as soon as they feel able as long as graft function and health are satisfactory, and employment does not put either at risk. Help should be available for those recipients seeking employment.
- *Health education:* smoking is discouraged owing to the risk of enhanced cardiorespiratory and vascular complications. Exercise and activity are encouraged, although contact sports, such as rugby or karate, may put the graft at risk. Female patients should have regular cervical smears and breast examinations because of the increased risk of malignancy. Male patients should be monitored for potential malignancies and encouraged to perform testicular self-examination.
- *Psychological health:* psychological support should be available to help with sexual problems, body image problems and marital problems.
- *Social needs:* help and advice should be available for social needs, such as benefits, housing and return to work.

PANCREAS–KIDNEY TRANSPLANTATION

Pancreatic transplantation is of proven clinical benefit for patients with type 1 diabetes who are undergoing renal transplantation, and is usually carried out at the same time (simultaneous pancreas–kidney transplant; SPK). The procedure has a slightly increased mortality and morbidity risk owing to the complexity of the surgery and the additional immunosuppression, but the long-term benefits outweigh these risks (Friedman et al 2001). SPK transplantation increases 10-year survival in diabetics compared to cadaveric renal transplant alone (Sollinger et al 1998). Pancreatic transplantation enables discontinuation of insulin and retardation of the complications of diabetes. Immunosuppression for kidney–pancreas transplantation is similar to that for kidney alone. Islet cell transplantation is yet to be established as a routine practice.

The pancreas is a fragile gland and easily damaged by trauma, poor perfusion or duct obstruction. Complications include pancreatitis, pseudocyst and leakage of digestive pancreatic enzymes.

Table 12.4 from UK Transplant (2006) shows pancreatic transplant activity. Overall, 34% of patients on the waiting list for a simultaneous kidney–pancreas transplant had received one by 31 March 2005.

Surgical placement of the pancreas is determined by the need to allow drainage of the pancreatic enzymes. This may be either into the bladder, with vascular connections to the external iliac artery and vein, or into the duodenum. Enteric drainage appears to confer a long-term benefit over bladder drainage, avoiding the problems associated with bladder drainage, such as dysuria, haematuria, metabolic acidosis (Lo 2001). The major advantage of urinary drainage, however, is the ability to detect pancreas rejection early by monitoring amylase excretion in the urine, and rejection is the most common cause of graft loss. Transplantation of a pancreas and a kidney from the same donor allows manifestations of kidney allograft rejection to guide treatment as kidney graft rejection is believed to precede or parallel pancreas rejection. Other causes of pancreas graft loss include vascular thrombosis, pancreatitis and infection. Vascular thrombosis may occur, in part, because of the low circulatory flow through the pancreas but can also accompany pancreatitis or rejection. Hyperamylasaemia is common after transplantation and may be either asymptomatic or indicative of symptomatic pancreatitis. Patients with a neurogenic bladder can develop 'reflux pancreatitis' from inadequate bladder emptying. Surgical problems related to exocrine pancreatic drainage and allograft pancreatitis are usually due to leakage or fistula formation leading to fluid collections, pseudocysts or abscesses surrounding the pancreatic graft.

In the post-transplant period, urinary tract infections are common and pancreatic enzyme activation can lead to 'chemical' cystitis or urethritis. In several cases, patients may develop urethral stricture or disruption, haematuria or perforation of the bladder or duodenum.

Finally, because of the loss of pancreatic secretions rich in sodium and bicarbonate into the urinary tract, pancreas transplant recipients are susceptible to metabolic acidosis and dehydration. All recipients must increase fluid and salt intake, but may require additional oral bicarbonate supplementation (Hakim 2006).

In addition to freeing the recipient from insulin therapy, the complications of diabetes are stabilised. Patients with type 2 diabetes have relative contraindications for pancreatic transplant: they are usually older by the time end-organ damage develops, and by this time usually have significant vasculopathy. Obesity is also strongly associated with increased mor-

Table 12.4 Pancreas donors and transplants, 1 April 2004–31 March 2005 (2003–2004) and transplant list at 31 March 2005 (2004) in the UK, by centre. (From the National Transplant Database maintained on behalf of transplant services in the UK and Republic of Ireland)

Centre	Cadaveric heart-beating donors[a]			Cadaveric transplants[b]			Active transplant list
	SPK	Pancreas only	Total	SPK	Pancreas only	Total	
Cambridge	12 (4)	1 (1)	13 (5)	6 (3)	0 (0)	6 (3)	2 (1)
Cardiff	2 (0)	0 (0)	2 (0)	2 (0)	2 (0)	4 (0)	5 (0)
Edinburgh	16 (6)	0 (0)	16 (6)	16 (9)	0 (2)	16 (11)	12 (9)
Liverpool	3 (5)	0 (0)	3 (5)	4 (5)	1 (0)	5 (5)	17 (17)
Manchester	19 (11)	0 (0)	19 (11)	17 (6)	1 (7)	18 (13)	35 (34)
North Thames (St. Mary's)	10 (14)	1 (0)	11 (14)	6 (7)	2 (2)	8 (9)	27 (12)
Newcastle	8 (7)	0 (0)	8 (7)	3 (3)	0 (1)	3 (4)	6 (3)
Oxford	24 (18)	0 (0)	24 (18)	14 (5)	1 (0)	15 (5)	1 (2)
South Thames (Guy's)	12 (11)	0 (0)	12 (11)	11 (9)	0 (0)	11 (9)	27 (20)
Non-designated[c]	7 (14)	0 (0)	7 (14)	0 (0)	0 (0)	0 (0)	– (–)
Total	113 (90)	2 (1)	115 (91)	79 (47)	7 (12)	86 (59)	132 (98)

[a] Includes 11 (17) donors aged less than 12 or greater than 45 years in 2004–2005 (2003–2004).

[b] Includes 7 (10) transplants using organs from donors aged less than 12 or greater than 45 years in 2004–2005 (2003–2004).

[c] Includes donors from hospitals in non-designated areas; Northern Ireland, Birmingham, Coventry or the kidney Trent Alliance area.

SPK, simultaneous pancreas–kidney transplants.

Statistics prepared by UK transplants, fom the National Transplant Database maintained on behalf of transplant services in the UK and Republic of Ireland.

bidity and mortality after pancreas transplantation (Odorico et al 1998). Additionally, insulin resistance is thought to lead to overstimulation of the pancreas, resulting in loss of function (Sasaki et al 1998). Finally, the shortage of organs precludes routine pancreatic transplantation in type 2 diabetes patients despite encouraging results (Light 2001).

SUMMARY

A successful renal transplant can provide the best quality of life for those with established renal failure. As one patient, who received a transplant in 1972 when aged 9 years, has said: 'It is amazing that the special gift from the donor has enabled me to achieve my career and personal goals and has resulted in the creation of a new family – a gift for generations to come'.

ACKNOWLEDGEMENT

With grateful thanks to Patricia Franklin who was the original author of this chapter.

References

AlKhawar FS, Gerry V, Stimson GV, Warrens AN. Attitudes toward transplantation in UK. Muslim Indo-Asians in West London. Am J Transplant 2006; 5: 1326.

Barber KM, Hussey JC, Bond ZC, Falvey SJ, Collett D, Rudge CJ. The UK national potential donor audit. Transplant Proc 2005; 37: 568–570.

Bell MDD, Moss E, Murphy PG. Brainstem death testing in the UK – time for reappraisal? Br J Anaesthes 2004; 92: 633–640.

British Medical Association. Organ donation in the 21st century – a review. June 2000 (available at www.bma.org.uk).

British Transplant Society and Renal Association. United Kingdom guidelines for living donor kidney transplantation, 2005 (available at www.bts.org.uk and www.renal.org; accessed 10/03/06).

Brook NR, Nicholson ML. An audit over 2 years' practice of open and laparoscopic live-donor nephrectomy at renal transplant centres in the UK and Ireland. BJU Int 2004; 93: 1027.

Buckley PE. The delicate question of the donor family. Transplant Proc 1989; 21: 1411–1412.

Butler JA, Roderick P, Mullee M, Mason JC, Peveler RC. Frequency and impact of nonadherence to immunosuppressants after renal transplantation: a systematic review. Transplantation 2004; 77: 769–776.

Carlisle D. Life-giving FATWA. Nurs Times 1995; 91: 2.

Christopherson LK. Cardiac transplantation: a psychological perspective. Circulation 1987; 75: 57.

Collaborative Transplant Study www.ctstransplant.org/public/data.html (accessed 10/5/06).

Conference of Medical Royal Colleges and their faculties in the United Kingdom. Br Med J 1976; ii: 1187–1188.

Conference of Medical Royal Colleges and their faculties in the United Kingdom. Lancet 1979; ii: 1069–1070.

Conference of Medical Royal Colleges and their faculties in the United Kingdom. Br Med J 1991; i: 32.

Conference of Medical Royal Colleges and their faculties in the United Kingdom. Lancet 1998; i: 261–262.

Connerney I, Bartlett S. Depression, readmissions and quality of life in kidney transplant patients. Psychosom Med 2001; 63: 91–190.

Coulter M. The needs of family members in ICUs. Intens Care Nurs 1989; 3: 4–10.

Council of Europe. International figures on organ donation and transplantation. Matesanz R, Miranda B, eds. Transplant Newslett 2005; September: 10(1). www.coe.int/T/E/Social_Cohesion/Health/NEWSLETTER%202005.pdf (accessed 05/06).

Department of Health. Guidance on the microbiological safety of human tissues and organs used in transplantation. HSG (96) 26. London: NHS Executive, 1996, revised 2000.

Derweesh IH, Goldfarb DA, Abreu SC, Goel M, Flechner SM, Modlin C, Zhou L, Streem SB, Novick AC, Gill IS. Laparoscopic live donor nephrectomy has equivalent early and late renal function outcomes compared with open donor nephrectomy. Urology. 2005; 65: 862-866.

Dubovsky SL, Penn I. Psychiatric considerations in renal transplant surgery. Psychosomatics 1980; 21: 481–491.

Evans RW, Manninen DL, Garrison LP Jr et al. The quality of life for patients with end stage renal disease. N Engl J Med 1985; 312: 553.

Feest TG, Riad HN, Collins CH et al. Protocol for increasing organ donation after cerebrovascular deaths in a district general hospital. Lancet 1990; 335: 1133.

Fehrman-Ekholm I, Elinder C-G, Stenbeck M, Tyden G, Groth CG. Kidney donors live longer. Transplantation 1997; 64: 976–978.

Fellner CH, Marshall JR. Twelve kidney donors. JAMA 1968; 206: 2703.

Flowers JL, Jacobs S, Cho E et al. Comparison of open and laparoscopic live donor nephrectomy. Ann Surg 1997; 226: 483.

Friedman EA, Friedman AL, Sommer BG. Pancreas Transplantation. In: Morris PJ, ed. Kidney transplantation, 5th edn. London: WB Saunders, 2001.

Fuggle SV, Belger MA, Johnson RJ et al. A new national allocation scheme for adult kidney transplantation in the UK. Clin Transplant 1998; 107–113.

Galpin C. Body image in end stage renal failure. Br J Nurs 1992; 1: 21.

Garrison RN, Bentley FR, Rague GH et al. There is an answer to the shortage of organ donors. Surg Gynaecol Obstet 1991; 173: 391–396.

Giessing M, Turk I, Roigas J, Schönberger B, Loening SA, Deger S. Laparoscopy for living donor nephrectomy – particularities of the currently applied techniques. Transplant Int 2005; 18: 1019–1027.

Gilks WR, Bradley BA, Gore SM, Klanda PT. Substantial benefits of tissue matching in renal transplantation. Transplantation 1987; 43: 669–674.

Gjertson DW. Look-up survival tables for living-donor renal transplants: OPTN/UNOS data 1995–2002. Clin Transpl 2003; 337–386.

Glotz D, Antoine C, Julia P et al. Desensitization and subsequent kidney transplantation of patients using intravenous immunoglobulins (IVIg). Am J Transplant 2002; 2: 758.

Hakim NS. Pancreatic transplantation (available at www.endocrinesurgeon.co.uk; accessed 10/03/06).

Halloran P.F. A Call for revolution: a new approach to describing allograft deterioration. Am J Transplant 2002; 2: 195–200.

Harvard Medical School. Report of the ad hoc committee of Harvard Medical School to examine the definition of brain death. Definition of irreversible coma. JAMA 1968; 205: 337.

Hilton BA, Starzomski RC. Families decision making about living related kidney donation. Am Nephrol Nurs Assoc J 1994; 21: 346.

Human Tissue Act 2004. London: Department of Health and Social Security, 2004.

Human Tissue Authority. 2006 Code of Practice. Donation of organs, tissue and cells for transplantation code, 2 January 2006 (available at www.hta.gov.uk; accessed 15/03/06).

Jacobs C, Johnson E, Anderson K et al. Kidney transplants from living donors: how donation affects family dynamics. Adv Renal Ther 1998; 5: 89.

Jain N. Evolution and development of a renal transplant co-ordinator for the Asian community. EDTNA/ERCA J 1999; XX: 5.

Jeffrey RF, Woodrow G, Mahler J, Johnson R, Newstead CG. Indo-Asian experience of renal transplantation in Yorkshire: results of a 10-year survey. Transplantation 2002; 73: 1652–1657.

Jofre R, Lopez-Gomez JM, Moreno F et al. Changes in quality of life after renal transplantation. Am Kidney Dis 1998; 32: 93.

Kemph JP. Renal failure, artifical kidney and kidney transplant. Am J Psychiatr 1966; 122: 1270.

Klein J. Natural history of the major histocompatibility complex. New York: John Wiley, 1986.

Kuo PC, Johnson LB. Laparoscopic donor nephrectomy increases the supply of living donor kidneys: a center-specific microeconomic analysis. Transplantation 2000; 69: 2211–2113.

Lee MA, Devaney A. Immunosuppression after adult renal transplant. Pharmaceutical Journal 2001; 266: 754-758.

Lee WC, Wu MJ, Cheng CH, Chen CH, Shu KH, Lian JD. Lamivudine is effective for the treatment of reactivation of hepatitis B virus and fulminant hepatic failure in renal transplant recipients. Am J Kidney Dis 2001; 38: 1074–1081.

Levey AS, Hon S, Bush HL Jr. Kidney transplantation from unrelated living donors: time to reclaim a discarded opportunity. N Engl J Med 1986; 314: 914.

Light JA, Sasaki TM, Currier CB, Barhyte DY. Successful long-term kidney–pancreas transplants regardless of c-peptide status or race. Transplantation 2001; 71: 152–153.

Li-Ming S; Ratner LE, Montgomery RA et al. Laparoscopic live donor nephrectomy: trends in donor and recipient morbidity following 381 consecutive cases. Ann Surg 2004; 240: 358–363.

Lo A, Stratta RJ, Hathaway DK et al. Long-term outcomes in simultaneous kidney–pancreas transplant recipients with portal–enteric versus systemic-bladder drainage. Am J Kidney Dis 2001; 38: 132–143.

Mathew TH. Recurrence of disease after renal transplantation. Am J Kidney Dis. 1998; 12; 85–96.

Meier-Kriesche H-U, Port FK, Ojo AO et al. Effect of waiting time on renal transplant outcome. Kidney Int 2000; 58: 1311–1317.

Miranda B, Vilardell J, Grinyó JM. Optimizing cadaveric organ procurement: the Catalan and Spanish experience. Am J Transpl 2003; 3: 1189.

Molter NC. Needs of relatives of critically ill patients. A descriptive study. Heart Lung 1979; 8: 332.

Mori/UKTCA/BACCN. Report of a 2 year study into the reasons for relatives' refusal of organ donation. Obtained from UKTCA secretariat. Newcastle upon Tyne: Royal Victoria Infirmary, 1995.

Morris PJ. ed. Kidney transplantation principles and practice. London: Saunders, 2001.

Morris PJ, Johnson RJ, Belger MA et al. Analysis of factors that affect outcome of primary cadaveric renal transplantation in the UK. Lancet 1999; 345: 1147–1152.

Morris PLP, Jones B. Transplantation versus dialysis – a study of quality of life. Transplant Proc 1988; 20: 23.

Najarian JS, Chavers BM, McHugh LE et al. Twenty years or more of follow up living donors. Lancet 1992; 340: 807.

National Institute for Clinical Excellence. Immunosuppressive therapy for renal transplantation in adults. Technology Appraisal 85, September 2004 (available at www.nice.org.uk/TA085guidance; accessed 10/03/06).

Nelson PW, Landreneau MD, Luger AM et al. Ten-year experience in transplantation of A2 kidneys into B and O recipients. Transplantation 1998; 65: 256–260.

New W, Solomon M, Dingwall R et al. A question of give and take. Research report no. 18. London: King's Fund Institute, 1994.

Novitzky D. Selection and management of cardiac allograft donors. Curr Opin Organ Transplant 1998; 3: 51–61.

Odorico JS, Becker YT, Van der Werf W et al. Advances in pancreatic transplantation: the University of Wisconsin experience. In: Cecka JM, Teresaki PI, eds. Clinical transplants 1997. Los Angeles: UCLA Tissue Typing Laboratory, 1998.

ONT (Organizacion Nacional de Trasplantes) Donantes de órganos en España. www.ont.es/estadisticas (accessed 10/05/06).

Pallis C. Brain stem death: the evolution of a concept. In: Morris PJ, ed. Kidney transplantation, principles and practice, 4th edn. London: Saunders, 1994: 71–85.

Park GR. Death and its diagnosis by doctors. Br J Anaesthes 2004; 92: 625–628.

Penn I. Evaluation of transplant candidates with pre-existing malignancies. Ann Transplant 1997; 2: 14–17.

Ross LF, Rubin DT, Siegler M, Josephson MA, Thistlethwaite JR, Wordle ES. Ethics of a paired-kidney-exchange program. N Engl J Med 1997; 336 1752–1755.

Ross LF, Woodle ES. Ethical Issues in increasing living kidney donations by expanding kidney paired exchange programmes. Transplantation 2000; 69: 1539–1543.

Royal London Hospital. Immunosuppression protocol. In: Fan S, ed. Hitchhiker's guide to the renal unit, London: Renal Unit 2005.

Rudge CJ, Fuggle SV, Burbidge KM. Geographic disparities in access to organ transplantation in the United Kingdom. Transplantation 2003; 76: 1395–1398.

Russell S, Jacob RG. Living related organ donation: the donor's dilemma. Patient Educ Counsell 1994; 21: 89.

Sasaki TM, Gray RS, Ratner RE, Currier C, Aquino A, Barhyte DY, Light JA. Successful long-term kidney–pancreas transplants in diabetic patients with high C-peptide levels. Transplantation 1998; 65: 1510–1512.

Schweitzer EJ, Wilson JS, Fernandez-Vina M et al. A high panel-reactive antibody rescue protocol for cross-match-positive live donor kidney transplants. Transplantation 2000; 70: 1531–1536.

Simmons RG, Klein SD, Simmons RL. The gift of life: the social and psychological impact of organ transplantation. New York: John Wiley, 1977.

Simmons RG, Hickley K, Kjellstrand CM et al. Donors and non donors: the role of the family and the physician in kidney transplantation. Semin Psychiatr 1971; 3: 102.

Smith MD, Kappell DF, Province MA et al. Living related kidney donors: a multicentre study of donor education, socioeconomic adjustment and rehabilitation. Am J Kidney Dis 1986; 8: 223.

Soin R, Friend PJ. Renal xenotransplantation. In: Morris PJ, ed. Kidney transplantation principles and practice, 5th edn. New York: Saunders, 2001.

Sollinger HW, Odorico JS, Knechtle SJ, D'Alessandro AM, Kalayoglu M, Pirsch JD. Experience with 500 simultaneous pancreas–kidney transplants. Ann Surg 1998; 228: 284–296.

Surman OS. Psychiatric aspects of organ transplantation. Am J Psychiatr 1989; 146: 972.

Terasaki PI, Cecka JM, Gjertson DW et al. High survival rates in kidney transplants from spousal and living unrelated donors. N Engl J Med 1995; 333: 333.

Thiel GT, Nolte C, Tsinalis D. The Swiss organ living donor health registry (SOL-DHR). Ther Umsch 2005; 62: 449–457.

Troppmann C, Debra B, Ormond DB, Perez RV. Laparoscopic (vs. open) live donor nephrectomy: a UNOS database analysis of early graft function and survival. Am J Transplant 2003; 3: 1295.

UK code of practice. A code of practice for the diagnosis of brain stem death prepared by a working party established through the Royal College of Physicians on behalf of the Academy of Medical Royal Colleges at the Health Department. London: Department of Health, 1998.

UK Transplant. Living kidney donation questions and answers. www.uktransplant.org.uk (accessed 10/03/06).

UK Transplant statistics. Available at www.uktransplant.org.uk (accessed 10/05/06).

Vincenti F. Immunosuppression minimization: current and future trends in transplant immunosuppression. J Am Soc Nephrol 2003; 14: 1940–1948.

Vlaminck H, Maes B, Evers G, Verbeke G, Lerut E, Van Damme B, Vanrenterghem Y. Prospective study on late consequences of subclinical non-compliance with immunosuppressive therapy in renal transplant patients. Am J Transplant 2004; 4: 1509–1513.

Wakeford RE, Stepney R. Obstacles to organ donation. Br J Surg 1989; 76: 35–39.

Waller JR, Hiley AL, Mullin EJ, Veitch PS, Nicholson ML. Living kidney donation: a comparison of laparoscopic and conventional open operations. Postgrad Med J 2002; 78: 153–157.

Wilkinson P. A qualitative study to establish the self perceived needs of family members of patients in a general intensive care unit. Intens Crit Care Nurs 1995; 11: 77–86.

Wilson CH, Bhatti AA, Rix DA, Soomro NA. Comparison of laparoscopic and open donor nephrectomy: UK experience. BJU Int 2005; 95: 131–135.

Chapter 13

Clinical practice guidelines and nursing audit

Nicola Thomas

CHAPTER CONTENTS

- To understand the process of setting, delivering and monitoring practice guidelines
- To identify the elements of the National Service Framework for Renal Services
- To evaluate the different national and international clinical guidelines which are available to the renal nurse
- To plan and evaluate the components of a clinical audit of renal care

LEARNING OUTCOMES FOR THIS CHAPTER

INTRODUCTION

In 1998, the Secretary of State announced specific measures to ensure that 'all patients should receive a first class service' (Department of Health 1998). This document highlighted that there are unacceptable variations in performance and practice, and in clinical outcomes. The previous chapters in this book have to some extent highlighted the inequalities in renal care (lack of autonomous renal services in some parts of the country; low acceptance rates for renal replacement therapy, particularly for older people; and poor numbers of specialist nurses) across the UK.

This chapter will explore the ways in which renal nurses can promote a high-quality service, through understanding of the clinical governance framework, knowledge of clinical standards and audit, and evaluation of best practice guidelines. Nurses have a vital role to play in the promotion of quality care in the renal specialty and are in a key position to understand the needs of individual patients and their carers.

SETTING, DELIVERING AND MONITORING STANDARDS OF CARE

Over the past 15 years, the renal specialty has seen the emergence of a number of national and international standards for renal care. When the government's way of setting clear national standards was announced in 1998, the main strategy for this was through National Service Frameworks (NSFs) and through a National Institute for Clinical Excellence (NICE). In July 2001, the work commenced on the NSF for kidney disease with the announcement of the co-chairs of the external reference group. In early 2004 and early 2005 the National Service Framework for Renal Services was published. This was the first NSF to be published in two parts.

NATIONAL SERVICE FRAMEWORKS

As outlined in the Department of Health (1997) paper 'The new NHS', the government will work with the professions and representatives of users and carers to establish clearer, evidence-based NSFs for major care areas and disease groups. In this way, patients will get greater consistency in the availability and quality of services, right across the National Heath Service (NHS). The government uses them as a way of being clearer with patients about what they can expect from the NHS.

So, the NSFs:

- set national standards and define service models
- put in place programmes to support implementation
- establish performance measures against which progress within an agreed timescale will be measured.

In 2001, the Kidney Alliance produced some service standards and recommended the structures that were necessary to deliver them in the new NHS. Many saw these standards as paving the way for the Renal NSF.

Part One of the NSF for Renal Services (2004) set five standards and identified 30 markers of good practice, which will help the NHS and its partners manage demand, increase fairness of access and improve choice and quality in dialysis and kidney transplant services. Part Two of the NSF for Renal Services (2005) set four quality requirements and identified 23 markers of good practice to help the NHS limit the development and progression of chronic kidney disease, minimise the impact of acute renal failure, and extend palliative care to people dying with kidney failure. Each of these documents is discussed in further detail in relevant chapters of this book.

In September 2005, a summary of progress to date towards achieving the standards and early actions set out in the Renal NSF, together with a review of the modernisation programme supporting delivery of the NSF, was published by the Department of Health (2005).

In order for renal units to learn from each when implementing aspects of the NSF, 'action learning sets' were established. Action learning sets bring together key individuals in service delivery in small dynamic groups to learn with others by probing, understanding and action. Learning sets in the areas of non-emergency patient transport for dialysis patients, in urban and rural areas, information and prevention of chronic kidney disease in primary care, and the extension of palliative care to renal services were established. In January 2006 a sharing event was convened and the day provided a summary of the work of the learning sets to date. Box 13.1 shows the four different learning sets and the renal units or renal networks leading each set.

Of particular note has been the learning set which has attempted to improve one of the most difficult aspects of dialysis for patients – transport. During the sharing event, some key achievements on improving transport were noted by the Cheshire and Mersey action learning set. By involving a patient representative, ambulance service managers, commissioners and renal nurses and managers, they undertook a comprehensive survey of good practice and current transport services across England. The group carried out patient interviews and held Listening and Sharing Events. The key challenge is now 'making it happen' and moving from a provider to patient/commissioner-led transport service (Scott 2006).

In June 2006 the NSF for Renal Services: Working for Children and Young People was published (Department of Health 2006). This document relates specifically to the care of children and young people in greater detail. It also brings together the recommendations from the NSF

Box 13.1   Renal learning sets

Palliative care
- Greater Manchester
- West Midlands

Information and prevention of chronic kidney disease in primary care
- Brighton
- Leicester

Non-emergency transport to and from hospital dialysis
- Durham and North Tees
- Cheshire and Merseyside

for Children, Young People and Maternity Services, to make an accessible, user-friendly document for all those with an interest in services for children and young people with kidney disease.

There are many other related projects and documents that have been published following publication of the NSF for Renal Services. These include a toolkit for commissioners, the information strategy, the report of a workforce modernisation project, a summary of guidance on haemodialysis away from home, advice on renal-specific, and more general, management of medicines. All of these documents can be found on the renal pages of the Department of Health website (www.dh.gov.uk/ PolicyAndGuidance/HealthAndSocialCareTopics/Renal/fs/en).

NATIONAL INSTITUTE FOR HEALTH AND CLINICAL EXCELLENCE (NICE)

NICE produces and disseminates clinical guidelines based on relevant evidence, associated clinical audit methods and information on good practice. The Institute identifies new and existing health interventions, collects evidence, considers the implications for clinical practice, disseminates the findings, implements at a local level and monitors the impact. To date, the guidelines produced by NICE that are specifically relevant to renal practice are to be found in Table 13.1.

DELIVERING QUALITY STANDARDS

Once the NSFs for specific specialities were to be published, the Department of Health (1998) asserted that 'we need consistent action locally to ensure that national standards and guidance are reflected in the delivery of services'. That action will be guided by a single robust framework – a new system of clinical governance – to monitor healthcare at a local level.

Table 13.1
National Institute for Health and Clinical Excellence (NICE): renal-specific guidance.

Date of publication	Topic
February 2002	Type 2 diabetes – renal disease
September 2002	Renal failure – home versus hospital haemodialysis
September 2004	Renal transplantation – immunosuppressive regimens (adults)
April 2006	Renal transplantation – immunosuppressive regimens for children and adolescents
September 2006	Anaemia management in chronic kidney disease
December 2006	Hyperparathyroidism – cinacalcet HCl
September 2008	Chronic kidney disease

HCl, hydrochloride. For further details look on the NICE website (www.nice.org.uk).

CLINICAL GOVERNANCE

Clinical governance can be defined as a framework through which NHS organisations are accountable for continuously improving the quality of their services and safeguarding high standards of care by creating an environment in which excellence in clinical care will flourish. Central to this initiative is the understanding that everyone in clinical care is responsible for delivering a high-quality service (Middleton & O'Donaghue 2001). The main components of clinical governance are shown in Box 13.2.

So what does all this mean for renal nurses? It could be argued that many of these suggested systems are already in place, but they do not necessarily work within an integrated and cohesive framework. This chapter will now go on to explore the ways in which renal nurses can contribute to improving the quality of patient care and work within a true partnership with patients, doctors and other members of the interprofessional team. As the Royal College of Nursing has recognised, nurses have a key role in implementing clinical governance and maximum use should be made of their skills and expertise to improve quality.

CLINICAL EFFECTIVENESS

Clinical effectiveness is about doing the right thing in the right way and at the right time for the right patient (Royal College of Nursing 1996). The NHS Executive (1998) described several key activities needed to support clinically effective practice and these include:

- selecting a particular aspect of practice to question or examine
- finding out from the literature and professional networks and other sources what is best practice and critically appraising the available literature and sources

---

Box 13.2   Main components of clinical governance (NHS Trusts)

- Clear lines of responsibility and accountability for the overall quality of clinical care
- A comprehensive programme of quality improvement activities, e.g. audit, evidence-based practice, continuing professional development, effective monitoring of clinical care
- Clear policies aimed at managing risks
- Procedures for all professional groups to identify and remedy poor performance, e.g. critical incident reporting, complaints procedures, staff supported to report any concerns about colleagues' professional conduct

Source: Department of Health (1998). Crown copyright material is reproduced with the permission of the Controller of HMSO and the Queen's Printer for Scotland.

- implementing and/or learning how to provide best-known clinical practice
- confirming that you are providing best practice on a day-to-day basis
- changing practice to make improvements, if necessary.

In renal nursing practice, we are fortunate to have a variety of clinical standards and guidelines to help us achieve clinically effective practice. In other words, many of the clinical guidelines that are available have been based on research evidence or expert opinion, so we do not have to examine all aspects of our care, as it has already been done for us. There now follows a review of the most important clinical standards and guideline documents available for renal nurses.

CLINICAL STANDARDS AND BEST PRACTICE GUIDELINES

HISTORICAL OVERVIEW

In 1990, the European Dialysis and Transplant Nurses' Association/ European Renal Care Association (EDTNA/ERCA) commenced work on writing European clinical standards and in 1995 published European Standards for Nephrology Nursing Practice (Van Waeleghem & Edwards 1995). This document was published alongside the European core curriculum for a postbasic course in nephrology nursing (Kuentzle & Thomas 1995), as part of the Association's strategy for the development of quality care in Europe (Kuentzle et al 1997). These standards formed one of the first publications that recommended specific guidelines for renal nursing practice. An outline of the key components is shown in Box 13.3.

Box 13.4 shows an example of one of the standards – discontinuation of treatment (dialysis). As can be seen from the example, these stand-

---

Box 13.3 European Dialysis and Transplant Nurses' Association/ European Renal Care Association (EDTNA/ERCA) European standards for nephrology nursing practice. (From Van Waeleghem & Edwards 1995, with permission)

Fundamental aspects of care
- Conservative management
- Education of staff
- Psychological support
- Discontinuation of treatment

Specific treatment modalities
- Haemodialysis
- Peritoneal dialysis
- Paediatric renal replacement
- Acute renal failure
- Transplantation

Box 13.4   Discontinuation of treatment

Standard statement

Nephrology patients and their families will be positively supported when decisions to discontinue treatment are made, whether by themselves, by members of the family, or by the multidisciplinary team, in order that the patient may die with dignity.

Structure criteria

1. The multidisciplinary team will provide appropriate bereavement and counselling support for patients and their families.
2. The nephrology nurse will have access to courses on bereavement and counselling skills.

Process criteria

1. The nephrology nurse will assess, plan and implement the most appropriate care to meet the needs of patients and their families during the dying and grieving process.
2. The nephrology nurse will refer patients and their families for bereavement counselling, as necessary.
3. The nephrology nurse will give patients and their families information about external agencies that provide bereavement counselling.

4. The nephrology nurse will ensure that the care environment is relaxing, non-judgemental, and provides patients and their families with maximum privacy.
5. The nephrology nurse will document all planned care and support, identifying the patients and/or families with special needs.

Outcome criteria

1. Patients and/or their families state that they were supported and encouraged to discuss their fears about, and adjustment to, impending death, and the processes of grieving and bereavement.
2. There is evidence that patients and their families have had access to bereavement counsellors and/or external agencies, as necessary.
3. The nephrology nurse has documented and evaluated the ongoing support for and interactions with the patient in the care plans.
4. Liaison between bereavement counsellors and/or external agencies and the nephrology team is documented as effective and appropriate.

---

ards are based on the Dynamic Standard Setting System as first described by Kitson for the Royal College of Nursing in 1990. These standards are broadly to allow for differing renal care practices across Europe and have been made more specific for local use. They were based on opinion, as a group of experienced healthcare professionals came together in a working group to define specific levels of practice.

In 1995, the EDTNA/ERCA developed a Research Board, which carries out a collaborative research project each year. In past years, topics for the collaborative research project have been vascular access (Van Waeleghem et al 2000), dietary advice (Nevett et al 2000) and water treatment (Lindley et al 2000). As a result of these European surveys into clinical practice, evidence-based clinical guidelines on water quality (2002) and nutrition (2002) have been developed; for further information, visit the EDTNA/ERCA website at www.edtna-erca.org. The Association has also managed and published results of the European Practice Database (EPD). The European Practice Database project is designed to provide a new European registry of multiprofessional practice. The aim of the project is capture data on the variation in practice both within and between countries. The pilot project of the EPD was successfully launched (December 2002) in each of the participating countries (North East Italy,

Czech Republic and Northern England) with a high response rate and the data collected was of good quality. The group 2 countries (Greece, Norway, Scotland and Belgium) did even better, with participation rates of between 65% and 91% (December 2003). Results have been published on infection control (De Vos et al 2006); hepatitis C (Zampieron et al 2006) and transplant practice (Kafkia et al 2006).

KDOQI

Some guidelines have been developed on consultation with expert groups, whilst others have been developed on opinion and evidence. An example of these is the KDOQI guidelines (Kidney Disease Outcome Quality Initiative; originally called DOQI or Dialysis Outcome Quality Initiative). KDOQI provides evidence-based clinical practice guidelines developed by volunteer physicians and healthcare providers for all stages of chronic kidney disease and related complications, from diagnosis to monitoring and management. KDOQI guidelines not only address dialysis but all stages of chronic kidney disease.

To date, the National Kidney Foundation (NKF) has published ten sets of KDOQI guidelines. The KDOQI Clinical Practice Guidelines for Chronic Kidney Disease: Evaluation, Classification and Stratification (2002) serve as the centrepiece of KDOQI. The classification outlined in these guidelines constitutes the basis for recent interventional guidelines for chronic kidney disease.

The core principles of the KDOQI guideline development process are:

- scientific and methodologic rigour using an evidence-based approach
- an interdisciplinary approach
- independence of work groups to facilitate an unbiased approach to guideline development, without the influence of organisations or industry
- openness of the guideline development process; draft guideline statements are subjected to a three-stage review process that invites comment from groups that the guidelines will affect.

Since the original development of the KDOQI guidelines in haemodialysis and peritoneal dialysis, there have been developments in certain areas of care, such as anaemia management. A list of published KDOQI guidelines is shown in Box 13.5.

RENAL ASSOCIATION

Within the UK, the Renal Association published the third edition of 'Treatment of adult patients with renal failure – recommended standards and audit measures' in 2002. From mid-2006, the clinical practice guidelines of the UK Renal Association have been being published in modular form. Table 13.2 shows the upcoming modules and their expected publication dates.

Modules are written in conjunction with representatives from relevant stakeholder organisations and will be available for public consul-

---

Box 13.5   Published Kidney Disease Outcome quality Initiative (KDOQI) guidelines

- Clinical practice guidelines for cardiovascular disease in dialysis patients
- Clinical practice guidelines on hypertension and antihypertensive agents in chronic kidney disease (*American Journal of Kidney Diseases,* May 2004)
- Bone metabolism and disease in chronic kidney disease (*American Journal of Kidney Diseases,* October 2004)
- Bone metabolism and disease in children with chronic kidney disease
- Clinical practice guidelines for chronic kidney disease: evaluation classification and stratification (*American Journal of Kidney Diseases,* February 2002)
- Managing dyslipidemias in chronic kidney disease (*American Journal of Kidney Diseases,* April 2003)

- Clinical practice guidelines for managing dyslipidemias in kidney transplant patients (*American Journal of Transplantation* Vol. 4, Suppl. 7, 2004)
- Hemodialysis adequacy update (*American Journal of Kidney Diseases,* January 2001)
- Peritoneal dialysis adequacy update (*American Journal of Kidney Diseases,* January 2001)
- Treatment of anemia of chronic renal failure update (*American Journal of Kidney Diseases,* January 2001)
- Vascular access update (*American Journal of Kidney Diseases,* January 2001)
- Nutrition in chronic renal failure (*American Journal of Kidney Diseases,* June 2000)

For further information, visit www.kidney.org/professionals/doqi

---

	Module	Status
1	Chronic kidney disease	Final version 10/04/07
2	Complications	Draft 07/01/07
3a	Haemodialysis	Final version 26/03/07
3b	Peritoneal dialysis	Final version 15/05/07
4	Transplantation	Draft 15/05/07
5	Acute renal failure	In preparation

Table 13.2
Renal Association clinical practice guidelines

tation before being finalised. The Transplantation module will focus on transplant medicine and is being written in conjunction with the British Transplantation Society. Separate paediatric guidelines will be produced and incorporated.

For further information on the Renal Association guidance, visit the website (www.renal.org/).

EUROPEAN BEST PRACTICE GUIDELINES

The European best practice guidelines (EBPG) are published on behalf of the European Renal Association/European Dialysis and Transplant Association. Best practice guidelines for anaemia in patients with chronic renal failure; European best practice guidelines for haemodialysis and European best practice guidelines for transplantation have been published. See the website (www.ndt-educational.org/guidelines.asp) for more information.

EVALUATION OF GUIDELINES

There are numerous local, national and international guidelines that renal nurses can access for achieving clinically effective practice, although Mead (2000) questions how useful these guidelines can actually be in promoting good practice. She summarises her debate with the following recommendations:

- guidelines are guides, not rules
- practitioners must critically appraise the included evidence
- national guidelines must be adapted to local circumstances
- it is vital to ensure judicious and selective guideline development.

It is helpful to have a checklist to evaluate how useful guidelines are to a local renal nursing team. The following questions could be used for evaluation.

- Are the guidelines based on evidence, expert opinion or both?
- What is the quality of the evidence? (Well-conducted clinical studies, reports, opinions, clinical experience of respected professionals.)
- Are the guidelines specific enough?
- Are the guidelines local, national or international?
- Have patients been involved in the development?
- Do the guidelines measure nursing?

The last point is difficult to evaluate, as of course nurses do not work in isolation and therefore all members of the multiprofessional team contribute to patient outcome. But it is important that nurses recognise that it is nursing that they have to measure, and not necessarily the easier-to-measure variables such as blood pressure, potassium level, Kt/V and haemoglobin levels. What matters to patients is the depth of the communication, the skill of the teaching and the quality of their life, and although it is recognized that all of these are very difficult to measure, surely nurses must strive to evaluate these as part of the audit process.

NURSING AUDIT

The NHS Executive (1998) described how to design and carry out a clinical audit. See Figure 13.1 for an overview of this process.

For renal nurses, it has been shown that, although there are many national and international guidelines available, one of the difficulties is how to select topics for audit that really matter to patient care. It is recognised that quality-of-life instruments may be one way of measuring more qualitative outcomes, but that in itself is challenging as 'there are no agreed methods of assessment upon which audit of this aspect of renal care can be based' (Renal Association 1997). Nurses are often taking the lead in auditing patient experience and some local audit teams

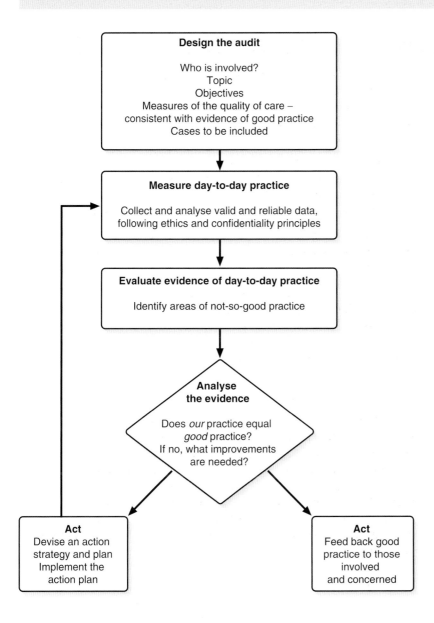

Figure 13.1
How to de sign and carry out a clinical audit. (From NHS Executive 1998.)

and endeavouring to audit topics related to the NSF. An example of such an audit is that carried out on behalf of the Pan Thames Renal Audit Group (PTRAG) into pre-dialysis care. This audit evaluated how far the NSF (Part One) was being achieved in the 13 Pan Thames renal units and made specific practice recommendations to units and commissioners following analysis of findings. Further information can be found on the NHS website (nww.esussex.nhs.uk/aiau/docs/specialised/index asp). (Please note this website can only be accessed from an NHS computer.)

SUMMARY

Increasingly, renal nurses are being asked to present clinical audit findings on behalf of the multiprofessional team, and it is important to remember that patients are also to be included in the audit cycle. There are international (European Kidney Patients' Foundation; CEAPIR), national (National Kidney Foundation; NKF) and local patients' associations that are ready to participate. Renal nurses are contributing to the culture of continuous quality improvement in patient care and have a very important role to play in implementation of clinical governance.

References

Department of Health. The new NHS. London: HMSO, 1997.

Department of Health. A first class service. Quality in the new NHS. London: HMSO, 1998.

Department of Health. National service framework for renal services. Part 1: Dialysis and transplantation. London: HMSO, 2004.

Department of Health. National service framework for renal services. Part 2. London: HMSO, 2005.

Department of Health. The national service framework for renal services: working for children and young people. London: HMSO, 2006.

De Vos JY, Elseviers M, Harrington M, Zampieron A, Vlaminck H, Ormandy P, Kafkia T. Infection control practice across Europe: results of the EPD. EDTNA ERCA J 2006; 32: 38–41.

Kafkia T, De Vos JY, Elseviers M, Zampieron A, Ormandy P, Harrington M. Transplant practice in Europe: selection of patients. EDTNA ERCA J 2006; 32: 33–37.

KDOQI (2002) Clinical Practice Guidelines for Chronic Kidney Disease: Evaluation Clasification and Statification. American Journal of Kidney Disease. 39 (2 suppl) S1–266.

Kidney Alliance. End-stage renal failure. A framework for planning and service delivery. Kidney Alliance, 2001.

Kitson A. The dynamic standard setting system. RCN standards of care paper. London: Royal College of Nursing, 1990.

Kuentzle W, Thomas N (eds). European core curriculum for a post-basic course in nephrology nursing. Ghent: European Dialysis and Transplant Nurses Association/ European Renal Care Association, 1995.

Kuentzle W, Thomas N, Hartley-Jones J. Developing a strategy for the quality of renal care in Europe. Jpn J Clin Dial 1997; 13: 21–25.

Lindley L, Lopot F, Harrington M et al. Treatment of water for dialysis: a European survey. EDTNA ERCA J 2000; XXVI: 22–27.

Mead P. Clinical guidelines: promoting clinical effectiveness or a professional minefield? J Adv Nurs 2000; 31: 110–116.

Middleton R, O'Donaghue D. Clinical governance in the field of renal medicine. Br J Renal Med 2001; 6: 17–20.

Nevett G, Nagel C, Elseviers M et al. Provision of dietary advice in selected centers across Europe. EDTNA ERCA J 2000; XXVI: 34–40.

NHS Executive. Achieving effective practice. A clinical effectiveness and research information pack for nurses, midwives and health visitors. London: HMSO, 1998.

Pan Thames pre-dialysis audit, 2004. http://nww.esussex. nhs.uk/aiau/docs/specialised/index asp.

Renal Association. Treatment of adult patients with renal failure. Recommended standards and audit measures. Bristol: Renal Association, 1997.

Renal Association. Treatment of adult patients with renal failure. Recommended standards and audit measures, 2nd edn. Bristol: Renal Association, 2002.

Royal College of Nursing. Clinical effectiveness. A Royal College of Nursing guide. London: Royal College of Nursing, 1996.

Royal College of Nursing. Improving quality of care – RCN guidance for nurses on clinical governance (available at www.rcn.org.uk/services).

Scott J. Learning set (transport). In: Implementing the renal NSF. The renal action learning sets: sharing the work in progress. Post conference report. London: HMSO, 2006: 5.

Van Waeleghem JP, Edwards P. European standards for nephrology nursing practice. Ghent: European Dialysis and Transplant Nurses Association/European Renal Care Association, 1995.

Van Waeleghem JP, Elseviers M, Lindley L. Management of vascular access in Europe, Part 1. EDTNA ERCA J 2000; XXVI: 28–33.

Zampieron A, Jayasekera H, Elseviers M, Lindley E, De Vos JY, Harrington M, Ormandy P. Sero-conversion of HCV negative patients: a European study on the epidemiology and management of HCV haemodialysis patients. EDTNA ERCA J 2006; 32: 45–50.

Chapter 14

Future trends in renal nursing

Jean-Yves De Vos

- To identify the challenges that renal nurses may face in the future
- To find solutions to cope with the healthcare needs of tomorrow
- To evaluate the ways in which renal replacement therapies will look in the future
- To analyse the challenges facing renal nurses in the 21st century.

LEARNING OUTCOMES FOR THIS CHAPTER

INTRODUCTION

Forty years ago, patients with kidney failure faced a brief future. Now, renal failure can often be treated successfully for several decades with dialysis techniques or transplantation. Although the technology existing to date is simple and on the whole well supported, dialysis treatments may last for hours and often involve additional hours of travel to and from dialysis centres, 3 or more days a week for the rest of an individual's life.

For the year 2000, the number of dialysis patients treated worldwide was estimated to be over 1.3 million (US Renal Data System (USRDS) 2004).

Advances in immunosuppressive therapy, better surgical and medical insight and management of transplanted renal failure patients have led and will continue to lead towards improved survival of patients with renal failure.

In addition, the improved care of patients who are dependent and will remain dependent on dialysis techniques, together with structural, molecular and pharmacological developments, continue to enhance the efficacy and safety of dialysis.

Recent successes in harvesting and expanding renal cells *in vitro* and the development of biologically active synthetic materials allow for the creation of three-dimensional functioning renal units, which in the future may be applied *ex vivo* or *in vivo* for partial or full replacement of kidney function – the bioartificial kidney. Even the generation of human tissues and organs through genetic engineering in specialised laboratories, along with the possibility of organ printing, may become reality in this century.

However, despite all these promising future initiatives, in view of the ever-increasing number of patients with renal failure and the increasing costs related to this, all these new innovations will not necessarily solve everything. As discussed in Chapter 1, there will not be enough facilities to meet the demand for care owing to funding and staff shortages. This has led to a possibly arbitrary selection of patients with renal failure needing treatment.

Even for those who will receive treatment, satisfactory results will be diminished as a consequence of overutilisation of existing facilities and staff. This includes potentially dangerous and indiscriminate reduction of session lengths, and limitation on the use of advanced and sophisticated materials and techniques. With such frightening prospects, dialysis treatments that are widely available and which give excellent patient outcomes at a reasonably low cost will be essential (Amiel & Atala 1999, Zickler 1998).

WHO WILL NEED RENAL REPLACEMENT IN THE FUTURE?

In 2002, the prevalence of established renal failure (ERF) per million population (pmp) was 11 107 for Europe, 419 263 for the USA, 28 061 for Canada and 219 966 for Japan (USRDS 2004). There are many reasons for this increase; for example, patients are often treated for decades because of better insight into treatment opportunities and improved development of treatment modalities. Also, as a consequence of these medical and technical improvements, patients with larger and multiple pathologies are being treated. This includes older patients and those with diabetes.

The number of older patients has continued to increase over time, as people live longer than in the past owing to better healthcare provision and better working conditions, at least in industrialised countries; the number of people over 65 years is increasing by 7–8% per year. As people grow older, one consequence is that they are more prone to multiorgan failure, and caring for these complex needs is one of the many challenges facing renal nursing today.

The European demographic profiles by age of chronic dialysis patients at present are: ≈10% 15–45 years; ≈30% are 46–65 years; and ≈58% are over 65 years. About 10% of the over-65 group are over 80 years according to the European Renal Association/European Dialysis and Transplant Association (ERA/EDTA) Registry Report (ERA/EDTA Registry 2006).

The median age of patients starting renal replacement therapy in England has increased from 63.3 in 1998 to 64.7 in 2004, and this compares with a much greater increase in Wales from 62.5 in 1998 to 68.7 years in 2004. Over the same time the percentage of patients aged over 75 years has risen from 18% to 25% (UK Renal Registry 2004).

Patients with diabetes are also increasing in number. At present, they make up around 20–25% of dialysis patients in Europe, and over 44% in the USA. There are also striking increases for other countries – towards 39% for Japan, 48.6% for Malaysia, 48.0% for the Canary Islands and 46.2% for Turkey (Organisatie van Paramedici der Dialyse en Transplantie afdelingen (ORPADT) 2003, USRDS 2004). However, in the UK, the proportion of patients with diabetic renal disease as the cause of ERF has remained unchanged between 1999 and 2004 (19.0% in 2000 and 2004) but, owing to the increase in the overall acceptance rate during this period, there has been an increase in the acceptance rate of patients with diabetic renal disease from 17 to 20 pmp.

These special groups of patients need very different and often more complicated care than those who are younger. More complex care means advanced caring skills, increased care time and higher costs.

WHO WILL CARE FOR THOSE WITH RENAL FAILURE?

It is clear that the need for broader care skills and time per patient will be the major challenge when treating the increasing numbers of patients with more complicated renal failure owing to age and multiple organ failure. At present, there is projected to be a shortage of nurses and doctors within the industrialised countries worldwide, at a time when numbers of patients are increasing yearly and pathology is demanding extra care. A survey of renal units carried out for the Kidney Alliance in 1999/2000 showed that, of the 55 renal units surveyed, only four stated that recruitment and retention of nurses was not a problem (Kidney Alliance 2001). By 2006, times had changed, with anecdotal evidence suggesting that up to 80% of newly qualified nurses are unemployed. This is partly because some trusts imposed recruitment freezes owing to mounting deficits. The challenge is for experienced nurses to prove their effectiveness in providing better outcomes for patients who need specialist care. In 2006, the NHS deficit had reached £512m and huge job cuts were expected.

An increase of 7–10% per year of those on dialysis means that in 10–15 years' time we will treat double the number of patients that are treated today.

What can be done about the shortage of nurses? There was much publicity concerning the lack of nurses in the UK and in Europe in the late 1990s (Kennedy 1999). Strategies include recruitment from overseas, although this in itself was not without problems (Mahoney 2001), continuing education for those who are new to renal care, and the overall challenge of improving working conditions and the social and financial recognition of the profession.

Another route might be to employ more healthcare support workers into the renal specialty, although specialist in-service education is essential for this group of healthcare workers. There has been much debate in the UK about the employment of healthcare support workers and many renal units are now using non-registered practitioners to take on specialist nursing skills (Kidney Alliance 2001), such as cannulation of fistulae. Many clinical nurse managers are having to evaluate the effects of a changing nursing skill-mix and are re-evaluating the roles of the healthcare assistant (Thornley 2000).

A renal nurse working in today's healthcare environment needs additional skills owing to the changed profile of the patients to be cared for – older people and those with co-morbid conditions, such as diabetes, heart disease and cancer.

At present, staff/patient ratios within Europe are about one nurse per four patients in the best situation and up to one nurse per six patients in chronic haemodialysis programmes. Staff/patient ratios for chronic peritoneal dialysis programmes and home haemodialysis programmes are much more widely spread within Europe, even within a single country (European Practice Database (EPD) 2002–2004, ORPADT 2003, Ansell & Feest 2001).

The British Renal Society established a multiprofessional National Renal Workforce Planning Group in January 2001 (National Renal Workforce Planning Group 2002) to prepare recommendations for establishments and staffing levels across each professional group involved in renal healthcare. Table 14.1 shows the 2001 establishment and 2010 projected requirement for qualified renal nurses. Clearly the number of renal nurses required by the end of the first decade of the 21st century is a big challenge for all renal units.

Staff/patient ratios have not really changed over the years, whilst patient care has differed enormously. Technical advances, such as controlled ultrafiltration, fully automatically controlled dialysis equipment and automated peritoneal dialysis devices have facilitated easier control of the treated patient, but this still does not balance with the more complicated care needs of patients.

At present and in the future, renal care centres will be needed to train or employ multispecialised renal care nurses to deal with the new patient profile. There will be a need for nurses with extra skills in addition to renal care skills, which are already essential. This includes knowledge

Table 14.1
Renal workforce requirements for qualified renal nurses in the United Kingdom.

	2001 Establishment	2010 Requirement
Haemodialysis	2330	4223
Peritoneal dialysis	250	524
Ward-based	1834	4760

> **Box 14.1   Competency RenOP3**
>
> **RenOP3: Enable patients and their families to understand established renal failure and its treatment**
> This competence is about helping patients understand what is happening to them and their bodies and to prepare them for what they can expect in the course of their established renal disease.

and regular updating on care and treatment of diabetes mellitus, older adults, wound care, infection control, psychosocial support and other pertinent issues. Collaboration with primary care to manage the increasing numbers of patients with chronic kidney disease is also crucial.

It is possible that a national competence framework will support this new way of working. 'Skills for Health' works with employers and other stakeholders to ensure that those working in the sector are equipped with the right skills to support the development and delivery of healthcare services. The Renal Framework contains 114 competencies and an example of one of the competencies is shown in Box 14.1. There will be a need to invest in allowing renal care workers to follow specific courses and conferences nationally and internationally. Renal care nurses will become more multidisciplinary in future. At least, they should have a knowledge of the total care needed for the new renal care patient, but importantly, they should work closely with skilled and educated specific care workers, such as dietitians, social workers, technicians, medical doctors, psychologists and podiatrists.

SOCIOECONOMIC CHALLENGES

Renal failure patients represent less than 1% of the population needing medical care while at present they consume over 5% of total medical expenditure (Editorial Spotlight 2000). There is no doubt that caring for more patients will open debate on what such treatment will cost in future, and if society will still be able to afford it.

Healthcare resources all over the world are restricted in relation to economic welfare, and each society will have to define how much can be spent for what purpose. There may be a lack of resources, not only because of the higher number of renal care patients with often more complex pathologies to be treated in the next decades, but also because of the ever-increasing costs when using newer but more expensive techniques and equipment.

Renal care workers will play an important role, in collaboration with authorities, private insurance companies and renal care industries, in planning for the best use of available resources. There will also be a need for multidisciplinary leadership from nephrologists, nurses, social workers, dietitians and patients. We will have to decide together which patient requires which renal replacement according to the individual profile of each patient.

ADVANCES IN RENAL REPLACEMENT THERAPIES

This section explores challenging future perspectives that could help the next generation to cope with the socioeconomic difficulties encountered when treating those with renal failure.

EXTRACORPOREAL TREATMENTS

There have been improvements in recent years in technical advances, such as ultrafiltration control, blood volume control, blood temperature monitoring, electrolyte profiling, ultrafiltration profiling, online efficiency measurements and individualised treatments. Over the next decades, the evolution of the effective use of biofeedback systems, in which biosensor technology will enable automatic steering of an individual's treatment according to biological needs, is anticipated. Further reading can be found in Grassmann et al (2000). However, it is believed that these often costly new innovations will not solve all the challenges of renal healthcare (Parker 2000).

Costs of in-centre dialysis have risen progressively during the last 20 years owing to a series of improvements in dialyse composition (better but more expensive water treatment and concentrate production), newer but more expensive membranes, more sophisticated equipment, increased use of more expensive techniques, such as haemofiltration and haemodiafiltration, staffing, transportation, and other issues. As well as cost, there is the problem of increased numbers of patients and, in the UK, dialysis services are under intense pressure. In a recent survey of provider trusts (Kidney Alliance 2001), 31 out of 56 autonomous centres reported their dialysis programmes as 'tight, bordering on clinical compromise'.

Although home haemodialysis has declined dramatically over the last 20 years, from 41% in 1983 to 3.2% in 1998 in the UK (Ansell & Feest 2001), many studies (Kenley et al 1995) have suggested that it offers the optimum dialysis in terms of outcome. Improvement in quality of life of some selected groups of patients, such as younger people in employment, is attested to by the revival of home haemodialysis, more specifically, short daily dialysis or long nocturnal dialysis, in which treatment frequency can be increased (Hombrouckx et al 1989, Kenley et al 1995, Kjellstrand & Ing 2000).

One of the reasons for the superior cost-effectiveness of home therapy is the reduced need for staffing and lower overhead costs in general. Studies have shown that treatment costs for a home dialysis patient are about half those for an in-centre patient. In some cases the reported savings are even greater (Kenley et al 1995). To date, less than 0.5% of European dialysis patients perform home haemodialysis, but 10.6% of Australian patients and 14.1% of New Zealand patients perform home haemodialysis, probably owing to the distances to renal centres (USRDS 2004).

DAILY DIALYSIS

The present commonly used haemodialysis schedules of 3–6 h three times a week is only a pragmatic compromise between the observation that it sustains patients reasonably well for long periods of time while twice a week did not (Kjellstrand & Ing 2000). Studies have shown that, if the frequency of dialysis is increased while total dialysis time per week is kept stable, this may lead to improved haematocrit, blood pressure control and general patient well-being, as well as the possibility of reducing or stopping some medication, such as antihypertensive therapy (see Case study 14.1).

There is no doubt about the medical superiority of daily dialysis compared to thrice-weekly dialysis schedule. At present there are no more obstacles for a wider application of this superior dialysis mode since some dialysis industries now offer basic but reliable dialysis machines for use at home (Kjellstrand & Ing 2000). For many, home therapy means improved quality of life, independence and flexibility, personalised dialysis and an active professional and social lifestyle.

PERITONEAL DIALYSIS

Another home therapy modality is peritoneal dialysis (see Ch. 8). Some promising future aspects are now explored.

Peritoneal dialysis is currently the dialytic treatment with the best cost–benefit ratio. However, it is used worldwide in fewer than 15% (5–50%, varying from country to country) of end-stage renal disease treatments in the vast majority of countries (USRDS 2004). The main factors limiting a wider dispersion and a longer duration of peritoneal dialysis treatment are the fear of infection complications, the progressive reduction in purifying efficiency, and the ability to maintain fluid balance and acceptable clearance over time. In future, better prevention of infection will be developed through newer and better techniques, and the possible use of vaccines against microorganisms that are frequently implicated in peritonitis (Amiel & Atala 1999, Shapiro 1979, Zickler 1998).

The use of new peritoneal dialysis fluids and continuous flow peritoneal dialysis has also been explored. Long-term (greater than 6 months) exposure to new peritoneal dialysis fluids with physiologic pH, lower lactate concentrations, or lower concentrations of glucose degradation products results in improved leukocyte cytokine release, ultrafiltration and mesothelial cell mass, respectively. Continuous flow peritoneal dialysis allows efficient removal of small molecules using dialysate with a lower glucose concentration and possibly less glucose degradation products.

Recent technical advances include the creation of a double-lumen peritoneal dialysis catheter, and methods of monitoring intra-abdominal pressure and ultrafiltration.

Although initial reports with biocompatible peritoneal dialysis fluids are promising, the efficacy of these new solutions in preventing long-term peritoneal dialysis failure is unproven to date. With respect to continuous flow peritoneal dialysis, substantial technical improvements are required before this technique can be widely accepted (Stigant & Bargman 2002).

Case study 14.1   Daily dialysis

This case study highlights the experience with ultrashort daily home haemodialysis in patients with end-stage renal failure in a dialysis unit in Belgium. The unit's nephrologist is a strong believer in increasing the dialysis frequency for haemodialysis patients in order to achieve better quality of life and improved long-term outcome.

The first patient was a 66-year-old woman who had been on chronic dialysis for 15 years because of polycystic kidney disease. As a result of increasing problems of general well-being and polyneuritis, she accepted a change from 3–4 h a week to 5–2 h a week.

The ultrafiltration rate decreased from 875 mL h^{-1} to 750 mL h^{-1}. Cramps, hypotensive episodes, nausea and vomiting disappeared. Her blood pressure decreased from 150/90 mmHg to 120/80 mmHg without the need of antihypertensive therapy. Haematocrit rose from 28% to 36% without erythropoietin. Phosphate binders decreased from 6 g day^{-1} calcium carbonate to zero. Nerve conductivity improved from 33 m s^{-1} to 40 m s^{-1} after 6 months. Mean weekly Kt/V increased from 3.6 to 6.4.

The second patient was a 57-year-old woman suffering from polycystic kidney disease. She was treated 6 × 1 h 45 min a week from the beginning while awaiting kidney transplantation. Daily home haemodialysis was her first choice as she was still an active teacher and she lived with her husband, who was blind and needed her help. The ultrafiltration rate on dialysis was 660 mL h^{-1}. No cramps, hypotensive episodes or nausea were experienced. Blood pressure was kept at 120/70 mmHg without any antihypertensive therapy. Haematocrit was kept at 33% without the need for erythropoietin. No phosphate binders were needed. Nerve conductivity stayed at 47 m s^{-1}. Mean weekly Kt/V was 7.8.

Note: Be careful when comparing Kt/V values when different treatment frequencies are used. Weekly Kt/V values should not simply be divided by the number of sessions a week to obtain comparable values of objective dialysis dose.

Results

In the first patient, general well-being improved significantly, as did the biological parameters and nerve conductivity. Ultrafiltration needs per dialysis session were significantly lower than before, resulting in better dialysis tolerance and significantly lower dry body weight. Antihypertensive drugs were no longer needed.

In the second patient, general well-being was good from the beginning. There was no polyneuritis, good blood pressure control, low ultrafiltration needs and good biological parameters. She was able to continue teaching and supporting her blind husband.

In both patients no problems with vascular access (both native fistulae) were encountered despite the increased number of weekly punctures.

Conclusions
- Fewer dialytic complications (cramps, hypotensive episodes, nausea)
- Less need for medication: no or little erythropoietin, no phosphate binders, no antihypertensive drugs; only vitamins (D, B and folic acid) and some iron were needed
- Increased dialysis dose
- Increased or stable nerve conductivity (electromyogram)
- Better dialysis tolerance due to low ultrafiltration rates
- Better control of hydration status
- More physiological therapy due to daily elimination of solutes
- More stable and better metabolic condition.

GENETIC ENGINEERING

Within the domain of transplantation, tissue engineering following genetic engineering sounds like science fiction, but it is not any more. Much is expected from this domain (Williams 1997).

The aim is to produce cells (such as pancreatic beta cells) that could be used in specific applications *ex vivo* and *in vivo* in the near future (Aebisher et al 1999, Roberts 2000). It is believed that by the year 2020 some diseases could be eradicated by replacing the defective genes. Bioengineers are already able to generate specific cells in specialised biolaboratories. The principle would be to inject or transplant a biodegradable framework with human stem cells into the sick patient. After administering the growth factors, specific functioning cells or tissues or organs will develop within the human body, restoring normal function. This will definitely cause a revolution, as a limited number of people would then need chronic dialysis treatment, for a limited time before and during the process of regeneration.

Already there is a new trend among parents to save their newborn baby's umbilical cord blood as a potential source of stem cells for use within the family. These stem cells can then be used in the future by the bioengineer to generate desired specific cells, tissue or organs. What is important is that no immunosuppressive drugs would be required as cells and tissues would be recognised as the patient's own (Editorial Transplantation 2000).

At present, an implantable bioartificial kidney, consisting of a haemofilter and hollow-fibre dialyser wherein human proximal tubular renal cells have been grown on the outside of the fibres, has been constructed and clinically applied (Cutler 1997). Also pancreatic islet cells (beta cells) have been grown successfully but are still rapidly lost due to hypoxia. Isolation of the beta cells from pigs is another possibility. Isolation of human cadaver pancreas is possible, but due to the large numbers of organs (at least five) needed to isolate sufficient cells to treat one adult with diabetes for only a limited time, this is not the first choice (Editorial Spotlight 2000). Grafting a whole pancreas together with a renal graft offers a good alternative for those with diabetes mellitus and renal failure.

Organ printing – a computer-aided, jet-based, three-dimensional (3D), tissue engineering technique – may become an interesting new approach. However, assembly of vascularized 3D soft organs remains a big challenge. Organ printing involves three sequential steps: pre-processing or development of 'blueprints' for organs; processing or actual organ printing; and post-processing or organ conditioning and accelerated organ maturation. A cell printer that can print gels, single cells and cell aggregates has been developed. Layer-by-layer sequentially placed and solidified thin layers of a thermoreversible gel could serve as 'printing paper'. The combination of an engineering approach with the developmental biology concept of embryonic tissue fluidity enables the creation of a new rapid prototyping 3D organ printing technology, which will dramatically accelerate and optimise tissue and organ assembly (Mironov et al 2003).

SUMMARY

The future of renal care will initiate heated debate and raise many ethical questions. There is congestion in many renal units, and some areas of the country are without autonomous renal services or even satellite units. There are also huge difficulties in the recruitment and retention of nurses.

The way forward is to support continuous quality improvement through interprofessional working, where nurses are seen to contribute on an equal footing within the healthcare team. Evidence-based practice and clinical audit are moving the renal nursing profession forward, together with recent appointments of nurse consultants within the nephrology speciality.

Finally, all the associations involved in renal care must work together with those who have experienced the service to ensure that renal care is truly patient-centred.

References

Aebisher P, Lysaght MJ, Parenteau N et al. Special report on the promise of tissue engineering. Sci Am 1999; April: 37–65.

Amiel GE, Atala A. Current and future modalities for functional renal replacement. Urol Clin North Am 1999; Feb: 235–246.

Ansell D, Feest T. Second annual report of the UK Renal Registry (available: www.renalreg.com/report99) 3 October 2001.

Cutler DS. A look at potential ESRD treatment alternatives for the future. The bio-artficial kidney. Nephrol News Issues 1997; 11: 14–15.

Editorial. Spotlight. Dial Transplant 2000; 29: 514–518.

Editorial. Transplantation. Nephrol News Issues 2000; 14: 66.

European Practice Database (EPD). Comparison of renal care in Europe: centre and patient characteristics. Elseviers M, De Vos JY, Harrington M, Zampieron A, Ormandy P, Kafkia T. EDTNA/ERCA Journal XXXII, nr. 1 January-March 2006; 8–13.

European Renal Association/European Dialysis and Transplant Association (ERA/EDTA) Registry. ERA/EDTA Registry 2004 Annual Report. Amsterdam: Academic Medical Center, Department of Medical Informatics, July 2006.

Grassmann A, Uhlenbusch-Körwer I, Bonnie-Schorn E et al. Recent advances in dialysis fluid management and outlook-dialysis fluid of the future. In: Composition and management of hemodialysis fluids. Vienken J. Germany: Pabst Science Publishers, Miami FL., USA. 2000: 244–287, 306–307.

Hombrouckx R, Bogaert AM, Leroy F et al. Limitations of short dialysis are the indications for ultrashort daily auto dialysis. Trans Am Soc Artif Intern Organs 1989; 35: 503–505.

Kenley RS, Twardowski Z, Depner T et al. Will daily home hemodialysis be an important future therapy for ESRD? Semin Dial 1995; 8: 261–274.

Kennedy A. A problem shared: a Europe wide approach to the chronic nursing shortage. World Irish Nurs 1999; 7: 14–15.

Kidney Alliance. End-stage renal failure – a framework for planning and service delivery. Kidney Alliance, London: Munro Foreter, 2001.

Kjellstrand CM, Ing T. Daily hemodialysis: history and revival of a superior dialysis method (available: www.aksys.com/therapy/superior_method.asp).

Mahoney C. NHS foreign recruitment sparks attack by WHO. Nurs Times 2001; 97: 5.

Millar B. Situations vacant. Nurs Times 2000; 96: 24–25.

Mironov V, Boland T, Trusk T, Forgacs G, Markwald RR. Organ printing: computer-aided jet-based 3D tissue engineering, Trends Biotechnol 2003; 21: 57–61.

National Renal Workforce Planning Group. A multi-professional renal workforce plan for adults and children with renal disease, 2002 (www.britishrenal.org/workfpg/WFP_Renal_Book.pdf).

Organisatie van Paramedici der Dialyse en Transplantie afdelingen (ORPADT). ORPADT Questionnaire 1997. A survey of nephrology nursing care and treatments in Belgium. Nephrol News Issues 1998; 11: 53–56.

Parker TF. Technical advances in hemodialysis therapy. Semin Dial 2000; 13: 372.

Roberts M. Conference report on the American Society for Artficial Internal Organs (ASAIO) meeting. Dial Transplant 2000; 29: 663–692.

Shapiro FL. Hemodialysis and alternative treatments. A look into the near future. Nephron 1979; 24: 2-6.

Skills for Health (www.skillsforhealth.org.uk/).

Stigant CE, Bargman JM. What's new in peritoneal dialysis: biocompatibility and continuous flow peritoneal dialysis. Curr Opin Nephrol Hypertens 2002; Nov: 11.

Thornley C. A question of competence? Re-evaluating the roles of the nursing auxiliary and health care assistant in the NHS. J Clin Nurs 2000; 9: 451–458.

UK Renal Registry. Eighth annual report of the UK Renal Registry. Bristol: UK Renal Registry 2005.

US Renal Data System (USRDS). Annual Report 2004 (www.usrds.org).

Williams D. Engineering a concept: the creation of tissue engineering. Med Devices Technol 1997; 8: 8–9.

Zickler P. Perspectives on dialysis therapy. Biomed Instrument Technol 1998; 36: 627–630.

Index

Page references: italics refer to illustrations; b to boxes; c to case studies; t to tables